Pediatric Intensive Care

Pittsburgh Critical Care Medicine

**Published and Forthcoming Books in
the Pittsburgh Critical Care Medicine series**

Pediatric Intensive Care

Edited by

R. Scott Watson, MD, MPH
Professor of Pediatrics
University of Washington
Associate Division Chief, Pediatric Critical Care Medicine
Seattle Children's Hospital
Center for Child Health, Behavior, and Development
Seattle Children's Research Institute
Seattle, Washington

Ann E. Thompson, MD, MHCPM
Professor of Critical Care Medicine and Pediatrics
Vice Dean, School of Medicine
Vice Chair for Faculty Development, Department of Critical
    Care Medicine
University of Pittsburgh
Pittsburgh, Pennsylvania

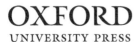

OXFORD
UNIVERSITY PRESS

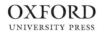

OXFORD
UNIVERSITY PRESS

Oxford University Press is a department of the University of Oxford. It furthers
the University's objective of excellence in research, scholarship, and education
by publishing worldwide. Oxford is a registered trade mark of Oxford University
Press in the UK and certain other countries.

Published in the United States of America by Oxford University Press
198 Madison Avenue, New York, NY 10016, United States of America.

CIP data is on file at the Library of Congress
ISBN 978-0-19-991802-7

9 8 7 6 5 4 3 2 1
Printed by Webcom, Inc., Canada

Series Preface

No place in the world is more closely identified with critical care medicine than Pittsburgh. In the late 1960s, Peter Safar and Ake Grenvik pioneered the science and practice of critical care not just in Pittsburgh, but around the world. Their multidisciplinary team approach became the standard for how intensive care unit care is delivered in Pittsburgh to this day. The Pittsburgh Critical Care Medicine series honors this tradition. Edited and authored largely by University of Pittsburgh faculty, the content reflects best practice in critical care medicine. The Pittsburgh model has been adopted by many programs worldwide, and local leaders are recognized as world leaders. It is our hope that, through this series of concise handbooks, a small part of this tradition can be passed on to the many practitioners of critical care the world over.

John A. Kellum
Series Editor

>

Contents

Contributors

Samina Afreen, MD
Division of Pediatric Infectious
Diseases
Children's Hospital of Pittsburgh
of UPMC
Pittsburgh, Pennsylvania

Michael Agus, MD
Division of Medicine Critical Care
Department of Medicine, Boston
Children's Hospital
Harvard Medical School
Boston, Massachusetts

Erik R. Barthel, MD, PhD
Pediatric Surgery
Children's Hospital Los Angeles
Los Angeles, California

Jeffrey J. Bednarski, MD, PhD
Department of Pediatrics
Division of Hematology & Oncology
Washington University School
of Medicine
St. Louis, Missouri

Robert A. Berg, MD
Hospital of the University of
Pennsylvania
Children's Hospital of Philadelphia
Philadelphia, Pennsylvania

Desmond Bohn, MB, FRCPC
University of Toronto
The Hospital for Sick Children,
Toronto
Toronto, Ontario, Canada

Sandra D. W. Buttram, MD
Phoenix Children's Hospital
Department of Child Health
University of Arizona College
of Medicine, Phoenix
Phoenix, Arizona

Joseph A. Carcillo, MD
University of Pittsburgh
Medical Center
Pittsburgh, Pennsylvania

**Ira M. Cheifetz, MD,
FCCM, FAARC**
Duke University Medical Center
Durham, North Carolina

Robert S. B. Clark, MD
University of Pittsburgh
Medical Center
Pittsburgh, Pennsylvania

Elizabeth Cleek, RN, MS
Division of Pediatric Surgery
Children's Hospital Los Angeles
Los Angeles, California

Jorge A. Coss Bu, MD
Texas Children's Hospital
Houston, Texas

Heidi J. Dalton, MD, MCCM
Pediatric ICU
Alaskan Native Tribal Health
Consortium
Anchorage, Alaska

Mark Davidson, MD
Royal Hospital for Sick Children,
Glasgow
University of Glasgow
Glasgow, Scotland, UK

Kathryn Felmet, MD
Department of Critical Care
Medicine
University of Pittsburgh
Medical Center
Pittsburgh, Pennsylvania

Joel E. Frader, MD
Northwestern University Feinberg
School of Medicine
Chicago, Illinois

Bradley P. Fuhrman, MD
Women & Children's Hospital
of Buffalo
Buffalo, New York

Dana Y. Fuhrman, DO
Division of Pediatric Critical
Care Medicine
Department of Critical Care
Medicine
University of Pittsburgh School
of Medicine
Children's Hospital of Pittsburgh
of UPMC
Pittsburgh, Pennsylvania

Barbara Gaines, MD
University of Pittsburgh School
of Medicine
Pittsburgh, Pennsylvania

**Catherine Goodhue,
MN, CPNP**
Division of Pediatric Surgery
Children's Hospital Los Angeles
Los Angeles, California

Iskra I. Ivanova, MD
Department of Anesthesiology
and Pain Medicine
University of Washington School
of Medicine
Seattle Children's Hospital
Seattle, Washington

Jan Hau Lee, MBBS, MRCPCH
Department of Paediatric
Subspecialties
KK Women's and Children's Hospital
Little India, Singapore

Joanna C. Lim, MD
Children's Hospital Los Angeles
Los Angeles, California

Lynn D. Martin, MD, MBA
University of Washington
School of Medicine
Seattle Children's Hospital
Seattle, Washington

**Marian G. Michaels,
MD, MPH**
Division of Pediatric Infectious
Diseases
Children's Hospital of Pittsburgh
of UPMC
Pittsburgh, Pennsylvania

Kelly N. Michelson, MD, MPH
Children's Hospital of Chicago
Northwestern University Fienberg
School of Medicine
Chicago, Illinois

Michael L. Moritz, MD
Division of Nephrology
Department of Pediatrics
University of Pittsburgh School
of Medicine
Children's Hospital of Pittsburgh
of UPMC
Pittsburgh, Pennsylvania

Vinay Nadkarni, MD, MS
Hospital of the University of
Pennsylvania
Children's Hospital of Philadelphia
Philadelphia, Pennsylvania

Eylem Ocal, MD
Department of Neurosurgery
University of Arkansas for Medical
Sciences
Little Rock, Arkansas

Renán A. Orellana, MD
Pediatrics and Critical Care
Baylor College of Medicine
Houston, Texas

Richard Orr, MD
Department of Critical Care
Medicine
University of Pittsburgh
Medical Center
Pittsburgh, Pennsylvania

Diana Pang, MD
University of Pittsburgh School
of Medicine
Pittsburgh, Pennsylvania

S. Sanjiv Pasala
Section of Pediatric Critical Care
Department of Pediatrics
University of Arkansas for Medical
Sciences
Little Rock, Arkansas

Peter P. Roeleveld, MD
Leiden University Medical Center
Leiden, The Netherlands

Anne-Michelle Ruha, MD
Banner Good Samaritan
Medical Center
Center for Toxicology and
Pharmacology Education and
Research
University of Arizona College
of Medicine, Phoenix
Phoenix, Arizona

Jorge G. Sainz, MD
El Paso Children's Hospital
El Paso, Texas

Stephen M. Schexnayder, MD
Section of Pediatric Critical Care
Department of Pediatrics
University of Arkansas for Medical
Sciences
Little Rock, Arkansas

Steven L. Shein, MD
Division of Pediatric Pharmacology
and Critical Care
University Hospitals Rainbow Babies
and Children's Hospital
Case Western Reserve University
School of Medicine
Cleveland, Ohio

Carmen Soto-Rivera, MD
Divisions of Endocrinology and
Medicine Critical Care
Boston Children's Hospital
Boston, Massachusetts

Philip C. Spinella, MD, FCCM
Washington University in St Louis
School of Medicine
St. Louis, Missouri

Robert M. Sutton, MD, MSCE

Hospital of the University of
Pennsylvania
Children's Hospital of Philadelphia
Philadelphia, Pennsylvania

**Ravi R. Thiagarajan,
MBBS, MPH**

Boston Children's Hospital
Harvard Medical School
Boston, Massachusetts

Jeffrey S. Upperman, MD

Division of General Pediatric
Surgery
Children's Hospital Los Angeles
Los Angeles, California

Hector R. Wong, MD

Cincinnati Children's Hospital
Medical Center
Cincinnati, Ohio

Vamsi V. Yarlagadda, MD

Cardiac Intensive Care Unit
Department of Cardiology
Boston Children's Hospital
Department of Pediatrics
Harvard Medical School
Boston, Massachusetts

Athena Zuppa, MD

Hospital of the University of
Pennsylvania
Children's Hospital of Philadelphia
Philadelphia, Pennsylvania

Chapter 1

Resuscitation and Stabilization

Vinay Nadkarni, Robert M. Sutton, and Robert A. Berg

Approximately 16,000 children (8–20/100,000 children/y) have a cardiopulmonary arrest event in North America each year: half out-of-hospital, with 3% to 12% survival to hospital discharge, and half in-hospital, with 27% to 48% survival to hospital discharge (see Box 1.1). Approximately 2% to 6% of all children admitted to pediatric intensive care units and 4% to 6% of children admitted to cardiac intensive care units experience a cardiac arrest. With implementation of early warning scores and rapid response teams, more than 95% of pediatric cardiac arrests occur in intensive care areas, not in wards. With advances in early detection and response, survival from pediatric cardiac arrest has improved substantially during the past 25 years. About 75% of cardiac arrest survivors have good neurological outcome, and more than 90% who survive to discharge are alive 1 year later.

Key Messages

- The four phases of cardiac arrest and cardiopulmonary resuscitation (CPR) are (1) prearrest, (2) no flow (untreated cardiac arrest), (3) low flow (CPR), (4) postresuscitation (see Figure 1.1).
- The most common precipitating event for cardiac arrests in children is respiratory failure, progressing to bradycardia and then pulseless electrical activity, or asystole; therefore, support of oxygenation and ventilation is a high priority before loss of pulses.
- The most treatable form of sudden cardiac arrest is witnessed ventricular fibrillation, with prompt recognition, CPR, and defibrillation shock.
- High-quality CPR requires you to
  1. Push hard, push fast (approximately 100–120 times per minute)
  2. Allow full chest recoil between compressions
  3. Minimize interruptions
  4. Avoid overventilation (rescue breaths at approximately 10 times per minute)
- Good-quality CPR is tiring. Switch chest compressors approximately every 2 minutes.

Box 1.1 Overview of Pediatric Cardiac Arrest

Out-of-Hospital Pediatric Cardiac Arrest
Respiratory etiology
Poor outcome (3%–12% survival to discharge, with ~66% good neurological outcome)
Rare witnessed, monitored, or shockable initial rhythms

In-Hospital Pediatric Cardiac Arrest
Combined respiratory and cardiac etiology
Seventy percent survive event, 27% to 48% survive to discharge (~75% good neurological outcome)
Commonly witnessed, monitored, and shockable (10%–15% initial rhythm)

- Rapid vascular access can be obtained with an intraosseous (IO) needle to deliver epinephrine at a 0.01-mg/kg/dose.
- Feedback on depth of compressions, end-tidal carbon dioxide target >20 mm Hg, and diastolic blood pressure >25 mm Hg can be used to guide quality of chest compressions and vasopressor administration during CPR.
- Attention to meticulous postresuscitation care can improve survival outcomes—specifically, (1) avoid hypotension, (2) manage targeted temperature to avoid hyperthermia, (3) normalize ventilation, (4) titrate oxygen to avoid hyperoxia or hypoxia (usual target 94%–99% oxygen saturation), (5) identify and treat seizures, and (6) avoid hypoglycemia and hyperglycemia.
- Consider family presence during resuscitation with appropriate dedicated support/guidance provided to family members.

Prearrest Phase

The prearrest phase focuses on early recognition and prevention of progression of relevant preexisting conditions (e.g., sepsis, pulmonary hypertension, shock, electrolyte abnormality, severe hypothermia, abdominal competition with breathing) to become precipitating events (e.g., respiratory failure, hypotensive shock, pulmonary hypertension with hypoxemia). Children who experience an in-hospital cardiac arrest often have changes in their physiological status in the hours leading up to their arrest event. Rapid-response teams or medical emergency teams are in-hospital emergency teams designed specifically for this purpose. These teams respond to patients on general inpatient units who are at high risk of clinical decompensation and then transfer these children to more acute care areas, with the goal of preventing progression to full cardiac arrest.

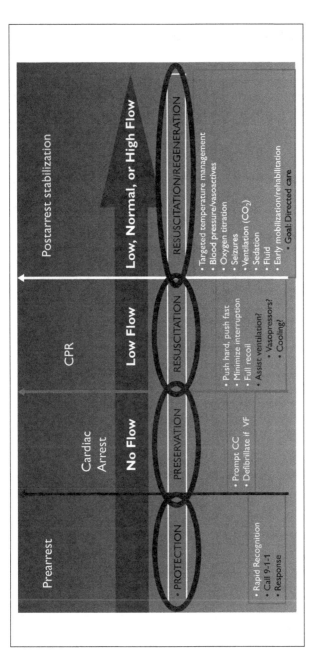

Figure 1.1 Four phases of cardiac arrest and cardiopulmonary resuscitation. CC, cardiac care; CO_2, carbon dioxide; CPR, cardiopulmonary resuscitation; VF, ventricular fibrillation.

No-Flow/Low-Flow Phase

Early recognition and transfer to high-intensity care areas shortens the no-flow phase of untreated cardiac arrest. Attach pads and recognize a shock-able rhythm rapidly (ventricular fibrillation [VF] and pulseless ventricular tachycardia). *For each minute of delay in defibrillation of a shockable rhythm, about 7% to 10% of lives are lost per minute.* The pediatric chest compression depth recommendation is at least one-third anterior–posterior chest depth, which is approximately 4 cm in infants and 5 cm in children. After children reach puberty, a depth of at least 5 cm, but no more than 6 cm, is recommended. Effective CPR optimizes coronary and cerebral perfusion pressures and cardiac output to critical organs. Important tenets of basic life support are push hard/push fast, allow full chest recoil between compressions, and minimize interruptions of chest compression. Achieving optimal coronary perfusion pressure, exhaled carbon dioxide concentration, and cardiac output during the low-flow phase of CPR is associated consistently with improved return of spontaneous circulation (ROSC) and improved short- and long-term outcome in both animals and humans. During the low-flow state of CPR, cardiac output and pulmonary blood flow are approximately 25% to 33% of that during normal sinus rhythm; therefore, much less ventilation is necessary for adequate gas exchange from the blood traversing the pulmonary circulation. Near-continuous blood flow is the priority, but adequate oxygenation and ventilation remain important for children because the etiology of most arrests is primarily respiratory compromise. Key common errors during resuscitation include overventilation (e.g., rapid, deep ventilations that increase pressure in the chest and impede venous return to the heart) and long interruptions (e.g., >10 seconds) of chest compressions for rhythm checks, charging of defibrillators, insertion of tracheal tubes, or change of chest compressors who are tiring.

Postarrest Stabilization Phase

The postarrest stabilization phase should focus attention on titration of oxygen, fluids, blood pressure, vasopressors, temperature, glucose, and seizure control in the minutes, hours, and days that follow return of spontaneous circulation. The immediate postresuscitation phase is a high-risk period for ventricular arrhythmias and critical organ (e.g., heart, brain, kidney) reperfusion injuries. The specific phase of resuscitation dictates the focus of care. Note that interventions that improve outcome during one phase may be deleterious during another. For instance, hyperventilation with high pressures and high oxygen may be beneficial during bradycardia with poor perfusion caused by hypoxia and impaired ventilation; but, when pulseless and with CPR in progress, the high pressure and rapid ventilations may impede venous return and decrease the likelihood of ROSC. Another example is intense vasoconstriction with higher dose epinephrine during the low-flow phase of cardiac arrest improves coronary perfusion pressure and the probability of ROSC; however, that same intense vasoconstriction during the early postresuscitation phase may increase left ventricular wall stress, myocardial strain and dysfunction, and arrhythmia potential.

Medications Used to Treat Cardiac Arrest

No single medication has been shown to improve survival outcome from pediatric cardiac arrest (Table 1.1). The main medication used during cardiac arrest is epinephrine (0.01 mg/kg/dose intravenous [IV] or intraosseous [IO]). Although there are special resuscitation circumstances when other medications such as antiarrhythmics (e.g., amiodarone, lidocaine, adenosine), calcium chloride, and sodium bicarbonate are used, medications are much less important than good circulation and oxygenation/ventilation to impact ROSC and survival outcomes.

Vasopressors

Epinephrine (adrenaline) is the primary resuscitative drug used for cardiac arrest resuscitation. Epinephrine is an endogenous catecholamine with potent α- and β-adrenergic effects. The α-adrenergic action (vasoconstriction) predominates at the doses used for cardiac arrest, which increases systemic, pulmonary, and coronary artery vascular resistance. The resultant increase in aortic diastolic blood pressure improves coronary perfusion pressure and myocardial blood flow, although it may reduce overall cardiac output. Epinephrine also increases cerebral blood flow transiently during CPR. However, evidence suggests that epinephrine can decrease local microcirculatory blood flow at a time when global blood flow is increased. Epinephrine also increases the coarseness of VF, increasing the likelihood of shock success. A study showed that, among

Table 1.1 Medications for Pediatric Resuscitation

Medication	Dose
Amiodarone	5 mg/kg IV/IO; may repeat twice up to 15 mg/kg; maximum single dose, 300 mg
Calcium chloride (10%)	20 mg/kg IV/IO (0.2 mL/kg); maximum single dose, 2 g
Epinephrine	0.01 mg/kg (0.1 mL/kg 1:10,000) IV/IO
Glucose	0.5–1 g/kg IV/IO
Lidocaine	Bolus, 1 mg/kg IV/IO; infusion, 20–50 μg/kg/min
Magnesium sulfate	25–50 mg/kg IV/IO over 10–20 min, faster in torsades de pointes; maximum dose, 2 g
Sodium bicarbonate	1 mEq/kg per dose IV/IO slowly

IO, intraosseous; IV, intravenous.

children with in-hospital cardiac arrest with an initial nonshockable rhythm who received epinephrine, delay in administration of epinephrine more than 5 minutes from time of cardiac arrest was associated with a decreased chance of survival to hospital discharge with a favorable neurological outcome. Note that although high-dose epinephrine (0.05–0.2 mg/kg) can improve myocardial and cerebral blood flow further during CPR and may increase ROSC, administration of high-dose epinephrine can worsen a patient's postresuscitation hemodynamics, and is associated with worse long-term neurological outcome. Thus, high-dose epinephrine is not recommended routinely for either initial or rescue therapy.

Alternative vasopressors, such as the long-acting endogenous hormone vasopressin, act on specific receptors that also mediate systemic vasoconstriction. However, vasopressin has a long half-life and can decrease splanchnic blood flow during and after CPR, and can increase myocardial afterload during the postresuscitation period. Thus, vasopressin is not a first-line agent in pediatric cardiac arrest.

Antiarrhythmic Medications: Lidocaine, Amiodarone, and Magnesium Sulfate

Administration of antiarrhythmic medications should not delay administration of shocks to a patient with a shockable rhythm (VF/ventricular tachycardia). However, after an unsuccessful attempt at electrical defibrillation, medications to increase the effectiveness of defibrillation should be considered. Epinephrine (0.01 mg/kg) is the first-line medication for both pediatric and adult patients in VF. If epinephrine and a subsequent repeat attempt to defibrillate are unsuccessful, lidocaine (1 mg/kg) or amiodarone (5 mg/kg) should be considered. There are limited data and experience with amiodarone use as an antiarrhythmic agent in children. Magnesium sulfate can be given, especially in torsades des pointes, usually in a dose of 50 mg/kg to a maximum of 2 g per dose.

Calcium

In the absence of a documented clinical indication (e.g., hyperkalemia, hypocalcemia, calcium channel blocker overdose, hypermagnesemia), the administration of calcium does not improve outcome from cardiac arrest. For these special resuscitation circumstances, calcium chloride (20 mg/kg/dose) or calcium gluconate (50 mg/kg/dose) is recommended. Despite lack of evidence for efficacy and association with potential harm, calcium is administered frequently during cardiac arrest. Note that routine calcium administration is associated with decreased survival and worse neurological outcomes.

Sodium Bicarbonate

The routine use of sodium bicarbonate is *not* recommended, and is associated with decreased survival and worse neurological outcomes. In special circumstances—such as hyperkalemia, severe acidosis that may depress the action of catecholamines, tricyclic antidepressant overdose, hypermagnesemia, or sodium channel blocker poisoning—sodium bicarbonate (1 mEq/kg/dose) may be considered. Note also that bicarbonate administration can elevate transiently the arterial and exhaled carbon dioxide load, and should not be used for management of respiratory acidosis.

Medications to Consider for Hyperkalemic Emergency/Cardiac Arrest

Consider the following medications in the following order:

Calcium chloride (10%) 20 mg/kg IV/IO or calcium gluconate 50 to 100 mg/kg IV/IO
Sodium bicarbonate 1 to 2 mEq/kg IV/IO
Glucose 0.5 to 1 g/kg IV/IO
Insulin 0.1 to 0.2 U/kg IV/IO
Albuterol aerosol
Kayexalate (potassium binder) with sorbitol (per rectum)

Postresuscitation Interventions

Targeted Temperature Management

Hyperthermia following cardiac arrest is common in children and is associated with poor neurological outcome. Neonatal trials of selective brain cooling and systemic cooling show promise in neonatal hypoxic–ischemic encephalopathy, suggesting that induced hypothermia may improve outcome. A large multicenter, prospective, randomized study of children age 2 days to 18 years who remained comatose after *out-of-hospital* cardiac arrest found a strong trend but no significant difference in survival with good functional outcome at 1 year and no additional complications in comatose patients who were treated with therapeutic hypothermia (32–34°C) compared with those treated with therapeutic normothermia (36–37.5°C). For infants and children remaining comatose after cardiac arrest, it is reasonable either to maintain 5 days of continuous normothermia (36–37.5°C) or to maintain 2 days of initial continuous hypothermia (32–34°C) followed by 3 days of continuous normothermia. Continuous measurement of temperature during this period is recommended and fever (temperature of 38°C or more) should be prevented and treated aggressively.

Blood Pressure Management

Titrate blood pressure after cardiac arrest to minimize high or low blood pressure during this high-risk period after resuscitation. Small observational studies after pediatric cardiac arrest show an association of worse survival to hospital discharge when children exhibited hypotension (less than the fifth percentile after ROSC). Maintain a systolic blood pressure of less than the 95th percentile for age. Continuous arterial blood pressure monitoring, with immediate access to inotropes (epinephrine, dobutamine) and vasopressors (epinephrine, norepinephrine), is recommended to identify and treat hypotension rapidly and effectively.

Postresuscitation Myocardial Dysfunction Management

Myocardial dysfunction and arterial hypotension occur commonly after successful resuscitation. The classes of agents used to maintain circulatory function (i.e., inotropes, vasopressors, and vasodilators) should be titrated carefully to the patient's cardiovascular physiology during the postresuscitation phase. Close goal-directed titration, and the use of invasive hemodynamic monitoring, may be appropriate.

Glucose Control

Both hyperglycemia and hypoglycemia after cardiac arrest are associated with worse neurological outcome. There is insufficient evidence to formulate a strong recommendation on the management of hyperglycemia in children with ROSC after cardiac arrest. If hyperglycemia is treated after ROSC in pediatric patients, blood glucose concentrations should be monitored carefully to avoid hypoglycemia, generally with a target glucose range of 80 to 180 mg/dL.

Seizure Surveillance and Control

Seizures are common after cardiac arrest—present in up to 30% of patients. Abnormal electroencephalographic background, burst suppression, and subclinical status epilepticus are all associated with worse neurological outcome. There is no current evidence that seizure prophylaxis or treatment of individual seizures or myoclonus improves outcome. However, close monitoring and treatment of status epilepticus are important postresuscitation goals.

Quality of Resuscitation and Stabilization

The quality of CPR performed during the resuscitation attempt is related directly to patient outcome. Early high-quality CPR is an important determinant of patient survival. The combination of focused bedside training, automated feedback defibrillator, frequent low-dose and high-frequency training, and environmental debriefing can improve guideline compliance, process of care, and outcomes.

Extracorporeal Membrane Oxygenation Cardiopulmonary Resuscitation

Extracorporeal membrane oxygenation cardiopulmonary resuscitation (E-CPR) has been used increasingly as a rescue therapy during CPR, especially for potentially reversible acute postoperative myocardial dysfunction or arrhythmias following cardiac surgery. Studies of E-CPR have demonstrated favorable early survival outcomes in children with primary cardiac disease when E-CPR protocols were in place at the time of the arrest. CPR and extracorporeal membrane oxygenation are not curative treatments. They are simply cardiopulmonary supportive measures that restore tissue perfusion until recovery from the precipitating disease process is achieved. As such, they can be powerful tools. Thus, E-CPR should be considered for children with cardiac arrest who have reversible conditions likely to recover or bridge to transplantation.

Summary

Outcomes from pediatric cardiac arrest and cardiopulmonary arrest events are improving. By focusing therapies strategically to specific phases of cardiac arrest and special, reversible resuscitation circumstances, there is great opportunity for successful cardiopulmonary and cerebral resuscitation in children.

Further Reading

Andersen LW, Berg KM, Saindon BZ, et al.; and American Heart Association Get With the Guidelines–Resuscitation Investigators. Time to epinephrine and survival after pediatric in-hospital cardiac arrest. *JAMA*. 2015;314(8):802–810.

Atkins DL, Berger S, Duff JP, et al. Part 11: pediatric basic life support and cardiopulmonary resuscitation quality: 2015 American Heart Association guidelines update for cardiopulmonary resuscitation and emergency cardiovascular care. *Circulation*. 2015;132(suppl 2):S519–S525.

de Caen AR, Berg MD, Chameides L, et al. Part 12: pediatric advanced life support: 2015 American Heart Association guidelines update for cardiopulmonary resuscitation and emergency cardiovascular care. *Circulation*. 2015;132(suppl 2):S526–S542.

de Caen AR, Maconochie IK, Aickin R, et al.; and Pediatric Basic Life Support and Pediatric Advanced Life Support Chapter Collaborators. Part 6: pediatric basic life support and pediatric advanced life support: 2015 international consensus on cardiopulmonary resuscitation and emergency cardiovascular care science with treatment recommendations. *Circulation*. 2015;132(suppl 1):S177–S203.

Institute of Medicine Report. *Strategies to Improve Cardiac Arrest Survival: A Time to Act.* Washington, DC: National Academies Press; 2015.

Lasa JJ, Rogers RS, Localio R, et al. Extracorporeal cardiopulmonary resuscitation (E-CPR) during pediatric in-hospital cardiopulmonary arrest is associated with improved survival to discharge: a report from the American Heart Association's Get With the Guidelines–Resuscitation (GWTG-R) Registry. *Circulation*. 2016; 133(2):165–176.

Moler FW, Silverstein FS, Holubkov R, et al.; and THAPCA Trial Investigators. Therapeutic hypothermia after out-of-hospital cardiac arrest in children. *N Engl J Med*. 2015;372:1898–1908.

Wolfe H, Zebuhr C, Topjian AA, et al. Interdisciplinary ICU cardiac arrest debriefing improves survival outcomes. *Crit Care Med*. 2014;42(7):1688–1695.

Chapter 2

Extracorporeal Life Support

Heidi J. Dalton, Mark Davidson, and Peter P. Roeleveld

Extracorporeal membrane oxygenation (ECMO) provides support for several days to weeks as a bridge to recovery or as a bridge to more definitive therapy (e.g., transplant or long-term support) for patients with severe respiratory or cardiorespiratory disease. Roller or centrifugal pumps are used to allow blood to pass from the patient's systemic venous circulation through a gas exchange device or "membrane lung" "before returning to the patient's venous or arterial circulation.

General guidelines and data on patient populations treated and overall outcomes are available on the Extracorporeal Life Support Organization website (www.elso.org). Recommendations can also be found from the Pediatric Acute Lung Injury Consensus Conference.[1] Reasonable criteria for use of ECMO follow.

Criteria for ECMO

1. *Exclusion*: patient for whom life-sustaining treatment is likely to be limited
2. *Inclusion*
    a. *Respiratory failure*
        i. Oxygenation index (OI)
            1. $OI = $ Mean airway pressure $\times FiO_2(100)/PaO_2$
            2. Consider ECMO for serial OI more than 25.
            3. OI values at 24 hours and worst in first 24 hours are associated with mortality (e.g., OI >16 at 24 hours is assocated with 28% mortality).
        ii. OI plus alveolar dead space (>30%) may help identify patients at high risk of mortality.
        iii. Mechanical ventilation less than 14 days (Longer duration of prior mechangical ventilation is a relative contraindication)
        iv. Consider P/F ratio less than 50 to 100.
        v. Inadequate gas exchange at conventional ventilator settings (CMV) (PIP <30 cm H_2O; PEEP ≥10 cm H_2O; FiO_2, 1.00)
        vi. Hypercapnia; inability to ventilate (persistent respiratory acidosis, pH <7.20)

vii. Consider high frequency, prone positioning, inhaled nitric oxide. If no response to escalating therapy within a few hours, consider ECMO.
viii. Severe air leak
b. *Cardiac failure/septic shock*
i. Inability to separate from cardiopulmonary bypass
ii. Persistent metabolic acidosis, elevated lactate, use of high-dose inotropes
iii. Use of venoarterial support in patients with aortic dissection or aortic insufficiency is not recommended.
c. *Extracorporeal cardiopulmonary resuscitation: ECMO initiated during cardiac arrest.* Consider involvement of extracorporeal cardiopulmonary resuscitation team after first dose of epinephrine without return of spontaneous circulation.

ECMO system components vary. Common components include the following.

ECMO Systems

1. *Roller pump or semiocclusive pumps* require gravity drainage and a longer circuit than a centrifugal pump. A venous reservoir (bladder or servoregulation system) helps limit negative pressure and hemolysis. Blood advances through the circuit by roller heads compressing tubing in the pump head casing. Prolonged pressure on tubing can lead to rupture. Occlusion of post-pumphead tubing can result in a rapid increase in pressure and tubing rupture.
2. *Centrifugal pumps*: The spinning centrifugal head draws blood into the pump head and dispels it tangentially. Occlusion does not cause high post-pumphead pressure.
a. Rotation (RPM) generates "suction" force for venous drainage. RPM must be high enough to generate forward flow; blood can drain *backward* from patient if forward flow is insufficient.
b. Loss of venous return can generate *high* negative pressure (–500 mm Hg) and hemolysis.
c. Adequate flow is dependent on preload and afterload!
d. The centrifugal pump head may trap air and emboli, but may instead distribute the air or particulate matter forward to patient. Risk of air emboli leads most centers to use an air detection device.

Choosing the mode of ECMO depends on a number of patient factors and equipment available.

Decision Tree for Mode of ECMO

Note: The use of ultrasound to establish size and patency of vessels being considered for cannulation may lessen waste of cannulas. Diameter (in millimeters) × 3 = French size (1 French = external diameter of 0.333 mm)

1. *Patient with cardiovascular instability*
   a. Venoarterial (VA) ECMO cannulation is most likely to provide adequate support
      i. If the chest is open, consider placement of cannulas in right atrium and aorta directly
         1. Allows maximal ECMO flow
         2. Bleeding may be greater than with other sites
      ii. Cervical VA ECMO: right internal jugular (RIJ) vein and right carotid artery
         1. Most common site for small infants (<10 kg)
         2. May be used in older patients. Shorter, larger diameter cannulas than are usually possible for femoral vein (FV) cannulation allow better venous return.
         3. There may be a greater risk of stroke higher than with femoral cannulation.
      iii. Femoral VA ECMO: FV and femoral artery (usually >15 kg or >2 years)
         1. Venous cannula
            a. Inserted to IVC/RA junction. A longer cannula adds resistance to flow and may restrict venous return.
            b. Venous engorgement of the limb distal to the cannulation site and compartment syndrome may develop.
         2. Short arterial cannula to limit resistance to flow
            a. Highly oxygenated blood into lower body
            b. In patients with respiratory dysfunction, poorly oxygenated blood ejected from the left heart may perfuse the brain, heart, and upper body preferentially to ECMO flow. Watch for the "red lower body/blue upper body syndrome." Follow arterial oxygen saturation with blood gases from the right radial artery or other means of following upper body saturations.
            c. Venous saturation obtained from the superior vena cava in femoral VA ECMO in patients with severe respiratory disease may be low and may serve as an indicator that additional upper body oxygenation is needed.
            d. Distal limb ischemia with a femoral arterial cannula can occur and demands close monitoring of perfusion
               i. Place the distal perfusion cannula down the femoral arterial vessel at the time of cannulation and "Y" into arterial return from the ECMO circuit.
               Or
               ii. Place the arterial line in the posterior tibial artery and "Y" into the arterial return from the ECMO circuit.
               iii. Neurovascular compromise can occur even with these methods, requiring amputation.

3. Modified femoral VA ECMO
   a. If there is inadequate upper body oxygen delivery, consider an additional venous cannula into the RIJ vein, "Y-ed" into the *arterial return* from the ECMO circuit. Divert a portion of the arterial blood flow into the RIJ cannula to improve oxygenation of the blood ejected to the upper body from the left heart.
4. Can transition to traditional use of RIJ vein, RIC artery if necessary.

2. Patients with respiratory dysfunction and hypoxemia or hypercapnia
   a. May benefit from venovenous (VV) ECMO, with blood withdrawn from and returned into the venous circulation. Adequate native cardiac function is essential.
   b. Common sites
      i. Two-site method:
         1. FV and RIJ vein
            a. Draining from the FV and returning to the RIJ vein limits recirculation.
            b. Cannula tips should be separated by 5 mm or more to reduce recirculation.
            c. Draining from the RIJ vein achieves the best blood flow but allows greater recirculation.
         2. Bilateral FVs
            a. One long and one short cannula helps avoid massive recirculation
            b. Less effective than RIJ vein placement, but good if it is needed for low blood flow only (e.g., hypercapnia)
      ii. Dual-lumen single cannula
         1. *RIJ vein*: Requires careful placement to avoid massive recirculation.
            a. Avalon cannula
               i. Proper placement at the SVC/RA or IVC/RA sites provides good venous return.
               ii. Oxygenated return from ECMO is directed toward the tricuspid valve and right ventricle, limiting recirculation.
               iii. Correct placement is difficult and should be supported with fluoroscopy demonstrating flow from ECMO circuit directed into tricuspid valve.
               iv. Initial confirmation of placement by echocardiogram (ECHO) can be helpful after cannula positioning.
            b. Other double lumen placement: drains SVC/RA and returns to RA; more recirculation than Avalon, easier to place
      iii. VV ECMO may have fewer neurological complications than VA support.

iv. Patients requiring vasoactive agents before ECMO may tolerate VV ECMO if cardiac dysfunction is secondary to poor oxygenation and/or high intrathoracic pressures.

Once cannulation is complete, ECMO flow is initiated.

Initiation of ECMO

1. Establish initial flow rate goal
   a. Determine cardiac index goal: CO/BSA
   or
   b. Infants: ECMO flow 100 to 150 mL/kg. Single-ventricle physiology and systemic to pulmonary artery shunts may require 200 mL/kg.
   c. Children: 70 to 100 mL /kg ECMO flow
   d. Adults: 50 to 70 mL/kg ECMO flow
   e. Increase flow over approximately 15 minutes. Follow arterial and venous oxygenation, blood pressure, and peripheral perfusion.
      i. Observe ECMO circuit venous return and arterial return pressures.
      ii. Active suction effect of centrifugal heads can create high negative pressure. Most manufacturers provide pressure-drop curves for each cannula across a range of flow rates. Selecting a cannula that provides the expected blood flow at a pressure drop of less than <100 mm Hg is recommended to avoid high negative pressure and hemolysis. Also, exposing the right atrium to pressures more negative than −20 mm Hg can result in damage to the intima. If the venous cannula chosen to provide the expected blood flow rate has a pressure drop of 40 mm Hg from inlet to outlet, the venous servo limit should be set at −60 mm Hg to provide adequate blood flow and to protect the right atrium from damage.
      iii. Arterial line pressures (postpump) are usually maintained at less than 350 mm Hg to prevent hemolysis (and risk of tubing rupture if using roller pump device).
2. When desired venous and arterial saturation levels are achieved, reduce ventilation to rest settings and decrease vasoactive agent dosing as tolerated.
   a. VA ECMO: venous saturation goals, 65% to 75%; arterial saturations, >90% (patient)
   b. VV ECMO: arterial saturations lower than with VA. Arterial saturations more than 80% are desired, but lower saturations may be acceptable if other indicators of adequate oxygen delivery are normal (mentation, hemodynamics, end organ perfusion).
3. Follow routine anticoagulation lab results as well as intermittent lab results for organ function.

Several points specific to ECMO management should be noted.

Special Points: VA ECMO

1. VA ECMO increases left-heart afterload. Inadequate ejection from LV can result in left atrial and pulmonary venous distention, pulmonary edema, and massive pulmonary hemorrhage.
2. Monitor adequacy of forward flow from LV by
   a. Pulse pressure (maintain some pulse pressure during ECMO). Systolic ejection indicates aortic valve opening and LV working; ECMO flow, itself, is usually nonpulsatile.
   b. ECHO provides evidence for aortic valve opening, ejection from LV, LV performance, LA dilation
   c. Chest X-ray to assess presence of pulmonary edema
   d. Suctioning frothy pulmonary edema is an ominous sign if present as a new finding.
3. If LV forward flow is inadequate
   a. Afterload reduction or low-level inotropy may help
   b. Establish drainage of left heart
      i. Closed-chest patients usually require atrial balloon septostomy in cardiac catheterization lab, which allows venous cannula to drain right and left atria.
      ii. Open-chest patients may benefit from placement of direct left-atrial vent catheter and "Y" into venous return to decompress LA.
      iii. In patients with adequate pulmonary gas exchange, ECMO circuit venous saturation is increased by oxygenated blood from the native pulmonary veins/left atrium mixing with the venous return to the pump. Need to use venous saturation at a site not "contaminated" with left-heart return (e.g., femoral venous catheter).
4. Vessel reconstruction at decannulation (especially carotid and femoral artery) is often recommended, but data on long-term benefit are limited.

Special Points: VV ECMO

Concerns specific to ECMO management are noted in this section.

1. Recirculation
   a. Occurs when oxygenated blood returning from the ECMO circuit is drawn back into the drainage cannula without reaching the patient's systemic circulation.
   b. Results in high-circuit SvO_2 but limits systemic oxygenation.
   c. Can highlight cannula malposition.
   d. Impact of recirculation
      i. New signs of impaired oxygen delivery

ii. Increased ECMO flow increases circuit SvO_2 without an increase in patient's SaO_2

iii. On occasion, reducing ECMO flow decreases recirculation.

Special Points: Specific Cardiac Lesions

Management of patients with congenital heart defects on ECMO requires recognition of specific physiology.

1. Single-ventricle patients
   a. Initially, during full ECMO support, target normal arterial saturation.
   b. As the myocardium recovers and ECMO is weaned, saturations will decrease as the patient's mixed circulation becomes the predominant source of blood flow.
   c. Clipping the Blalock-Taussig shunt is not recommended unless pulmonary blood flow during ECMO is excessive and limits systemic flow. Clipping may be associated with lung ischemia, reperfusion injury, and increased risk of death.
2. ECMO may be considered in patients with a bidirectional Glenn or Fontan circulation with profound low cardiac output after excluding obstruction in the bidirectional Glenn or Fontan circuit. Outcome in these patients is inferior compared with other cardiac lesions supported with ECMO. A patient may require both SVC and IVC drainage.

Patient Management during ECMO

Although patient care must be individualize, some generally accepted elements of management follow.

1. *Ventilator settings*
   a. Reduce to "nontoxic" settings (e.g., PEEP, 5–15 cm H_2O; PIP, <25–30 cm H_2O; rate, 6–10; FiO_2, 0.21–0.5) *or* promote spontaneous breathing with pressure support or similar mode.
      i. Consider early tracheostomy if ECMO course likely to be prolonged.
      ii. Extubation is possible in both cardiac and respiratory failure patients.
   b. Dyspnea during weaning is common even with adequate pCO_2 and arterial oxygen saturations. If patient can tolerate changes, proceed with weaning.
   c. Expect low tidal volumes in patients with acute respiratory distress syndrome and poor compliance (e.g., 1–3 ml/kg). *Do not* increase vent settings to "recruit" poorly compliant lungs; await lung healing, which may take weeks.

2. *Prone positioning* may be done safely, but is not routine.
3. *Bronchoscopy* may be useful to assess pathology but should not be routine.
4. *Inotropes*: wean inotropic support as tolerated.
5. *Infection*: There is no indication for prophylactic antibiotics in patients on ECMO. Markers of blood stream infections, such as temperature lability and inflammatory markers are unreliable. Cultures for suspected infection and appropriate treatment should be instituted as needed.
6. *Renal*: Renal failure is associated with increased mortality. Almost all patients on ECMO receive diuretics. Renal replacement therapy to maintain fluid balance or support renal insufficiency via a hemofilter placed in an ECMO circuit or via conventional renal replacement therapy devices is recommended.
7. *Nutrition*: Nutritional support is essential. Most patients tolerate enteral nutrition.
8. *Pharmacology*: When therapeutic drug level measurements are available, they should be done to demonstrate adequate dosing.
9. *Neurology*: Baseline head ultrasound in neonates and serial examinations for the first few days of ECMO are recommended to identify bleeding or infarction. Keeping patients awake to monitor neurological status is optimal.
10. *Anticoagulation*: Heparin is the agent used most commonly. A bolus dose of 50 to 100 U/kg at cannulation is routine, followed by a continuous infusion (10–20 U/kg/h) after the anticoagulation goal is reached (activated clotting time, <300 seconds).
11. *Monitoring*:
    a. Activated clotting time: range, 160 to 220 seconds. Can be done at bedside.
    b. Anti-Xa: 0.30 to 0.7 U/mL. Usually checked every 4 to 8 hours or less.
    c. PTT: 1.5 to 2 times normal (not very reliable in neonates)
12. *Alternatives to heparin*:
    a. Argatroban (adapted from University of Michigan ECLS program)
        i. Dosing: 0.2 µg/kg/min and increase; maximum level, 10 µg/kg/min. Increase by 0.05 µg/kg/min every 45 minutes as needed.
        ii. Monitoring: aPTT, 1.5 to 2.5 normal.
    b. Bivalirudin (250 mg + sodium chloride 0.9% 250 mL) (adapted from Mayo Clinic ECLS program)
        i. Give IV 0.15 mg/kg/h. May start at 0.05 mg/kg/h if worried about bleeding.
        ii. Monitor via aPTT 1.5 to 2.5 normal
        iii. Adjust drip as follows:
        iv. aPTT less than goal: Increase infusion rate by 20%; recheck aPTT in 2 hours.
        v. aPTT within goal range: No change in infusion; recheck aPTT in 2 hours. If still within therapeutic range, may check aPTT every 12 hours to daily.

vi. aPTT more than goal: *Stop* infusion for 1 hour, then decrease infusion rate by 30%; recheck aPTT in 2 hours.

13. *Blood product replacement* (adapted from St. Louis Children's Hospital, with permission):
   a. Packed red blood cells (10–20 cc/kg) to maintain hemoglobin (usually 7–10 g/dL)
      i. Patients with impaired oxygenation on VV support may benefit from increased hemoglobin to increase oxygen carrying capacity.
   b. Platelets: 10–20 mL/kg; maximum, usually 2 U at a time
      i. Nonbleeding patient
         1. Maintain more than 100,000 if at high risk of intracranial bleeding.
         2. Maintain more than 50,000 if not at high risk of intracranial bleeding.
         3. In patients with persistent thrombocytopenia, assess for heparin-induced thrombocytopenia. If a result of a chronic condition, accept lower platelet count (levels 20,000–50,000 reported without bleeding).
      ii. Actively bleeding patient: usually maintain platelet count more than 100,000
   c. Fresh frozen plasma: 10–20 cc/kg; maximum, usually 2 U
      i. Nonbleeding patient: INR more than 2, reduce heparin dose if tolerated, consider FFP.
      ii. Bleeding patient: INR more than 1.7, reduce heparin dose if tolerated, consider FFP.
   d. Cryoprecipitate: 1 U/10 kg; maximum, 10 U
      i. Maintain fibrinogen more than 100.
   e. Massive bleeding: Follow massive transfusion protocol.
   f. Antithrombin III
      i. Replace if patient has required increasing heparin with little effect, significant thrombotic events, low anti-Xa levels.
      ii. Strict level not known, usually more than 50%.
      iii. Dosage (not well-validated in children):

$$\text{Bolus dose} = \left(\frac{\text{Goal} - \text{Measured activity}}{\text{Goal activity}} \right) \times \text{Total plasma volume}$$

14. *Recovery from underlying disease*:
   a. Evidenced by
      i. Improved cardiac performance via ECHO at lowered flows
      ii. Improved hemodynamic function
      iii. Improved gas exchange (PaO_2, $ETCO_2$) at constant ventilator settings, ECMO flow and FiO_2
      iv. Improved tidal volume and lung compliance, improving CXR

15. *Weaning from VA ECMO*:
    a. Procedure
        i. Increase ventilator settings to ones desired for removal from ECMO
            1. PIP, less than 28; PEEP, 5 to 10; rate appropriate for age; FiO_2, 0.5 or less
            2. Removal of patients from ECMO on no ventilator support is possible but uncommon.
        ii. Decrease ECMO circuit flow by 20 to 50 mL/min (faster if tolerated) to "idle" settings (at least 10 mL/kg/min). Follow hemodynamic function, acid–base status, gas exchange.
            1. If using centrifugal pump and hollow-fiber membrane lung, note that minimal flows (250–500 cc) increase risk of thrombosis/hemolysis. Consider increasing anticoagulation.
            2. Once at "idle" flow, clamp off VA circuit to obtain true "test" of cardiac and pulmonary performance. Need to assess patient gas exchange (especially CO_2 elimination) completely off support because even minimal ECMO flow removes CO_2 very efficiently. During clamped period, must reestablish flow through cannulas every 10 minutes to prevent clotting.
            3. Obtaining ECHO at low flow or clamped ECMO helps to assess cardiac function.
            4. If patient is hemodynamically stable with adequate gas exchange for 1 to 2 hours, decannulation may be indicated.
16. *Weaning from VV ECMO*:
    a. Procedure
        i. Increase ventilator settings as noted earlier.
        ii. Decrease FiO_2 and gas flow to oxygenator, and "cap" it by removing gas inflow line so that no CO_2 is removed or oxygen is added.
        iii. Because all blood flow is withdrawn and returned to the venous circulation, weaning ECMO flow is not essential, but decreasing flow gradually may help "condition" the heart to assume normal cardiac output and ventricular configuration. Maintaining adequate circuit flow to prevent thrombosis is essential. Total clamping off ECMO with VV support is *not* needed.
        iv. Monitor hemodynamic function and gas exchange.
        v. Decannulate if hemodynamic function and gas exchange are stable.
17. *Special points during weaning*:
    a. If patient has a left atrial vent, it must be clamped or removed to allow left heart filling during weaning.
    b. If patient has an atrial communication created during ECMO, filling the native ventricle at reduced ECMO flows (VA ECMO) may induce a right-to-left atrial shunt (or vice versa). Closure of the atrial communication after ECMO or, rarely, during ECMO before successful weaning may be necessary.

18. *Other points*:
    a. Cardiac patients on VA ECMO
        i. If patient is not improving within 24 to 72 hours, cardiac catheterization to identify correctable residual defects is appropriate.
        ii. Myocarditis/cardiomyopathy: Recovery can be prolonged. Consider changing to a longer term ventricular assist device after 1 week.
        iii. Discuss candidacy for heart transplant within 1 week for surgical patients and within several weeks for myocarditis or cardiomyopathy.
19. *Post-ECMO*:
    a. Maintain focus on hemodynamic function, gas exchange, and acid–base status.
    b. Heparin effect should be allowed to resolve spontaneously. Protamine is *not* recommended.
    c. Larger patients and older adolescents/adults may benefit from continued anticoagulation for deep vein thrombosis prevention.
20. *Follow-up recommended*:
    a. Brain magnetic resonance imaging before discharge
    b. Baseline and discharge Functional Status Scale to identify deficits and institute early intervention
    c. Pulmonary function tests as serial measures
    d. Neurological, developmental, pulmonary follow-up

Reference

1. Dalton HJ, Macrae DJ, for the Pediatric Acute Lung Injury Consensus Group. Extracorporeal life support in children with pediatric acute respiratory distress syndrome: Proceedings from the Pediatric Acute Lung Injury Consensus Conference. *Ped Crit Care Med.* 2015:16:S111–S117.

Further Reading

Angerstrand CL, Burkart KM, Abrams DC, Bacchetta MD, Brodle D. Blood conservation in extracorporeal membrane oxygenation for acute respiratory distress syndrome. *Ann Thorac Surg.* 2015;99(2):590–595.

Barrett CS, Bratton SL, Salvin JW, et al. Neurological injury after extracorporeal membrane oxygenation use to aid pediatric cardiopulmonary resuscitation. *Pediatr Crit Care Med.* 2009;10:445–451.

Chen YS, Lin JW, Yu HY, et al. Cardiopulmonary resuscitation with assisted extracorporeal life-support versus conventional cardiopulmonary resuscitation in adults with in-hospital cardiac arrest: an observational study and propensity analysis. *Lancet.* 2008;372(9638):554–561.

Conrad SA, Grier LR, Scott LK, Green R, Jordan M. Percutaneous cannulation for extracorporeal membrane oxygenation by intensivists: a retrospective single-institution case series. 2015;43(5):1010–1015.

Dalton HJ, Butt WW. Extracorporeal life support: an update of Rogers' Textbook of Pediatric Intensive Care. *Pediatr Crit Care Med.* 2012;13(4):461–471.

Desai SA, Stanley C, Gringlas M, et al. Five-year follow-up of neonates with reconstructed right common carotid arteries after extracorporeal membrane oxygenation. *J Pediatr.* 1999;134:428–433.

Gow KW, Heiss KF, Wulkan ML, et al. Extracorporeal life support for support of children with malignancy and respiratory or cardiac failure: the extracorporeal life support experience. *Crit Care Med.* 2009;37(4):1308–1316.

Lequier L, Joffe AR, Robertson CMT, et al. Two-year survival, mental, and motor outcomes after cardiac extracorporeal life support at less than five years of age. *J Thorac Cardiovasc Surg,* 2008;136:976–983.

Moazami N, Moon MR; Lawton JS; Bailey M, Damiano RJr. Axillary artery cannulation for extracorporeal membrane oxygenator support in adults: an approach to minimize complications. *J Thorac Cardiovasc Srg.* 2003;126:2097–2098.

Pettignano R, Fortenberry JD, Heard ML, et al. Primary use of the venovenous approach for extracorporeal membrane oxygenation in pediatric acute respiratory failure. *Pediatr Crit Care Med.* 2003;4:291–298.

Piena M, Albers MJ, Van Haard PM; Gischler S, Tibboel D. Introduction of enteral feeding in neonates on extracorporeal membrane oxygenation after evaluation of intestinal permeability changes. *J Pediatr Surg.* 1998;33:30–34.

Rao AS, Pellegrini RV; Speziali G; Marone LK. A novel percutaneous solution to limb ischemia due to arterial occlusion from a femoral artery ECMO cannula. *J Endovasc Ther.* 2010;17(1):51–54.

Saini A, Spinella PC. Management of anticoagulation and hemostasis for pediatric extracorporeal membrane oxygenation. *Clin Lab Med.* 2014;34(3):655–673.

Scott LK, Boudreaux K, Thaljeh F, Grier LR, Conrad SA. Early enteral feedings in adults receiving venovenous extracorporeal membrane oxygenation. *J Parenter Enteral Nutr.* 2004;28:295–300.

Spurlock DJ, Toomasian JM, Romano MA, et al. A simple technique to prevent limb ischemia during veno-arterial ECMO using the femoral artery: the posterior tibial approach. *Perfusion.* 2012;27(2):141–145.

Thomas TH, Price R, Ramaciotti C, et al. Echocardiography, not chest radiography, for evaluation of cannula placement during pediatric extracorporeal membrane oxygenation. *Pediatr Crit Care Med.* 2009;10:56–59.

Turner DA, Rehder KJ, Bonadonna D, et al. Ambulatory ECMO as a bridge to lung transplant in a previously well pediatric patient with ARDS. *Pediatrics.* 2014;134(2):e583–e585.

Chapter 3

Transport of the Critically Ill Child

Kathryn Felmet and Richard Orr

All transports out of an emergency department (ED) or intensive care unit (ICU), whether inter-or intrahospital, subject patients to a high-risk environment with multiple distractions and limited resources. The goal during transport should be to prevent a decrement in the care the patient would have received had he or she been stationary, anticipating deterioration of the underlying disease and minimizing the risk of unplanned events while en route.

In the United States, the transfer of patients from one hospital to another is regulated by federal law. The Consolidated Omnibus Budget Reconciliation Act (commonly referred to the "COBRA" law) of 1986 and its 1989 amendment set the current legal standard for patient stabilization and transfer. To promote equal access to emergency treatment regardless of ability to pay, the Consolidated Omnibus Budget Reconciliation Act attributes responsibility for the patient's transfer to the referring hospital and physician. Violations can result in a number of penalties. However, studies of EDs in the United States reveal that many are not equipped to handle critically ill children. Only 5.5% of EDs have all recommended pediatric medical supplies, 12.4% have all recommended vascular access supplies, 23% have 24-hour access to a pediatric emergency medicine-trained physician, and only 62% have access to any pediatric-trained physician.

Hospitals cannot transfer patients unless the transfer is "appropriate," the patient consents to transfer after being informed of the risks of transfer, and the referring physician certifies that the medical benefits expected from the transfer outweigh the risks. Appropriate transfers meet the following criteria: (1) the transferring hospital must provide care and stabilization within its ability; (2) copies of medical records and imaging studies must accompany the patient; (3) the receiving facility must have available space and qualified personnel, and agree to accept the transfer; and (4) interfacility transport must be made by qualified personnel with the necessary equipment.

Risks of Transport

Transport carries numerous risks induced by limited resources and multiple distractions. In addition, it nearly always occurs when the disease process is

Table 3.1 Risks of Interfacility Transport and Potential Mitigating Strategies

Risk	Mitigating Strategies
Communication errors[a]	Communication protocols and/or checklists
Equipment failure	Protocols to verify equipment function, backup plans
Depletion of therapies en route (e.g., medication, oxygen)	Anticipation of needs, prudent use of resources, plan for alternative therapies or interruption of transport
Temperature stress (hot or cold)	Frequent temperature monitoring and use of patient warming/cooling measures as needed
Child fear/anxiety	Consider allowing parent to accompany patient
Motion and noise impede physical examination and monitor function	Use of monitors designed for transport
Lines/tubes become dislodged	Minimize the number of transfers, take extra care to secure equipment
Transport motor vehicle accident[b]	Encourage drivers to abide by speed limits (use of lights and sirens does not improve outcome)

a. Minimum of 3 care teams (referring, transport, receiving) leads to multiple hand-offs

b. EMS providers have an occupational risk of death similar to that of police and firefighters

in a state of evolution and its progression is a common cause of clinical deterioration during transport. When a patient is in shock, a state in which the outcome is dependent on time-sensitive resuscitation, the time lost by failure to advance care during the crucial first hours after presentation may worsen the ultimate outcome. Of nearly 20,000 air medical transports, significant adverse events (death, need for major resuscitative measures, hemodynamic deterioration, inadvertent extubation, or respiratory arrest) occurred in 1 of 20 transports. Baseline hemodynamic instability and assisted ventilation before transport were independent predictors of adverse events. Nonetheless, risks can be mitigated (Table 3.1).

Risks Specific to Air Medical Transport

The physical stresses of the environment itself are magnified during all modes of air transport. Barometric pressure changes from increasing altitude lower alveolar oxygen tension and increase the volume of gas entrapped in the bowel, sinuses, pleural space, and so on. At the altitudes used by rotorcraft (generally <2000 feet (610 meters) above ground level), changes in oxygen tension are insignificant and pressure changes have only a minor impact on the volume of most air-filled spaces. On fixed-wing flights, a cabin pressurized to 8000 feet (2400 meters) above sea level can increase the size of pneumothorax or interstitial emphysema by 30%. On all flights, the relatively small volume of air in a tracheal tube cuff may be subject to clinically significant pressure changes, risking severe airway injury. During helicopter transport, at a mean of just 2260 feet (690 meters), 98% of patients had tracheal tube cuff pressures >30 mm Hg; 72% had cuff pressures greater than 50 mm Hg. Therefore, tracheal tube cuff pressures must be measured and adjusted during flight for any patient undergoing transport by air. Similarly, air removed at altitude needs to be replaced during descent.

The stressors that increase the likelihood of patient deterioration during transport can impair the performance of the transport team as well. Noise, vibration, altitude, and cold can all impair response time and judgment. The added stress of long, sleepless shifts; intense work; and missed meals can amplify the problem. Air transport personnel must be sensitive to their own limitations and to the performance of their team members.

Helicopter Transport

Patients should be well stabilized before helicopter transport, and the threshold for intubation should be lower than that in those undergoing ground transport. Temperature decreases significantly with increasing altitude, particularly in a helicopter. The helicopter environment is noisy, so auscultation of blood pressure and breath sounds is difficult, if not impossible. Flight crews must rely on monitoring that does not depend on audible sounds, such as noninvasive blood pressure monitoring, capnometry, and pulse oximetry. Helicopters produce significant vibrations, making simple procedures such as intubation or restoring intravenous access quite difficult. Cabin size may limit access to the patient. Because physiological changes are easy to miss, and new interventions are rarely initiated, significant deterioration can occur even during relatively short flight times.

Fixed-Wing Transport

Cabin Pressure

Most fixed-wing flights maintain a cabin pressure equivalent to 6000 to 8000 feet (1830 to 2400 meters). In the United States, Federal Aviation Administration regulations mandate a cabin altitude less than 8000 feet. Atmospheric pressure drops from 760 mm Hg at sea level to 565 mm Hg at 8000 feet (2400 meters), with a corresponding decrease in the partial pressure of oxygen. Predicting PaO_2 at altitude is an inexact science; all that can be said conclusively is that those with a marginal PaO_2 at ground level are worse at cruising altitude. In practice, the impact of a cabin pressure in this range can usually be overcome with supplemental oxygen. Oxygen should be used prophylactically in patients who are sensitive to alveolar hypoxia (e.g., those with reactive pulmonary hypertension).

Ventilators

Ventilators are calibrated for performance at sea level. Ventilators that recognize and compensate for changes in barometric pressure are used commonly only by the military. Tidal volumes in volume control mode delivered by the LTV 1000 (Pulmonetic Systems Inc., Minneapolis, MN), commonly used in transport, vary 5% to 12% at simulated altitudes of 4000 feet and 8000 feet.

At 15,000 feet, tidal volumes delivered by the LTV may be 30% to 37% greater than set tidal volumes. Similar findings have been reported with the Drager Oxylog ventilator (Drager, Telford, PA). Ventilators that use pneumatic circuits for respiratory rate control may also deliver lower rates and increased tidal volumes at high altitude.

Acceleration and Deceleration

Acceleration and deceleration forces during takeoff and landing can cause clinically significant fluid shifts. In most aircraft, the stretcher must be positioned head forward. This position causes blood to pool in the legs during acceleration (takeoff) and in the head during deceleration (landing). In a patient with shock, raising the feet can minimize the decrease in cardiac output resulting from decreased venous return associated with takeoff. In a patient with increased intracranial pressure, the head should be raised higher during landing to minimize the increase in intracranial pressure.

Psychological and Social Factors

Finally, pressure on pilots to fly, competition among aeromedical services within a region, and failure to observe minimal weather safety standards can contribute to the potential for catastrophic accidents. Pilots should be encouraged to make decisions based on flight conditions, separate from patient care issues. In regions with competing aeromedical services, the services should act jointly to establish regional safety guidelines, minimum weather standards, and a quality assurance program that examines compliance.

Optimizing Safety and Patient Stabilization During Interfacility Transport: Goal-Directed Therapy Versus "the Golden Hour"

The referring physician is responsible, in consultation with the accepting physician, for determining when a patient is stabilized adequately for safe transfer and for choosing a mode of transport from among the available options. These two decisions represent the central controversies in pediatric interfacility transport, and some disagreement exists between pediatric specialists and adult-oriented emergency practitioners.

The decades-old concept of "the golden hour" is the idea that the amount of time between the moment of injury or severe illness and *arrival at a center* capable of delivering definitive care is among the most important determinants of survival. This concept has dominated decision making in transport medicine. Unfortunately, it is not based on evidence and is incorrect for many patients. Studies have found that time from scene departure to arrival at the hospital was not associated with survival in out-of-hospital cardiac arrest, and transport time (including scene time) was not associated with survival in trauma. The length of the golden hour does determine survival in a few disease processes (e.g., aneurysms requiring neurosurgical intervention, myocardial infarction, and thrombotic events requiring thrombolysis), but these are uncommon in children.

Respiratory failure and shock are the most common reasons for transport of pediatric patients. These conditions may benefit from greater stabilization before transport, even if this adds to the overall transport time. Pediatric guidelines recommend aggressive fluid resuscitation, initiation of inotropes if needed, and administration of antibiotics within the first hour after presentation. These are relatively straightforward interventions that can be initiated in community EDs and can be continued and refined in transport. When community physicians resuscitate aggressively and reverse shock successfully before a transport team arrives, patients have a ninefold increase in their odds of survival. Of course, the treating physician and transferring team must appreciate the urgent need and be sensitive to the sometimes subtle signs of shock in children.

In summary, the current literature defies the popular notion that stabilization before arrival at the receiving center wastes time and delays essential care. Recently, the golden hour concept has been reframed in pediatric transport to be time from presentation to initiation of appropriate treatment, not arrival at a tertiary/receiving center. Thus, appropriate treatments should be initiated as soon as possible at the referring facility and then should be continued and refined by the transport team.

Mode of Transport

Selecting a mode of transport involves deciding between ground versus air ambulance and determining the composition of the team to accompany the patient. Ground ambulance transport is the mainstay of interfacility transport in the United States. Inappropriate application of the golden hour concept may lead to referring physicians prioritizing speed of transport over taking needed time to stabilize the patient. Rather, physicians should choose the mode of transport that can best meet the patient's needs, which may not necessarily be the one that is the fastest. Although mode of transport is commonly determined by consensus between the referring and accepting physicians, the referring physician bears nearly all the legal responsibility.

Ground Versus Air

Air transport is an expensive alternative with several advantages. In general, air medical transport is associated with both shorter transport intervals and a greater medical capability of the transporting team. The decision to use air or ground transport should be based on the factors of time, distance, weather, traffic, geography, patient stability, and local resources.

The practical transport range for helicopter transfers is generally 150 miles from the craft's base of operations. Helicopters depend on certain minimum weather conditions, and changes in weather can make helicopter travel suddenly impossible. Some flight programs are able use rotorcraft in instrument-flight-rules missions, allowing transport of patients in weather conditions that would otherwise preclude helicopter transport. This method requires filing an Instrument Flight Rules flight plan, which may introduce delay.

For longer distance transports or in poor weather conditions, fixed-wing aircraft are used by many air medical services. Many of these aircraft are fitted with very sophisticated medical equipment.

Team Composition
Emergency Medical Service
Most interfacility transfers do not involve critically ill patients and can be accomplished safely by a local emergency medical service (EMS) under pre-defined protocols or with specific instructions from a command physician. In rural areas, use of a local EMS for interfacility transfer risks depleting a large geographic area of valuable medical resources for the duration of the transport. The referring physician, who has little control over the en-route phase of the transport, assumes a significant legal risk.

Because of the variable backgrounds of EMS staff, the transferring personnel may not be equipped or trained to provide the necessary care in every situation. In 2000, less than 5% of the instruction received by nationally registered paramedics was dedicated to pediatrics, and less than 10% of all EMS transports nationwide are for infants and children. This translates into three pediatric patients per month for 60% of the nation's paramedics. Without repeated reinforcement, cognitive and interventional skills deteriorate over time.

Referring Hospital Staff
In some situations, referring hospital staff may accompany a local ambulance service. The legal risk is reduced because the referring physician maintains tighter control over the patient's treatment during the transfer. Disadvantages of this option include the loss of personnel from the referring hospital.

Air Transport Teams
Patients may also be transferred by a regional retrieval system, most of which are centered around air medical transport. Because air medical transport systems are used to transferring sicker patients, the medical teams on these flights offer significantly greater medical capability compared with ground ambulance EMSs.

Air medical transport team members are trained to deal with out-of-hospital emergencies and are acclimated to the stress of working in a moving environment. The team routinely carries equipment to manage deterioration during transfer and has portable monitoring devices designed for use in moving environments. A command physician, usually based at the institution from which the team originates, provides recommendations for management until the team arrives.

Specialized Pediatric Teams
Pediatric or neonatal specialty teams provide an even greater level of expertise in the care of selected patients, although they are not available in all areas.

Because these teams tend to be based at tertiary care centers, time between decision to transfer and team arrival at the bedside may be longer than for a local EMS or regional air medical team. Specialty teams often perform additional stabilization maneuvers before leaving the referring facility. This practice has been criticized as prolonging bedside time and thus the overall transport time. Indeed, time at the bedside can be relatively long (97 minutes for neonates and 50 minutes for pediatric patients). However, this time can actually shorten the time until the patient begins receiving definitive care, because these teams bring the ICU to the patient. The use of pediatric specialized teams has been associated with improved hemodynamic stability, fewer preventable insults (leading to decreased overall costs), and an improvement in risk-adjusted mortality.

Lessons Learned from Improved Outcomes with Pediatric Specialized Teams

The improvement in outcome associated with the use of pediatric specialized teams likely stems from differences between respiratory mechanics and cardiovascular physiology in adults and children that are rarely reinforced by the experience of many adult-oriented emergency physicians. A better appreciation of these pediatric-specific issues would help patients even in areas in which pediatric teams are unavailable.

Respiratory Support
High peripheral airway resistance, small alveoli, and a compliant chest wall increase lower airway obstruction, atelectasis, work of breathing, respiratory muscle fatigue, and the risk of acute respiratory failure. Thus, many children benefit from the institution of mechanical ventilation before transport.

Cardiovascular Support
Shock in children can also be difficult to recognize. Infants and children have a greater capacity to increase systemic vascular resistance during shock states and tend to preserve blood pressure until very late in the evolution of shock. Consensus guidelines for pediatric shock resuscitation call for use of clinical signs as therapeutic endpoints that include age-specific targets for heart rate and blood pressure, and relatively subtle indicators of perfusion.

Transport within the Hospital

In-hospital transport of ICU patients occurs much more commonly than interfacility transport and also carries risks that may be life threatening. The transport environment causes physiological stress. Almost all transported patients experience temporary changes in vital signs requiring intervention, and unplanned events—including equipment failure—occur commonly. Fortunately, during the past two decades, the risks associated with in-hospital transport have decreased significantly.

Specific guidelines for intrahospital transport have been published by the American College of Critical Care Medicine, with general principles the same as those for interfacility transport. Transfer of critically ill patients to another location should be treated as an extension of intensive care. Patients should be stabilized before the trip, and potential causes of deterioration during transport should be included in planning. The need for additional sedation should be anticipated. Particular attention must be paid to maintenance of hypothermia in patients to whom this therapy has been applied. In the sickest patients, mechanical ventilation is superior to hand ventilation. Some studies have documented a decrease in unplanned events with a greater experience level of the accompanying physician.

Equipment taken on an in-hospital transport should include medications for emergency response, airway equipment (including a suction apparatus), and an E-sized oxygen cylinder with tubing of sufficient length. Monitoring should include electrocardiography, pulse oximetry, and the addition of capnography for patients who require mechanical ventilation. Invasive blood pressure monitors should be continued to minimize risk of hemorrhage from a disconnected line.

Conclusions

The decision to transport a patient, between or within hospitals, is predicated on the idea that the risks of transfer are outweighed by its benefits. Although this is nearly always true, transport of critically ill patients entails risk that can be mitigated by careful attention to detail.

In the United States, referring physicians have responsibility for the transport; but, in most cases, they have limited exposure to critically ill pediatric patients. Most pediatric patients with septic shock survive their acute illnesses, and emergency providers rarely witness development of organ dysfunction from seeds sown during the first few hours of the shock state. The accepting physician at a pediatric hospital plays an important role in advocating for the needs of sick children when they differ from a comparable adult.

Further Reading

Dellinger RP, Levy MM, Rhodes A, et al., and the Surviving Sepsis Campaign Guidelines Committee including the Pediatric Subgroup. Surviving sepsis campaign: international guidelines for management of severe sepsis and septic shock, 2012. *Intensive Care Med.* 2013;39(2):165–228.

Han YY, Carcillo JA, Dragotta MA, et al. Early reversal of pediatric–neonatal septic shock by community physicians is associated with improved outcome. *Pediatrics.* 2003;12:793–799.

Newgard CD, Schmicker RH, Hedges JR, et al. Emergency medical services intervals and survival in trauma: assessment of the "golden hour" in a North American prospective cohort. *Ann Emerg Med*. 2010;55(3):235–246.

Singh JM, MacDonald RD, Bronskill SE, Schull MJ. Incidence and predictors of critical events during urgent air-medical transport. *CMAJ*. 2009;181(9):579–584.

Stroud MH, Prodhan P, Moss M, Fiser R, Schexnayder S, Anand K. Enhanced monitoring improves pediatric transport outcomes: a randomized controlled trial. *Pediatrics*. 2011;127(1):42–48.

Warren J, Fromm RE, Orr RA, Rotello LC, Horst HM. American College of Critical Care Medicine guidelines for the inter- and intrahospital transport of critically ill patients. *Crit Care Med*. 2004;32(1):256–262.

Chapter 4

Procedures

Sanjiv Pasala, Eylem Ocal, and Stephen M. Schexnayder

Pediatric intensive care physicians are called on frequently to perform numerous bedside procedures that facilitate the care of the critically ill child. These procedures provide invasive monitoring, support organ function, deliver therapies, and aid in diagnostic and therapeutic interventions.

Intubation

Respiratory failure is a common diagnosis in the pediatric intensive care unit, making endotracheal intubation a fundamental skill for pediatric intensivist. As the body grows and develops, the airway undergoes many changes, making the understanding of anatomic differences in the airway important.

A history related to previous airway surgeries and trauma or known airway abnormalities is important. Perform a physical examination before the procedure, focusing on aspects of the patient's head, neck, and airway anatomy that may make endotracheal intubation difficult. It is important that you pay special attention to any limitations to opening of the mouth, loose teeth, or limited neck mobility. Any indication that the airway may be difficult to intubate requires further planning, specialized tools for difficult airways, and possibly assistance from anesthesia or otolaryngology colleagues.

Indications for endotracheal intubation include respiratory failure resulting from hypoxemia or hypoventilation, airway obstruction, acute lung injury, severe hemodynamic instability, neuromuscular weakness, and infectious processes. Severe traumatic brain injury or depressed level of consciousness with impairment of airway protective reflexes are also indications for endotracheal intubation.

Equipment

Most institutions have dedicated airway equipment carts or bags. Familiarity with the local equipment allows you to anticipate the need for specialized equipment. Also, check each piece of equipment for proper functioning before the procedure. The general equipment needed to perform intubation is listed in Box 4.1.

Technique

Place the patient in a flat, supine position with the head positioned at the head of the bed. In infants and younger patients, place a rolled towel behind the

Box 4.1 Equipment for Endotracheal Intubation

The following equipment is required for endotracheal intubation:
* Appropriate-size bag and mask
* Oxygen source
* Suction and suction tips/catheters
* Appropriate-size endotracheal tube and one size smaller, cuffed or uncuffed
* Appropriate-size stylet
* Appropriate-size laryngoscope blade, curved or straight (operator preference)
* Laryngoscope handle
* Appropriate-size oral airway
* Appropriate-size laryngeal mask airway
* Colorimetric end-tidal carbon dioxide detector
* Sedation, analgesia, anticholinergic, and neuromuscular blocking medications

shoulders to position the patient in the sniffing position. The external auditory meatus should be aligned with the anterior surface of the shoulder for optimal visualization. As the patient's body habitus approaches that of an adult, a folded towel may need to be placed behind the head. Positioning facilitates intubation by aligning the tracheal and oropharyngeal axes. The patient is preoxygenated with 100% oxygen to increase the time the patient maintains acceptable oxygen saturation levels during apnea. A nasogastric tube placed just after sedatives are administered allows decompression of gastric distention during bag mask ventilation. (In the case of the patient with a full stomach, any effort to decompress the stomach should be limited to time when the patient has intact airway reflexes.)

Administer the sedative and analgesic medications. When the patient is sedated, and assuming the patient is not expected to have a full stomach, confirm the ability to perform bag mask ventilation and then administer the neuromuscular blocking agent. After neuromuscular blockade is achieved, open the patient's mouth and advance the laryngoscope blade into the mouth. Lift the blade to visualize the airway. The curved blade should be placed in the valecula to lift the epiglottis, whereas the straight blade should be placed under the epiglottis to lift the epiglottis to expose the airway. Insert the tube into the mouth next to, but not through, the channel of the laryngoscope blade, and advance it into the airway between the vocal cords. Remove the laryngoscope and stylet, if used, from the endotracheal tube, taking care to prevent dislodgment of the endotracheal tube. Confirm correct placement of the endotracheal tube by colorimetric end-tidal carbon dioxide detection or capnography, equal chest rise, equal chest auscultation, mist in the endotracheal tube, and, ultimately, by chest radiography. Secure the tube, noting the depth landmark, and provide ventilation by bag or mechanical ventilator. If the patient desaturates before successful placement of the endotracheal tube, discontinue the attempt to intubate and resume bag mask ventilation. In cases of suspected increased intracranial pressure, remember that arterial carbon dioxide increases with increasing apneic time, and may require manual ventilation to prevent hypercapnia and critically increased intracranial pressure, even in the face of adequate oxygenation.

Complications

Minor complications after endotracheal intubation are common, but usually avoidable. They include lacerated gums or lips, irritation to the throat and upper airway, and chipped or dislodged teeth. More serious complications include laryngospasm, perforation of the trachea or esophagus, aspiration of gastric contents, dislocation or fracture of the cervical spine, and vocal cord injury. Main-stem intubation may result in no complications if recognized early; if unrecognized, the patient may experience atelectasis of the contralateral lung or ventilator-induced injury if full mechanical ventilation is delivered to one lung. Inability to secure the airway or unrecognized esophageal intubation can lead to severe hypoxemia, bradycardia, and cardiac arrest.

Arterial Catheter Placement

Frequent analysis of arterial blood samples is an important aspect in the management of the critically ill pediatric patient. Arterial samples allow for monitoring of oxygenation, ventilation, and acid–base status. Arterial catheters allow continuous monitoring of blood pressure in a patient with rapidly changing hemodynamics.

Indications for arterial catheter placement include the need for close hemodynamic monitoring or to confirm timely response to interventions. Arterial access is also indicated in a patient who requires multiple arterial blood samples to monitor gas exchange and acid–base status, and may allow for accurate sampling without resulting physiological changes from the stress of percutaneous blood sampling. Arterial catheters are indicated for continuous cerebral perfusion pressure monitoring in traumatic brain injury and other acute central nervous system problems.

Few absolute contraindications exist for the placement of an arterial catheter. The skin overlying the desired artery should be intact before attempting placement of an arterial catheter, and evidence of overlying skin infection is an absolute contraindication to placement. Other disruption of the skin, such as a burn, is a relative contraindication. Coagulopathic or anticoagulated patients are at greater risk of bleeding from arterial catheter placement attempts or from the site of the catheter. Assess collateral circulation before choosing a site for placement to minimize the risk of distal blood supply disruption, and do not place an arterial catheter in an extremity with compromised perfusion. Weigh the risks against the benefits of increased hemodynamic monitoring capabilities before attempting placement of an arterial catheter.

Equipment

Prepackaged arterial catheter kits are available commercially and may be preferred in individual institutions. The following is a list of supplies that are commonly used for the procedure:

• Appropriate-size catheter (catheter over needle, or needle and separate catheter with flexible wire)
• Chlorhexidine (preferred) or povidone–iodine
• Sterile towels
• Luer-lock connecter flushed with heparinized saline and additional heparinized saline in labeled syringes or cups
• Sterile gloves, sterile gown, and mask
• Suture
• Instrument tray with needle driver and scissors
• Clear occlusive dressing
• Pressure tubing and transducer primed with heparin-containing fluids with or without papaverine

Technique

Select the site, first considering the peripheral arteries of distal extremities based on ease of access, good collateral circulation, ease of site observation, and control of hemorrhage with direct pressure. Most common peripheral sites include the radial, dorsalis pedis, and posterior tibial arteries. In the case of inadequate peripheral sites, arterial catheters may be placed in the femoral or axillary arteries. There have been recent reports of using brachial arteries in pediatric patients with good success, but this artery has no collateral circulation. The temporal artery should be avoided because of poor collateral circulation and retrograde flow into the cerebral circulation with potential air embolism.

When the site has been selected, position and immobilize the extremity. In the case of the radial artery, slightly hyperextend the wrist, bringing the artery closer to the skin and straightening its course near the puncture site.

The following procedure and techniques can be used to place an arterial catheter in any selected site. Prepare the skin with chlorhexidine solution and drape the area with sterile towels. Topical anesthetics can be used before skin preparation and draping, or local anesthetics can be injected subcutaneously. Arterial catheters can be placed percutaneously using any of the three methods discussed next.

The first method involves using the Seldinger technique. Palpate the arterial pulse to pinpoint the location of the artery. Advance the introducer needle through the skin and anterior wall of the artery. After confirmation of continuous arterial blood flow from the hub of the introducer needle, pass a guidewire through the needle and advance it into the lumen of the artery. Remove the needle and advance a catheter over the guidewire into the artery. Remove the wire and attach a flushed Luer-lock connecter to the catheter. Confirm correct placement by aspiration of blood through the catheter and into the syringe attached to the connector. Flush the catheter and secure it using suture, tape, or a catheter securement device. Cover the site with a transparent occlusive dressing. At some centers, chlorhexidine-impregnated patches are placed over the site before applying the occlusive dressing.

The next method uses an over-the-needle catheter in a manner similar to placing a peripheral intravenous (IV) catheter. Locate the artery using palpation. Advance the catheter-over-needle through the skin and the anterior wall of the artery until arterial blood is seen. Advance the catheter and needle a few millimeters to ensure the catheter tip is in the lumen of the artery. With the needle held in position, advance the catheter over the needle into the lumen of the artery. When the catheter has been advanced to the hub, remove the needle. Flushing saline slowly through the catheter as it is advanced in the lumen of the artery may aid advancement of the catheter. Confirm correct placement with aspiration of arterial blood. Secure and dress the catheter.

The final percutaneous method also uses an over-the-needle catheter, but the technique involves transfixing the artery. In this method advance the needle through the skin and anterior wall of the artery. When there is a flash of arterial blood through the needle, advance the needle through the posterior wall of the artery and into the surrounding tissues, transfixing the artery. Remove the needle, leaving the catheter through the artery. Withdraw the catheter slowly into the lumen of the artery until arterial blood flows from the hub of the catheter. Advance the catheter into the lumen of the artery. Correct placement is confirmed again by aspiration of arterial blood through the catheter. Secure and cover the catheter.

The percutaneous techniques can be used in combination with bedside ultrasound guidance. Currently there is conflicting evidence regarding the success rate, puncture attempts, and length of procedure comparing the simple palpation technique with use of ultrasound guidance.[1,2]

Complications

Complications of arterial catheters include hemorrhage, thrombus formation, distal ischemia, emboli, and infection. A recent study showed an overall complication rate of 10.3% of arterial catheters in children. The most common complication was infection.[3] Infection of arterial catheters can be local or systemic and may be related to the length of catheter use and location in the femoral artery. It is important to assess the need for an arterial catheter daily and remove it as soon as it is no longer required for optimal care.

Central Venous Catheter Placement

The ability to monitor central venous parameters and gain stable venous access is a critical skill of the intensivist. Central venous catheters (CVCs) can be essential monitoring tools as well as therapeutic delivery devices.

Anticipate the need for central venous access to allow for a safe and controlled procedure.

Indications for CVCs include the need for stable and reliable venous access in a patient with limited peripheral venous access as well as the administration of medications and IV nutrition that require central delivery. Frequent blood sampling and access for providing extracorporeal support such as continuous renal replacement therapy are also indications. A CVC may be used to monitor central venous pressure and oxygen saturation.

Contraindications related to CVC placement are related to the site and are not absolute. Femoral CVCs placed in abdominal or pelvic trauma can lead to increased risk of complications. In patients with coagulopathies, the subcalavian vein involves more risk because of the difficulty in applying direct pressure. Avoid CVC placement through infected skin. As with any procedure, the risks and benefits should be considered before CVC insertion.

Equipment

Complete sterile barrier kits for CVC placement are available commercially. Choose the appropriate catheter for the size of the patient and the size of the target vein. Catheters are available commercially in multiple diameters, lengths, and number of lumens. Most catheters used for CVCs are made of plastic polymers and are also available with antibiotic or antiseptic coating.

Technique

Review the anatomy of the chosen vessel and surrounding structures (i.e., respective artery and nerve) at the insertion site. Sedation and analgesia enable the patient to tolerate the procedure comfortably. Even with the use of systemic agents, use of a local anesthetic is important in reducing the need for systemic agents. Adequate sedation and analgesia allow for easier and safer placement of the CVC.

Use full-barrier precautions during CVC insertion, including wearing a cap, mask, and sterile gown, and careful hand washing. The skin at the insertion site should be cleaned with chlorhexidine. Cover the entire patient and work surface with sterile drapes.

The Seldinger technique is appropriate for CVC insertion, regardless of the chosen site. Palpate the anatomic landmarks and locate the target vein. Advance an introducer needle with syringe attached through the skin into the lumen of the vein while aspirating on the syringe. Blood flows freely into the syringe when the needle tip is in the vein lumen. Stabilize the introducer needle and remove the syringe from the needle. Blood flow rate through the needle depends on the vein and needle size. Confirm that blood flow is not pulsatile. If there is concern that arterial placement has occurred, attach sterile saline-filled extension tubing to the needle and elevate it to estimate venous pressure. Pulsatile blood flow indicates arterial placement, regardless of the tubing elevation. Advance the J-shaped guidewire through the introducer needle into the lumen of the vein. The wire should pass with no resistance into the vein. If resistance is met while advancing, remove the wire and reposition the needle into the lumen of the vessel. If necessary, reattach the syringe to the introducer needle during repositioning to confirm free blood flow from the vein. If at any time the wire cannot be removed easily from the needle, remove the needle and wire together to avoid shearing the wire. When the guidewire is advanced well into the vein lumen, use a scalpel to widen the insertion site at the skin to allow for the dilator to pass. Remove the needle over the wire, using caution to keep the wire stationary. Pass the dilator over the wire and into the skin and soft tissue and just into the vessel wall to create a path for the catheter. Remove the dilator, again keeping the guidewire stable, and advance the CVC over the wire to a predetermined length into the vein lumen. Check all lumens for blood return and flush to prevent thrombosis.

Secure the catheter to the skin using sutures or a commercially available catheter securement device. Cover the site with a clear occlusive dressing. Some institutions place a chlorhexidine-impregnated patch at the skin entrance site of the CVC before the occlusive dressing.

The use of real-time bedside ultrasound during placement of CVCs is becoming standard practice in many centers. Before ultrasound, the location of the vessel was determined using anatomic landmarks only, but portable ultrasound devices with transducers designed to visualize vessels are now available. Ultrasound allows the operator to assess the patency and size of the vein before attempting CVC placement, allowing the delineation of variations from classically described anatomy. Using sterile sheaths, the ultrasound transducer can be used to locate the vessel and track the path of the needle as it is advanced into the lumen of the vein. Real-time ultrasound guidance allows visualization of surrounding structures to reduce complications such as accidental arterial puncture. Ultrasound-guided CVC placement decreases the complications and placement attempts in pediatric patients compared with the landmark-only approach.[4] The US Agency for Healthcare Research and Quality recommends real-time ultrasound guidance for CVC placement.

The landmark-based approach to central venous line placement remains an essential skill for the intensivist. Proper positioning is essential for both the landmark-based technique as well as for real-time ultrasound-assisted placement. For central venous line placement in the femoral vein, place the patient in a supine position, usually with a rolled towel under the hips to elevate the pelvis and straighten the course of the femoral vein. Abduct the leg slightly and rotate it externally. The femoral vein is located medial to the artery and nerve in the neurovascular bundle as it travels from the peritoneal cavity, under the inguinal ligament, and into the leg. Palpate the arterial pulse and insert the introducer needle 5 to 10 mm medial to the femoral artery and 1 to 2 cm below the inguinal ligament, reducing these distances in smaller patients. Hold the needle at a 30° angle from the surface of the leg and aim toward the umbilicus.

Positioning for accessing the internal jugular vein involves having the patient lying in the supine position with a rolled towel placed behind the shoulders to extend the neck. Trendelenburg positioning distends the internal jugular vein in some patients. Turn the patient's head to the contralateral side to expose the target vein. The sternocleidomastoid muscle separates into to bundles before attaching onto the clavicular head. The internal jugular vein traverses the anatomic triangle created by the separation of the sternal and clavicular heads of the sternocleidomastoid muscle. Hold the introducer needle at a 20° to 30° angle from the neck surface and advance the needle toward the ipsilateral nipple.

For the subclavian approach, position the patient in a flat, supine position with a rolled towel placed along the spine. The subclavian vein passes behind the clavicle and the sternum before joining the superior vena cava. Palpate the junction of the distal and middle third of the clavicle. At this site, the needle angle is almost flat against the chest and is directed toward the suprasternal notch. The needle passes along the inferior aspect of the clavicle and into the vein. The angle of the needle needs to remain as flat as possible to reduce the risk of pneumothorax.

Complications

Complications of CVC insertion include air embolism, arrhythmias, retained wire, and venous or arterial bleeding. When the insertion site is located in the internal jugular or subclavian artery, the complications can also include cardiac tamponade, hemothorax, pneumothorax, hydrothorax, and chylothorax. Complications arising after insertion include local and systemic infection, phlebitis, thrombosis, pulmonary embolism, vascular perforation, and bleeding.

Tube Thoracostomy

Tube thoracostomy for chest drainage is a common procedure in the pediatric critical care setting. Indications for tube thoracostomy include removing space-occupying material from the pleural space such as pneumothoraces, large parapneumonic effusions or empyemas secondary to infectious or malignant processes, hemothoraces or hemopneumothoraces in trauma patients, and chylothoraces in postoperative cardiac patients. Consideration of the nature of material to be removed from the chest may allow a smaller tube and/or less invasive techniques to be used.

There are no absolute contraindications to tube thoracostomy. If a patient is coagulopathic, attempt to correct the coagulopathy before the procedure to minimize bleeding complications. In the case of an emergent need for tube thoracostomy, perform the procedure with treatment of the coagulopathy in progress during or immediately after the procedure.

Equipment

Chest tube trays with sterile instruments are available at most institutions. The technique used to perform the tube thoracostomy dictates the equipment required. The following is a general list of equipment used in the techniques to be described:

- Appropriate-size chest tube
- Scalpel and blade
- Sterile gloves, towels, and gauze sponges
- Chlorhexidine solution
- Suture
- Instruments including needle driver, scissors, and curved (Kelly) forceps of various sizes
- Local anesthetic and in a labeled syringe with needle
- Chest tube drainage apparatus

Technique

Tube thoracostomy is painful; patients should receive sedation and analgesia for this procedure. In addition, use generous local anesthesia with 1% lidocaine (up to 0.5 mL/kg). The technique and tube selection are based on the material to be removed from the chest. Thin, transudative fluid can be removed with small-caliber pigtail catheters using a modified Seldinger technique for placement, whereas more viscous fluid may require a larger tube.

After providing sedation and analgesia, place the patient in a supine position. Alternatively, perform the procedure with the patient sitting up and leaning over a padded table. An assistant is usually necessary to help maintain the patient's position and monitor his or her cardiopulmonary status. Prepare the skin overlying the site with chlorhexidine and drape with sterile towels. Infiltrate the site with lidocaine, including the subcutaneous tissue, the periosteum of the rib, and the intercostal muscle. Advance the introducer needle, with a syringe attached, in the fourth or fifth intracostal space in the midaxillary line over the top of the rib to avoid the neurovascular bundle. Apply continuous suction to the syringe and advance the needle slowly until air or fluid is aspirated. Remove the syringe from the needle and advance the guidewire through the needle into the pleural space. Remove the needle over the guidewire and incise the skin with a scalpel. Pass the dilator over the wire and advance it to dilate the skin and subcutaneous tissue. Next, pass the chest tube over the guidewire and advance it into the pleural space. Remove the guidewire and connect the tube to the drainage apparatus. Secure the tube to the skin with sutures or a securement device. Pigtail catheters tend to be less painful to the patient after placement than larger thoracostomy tubes, but generally do not drain viscous fluids well (e.g., blood or pus).

Placing larger straight chest tubes requires a variation on this technique. After the guidewire is in the pleural space, pass progressively larger dilators through the skin and soft tissue. Finally, pass a straight tube over a dilator over the wire, and remove the dilator and wire. These tubes and dilators are available in commercially packaged kits.

The traditional technique of incision and blunt dissection for tube thoracostomy may be required to drain viscous fluids from the chest. After adequate sedation and analgesia, place the patient in the supine position. Prepare the skin over the site with chlorhexidine and drape with sterile towels. Inject a local anesthetic into the site. Incise the skin over the lower rib with the goal of inserting the tube in the fourth or fifth intercostal space in the midaxillary line. Dissect the soft tissue bluntly using the curved clamp until the superior border of the rib is reached. Then, push the clamp through the intercostal muscles and pleura. The end of the tube is attached to the clamp and inserted into the pleural space. A second clamp or hemostat applied to the distal tube reduces the free flow of liquid when the pleural space is entered. Open the clamp within the pleural space and advance the tube. The preferred position of the tube is anterior for pneumothoraces and posterior for effusions or blood. The tube is then attached to the drainage apparatus and secured to the skin using a horizontal mattress suture, purse-string suture, or securement device.

Complications

Several potential complications exist with placement of chest tubes. If tubes are forced into the pleural cavity, any structure in the chest may be injured. Placement of tubes into lung parenchyma is a relatively common complication and is more frequent with Seldinger technique-placed tubes in patients with poorly compliant or hyperinflated lungs. This can lead to the development of bronchopleural fistulas. Injury to vascular structures can occur with high placement of chest tubes. Computed tomographic scanning of the chest can reveal the exact placement of the tube within the chest.

Paracentesis

Paracentesis is a procedure for percutaneous aspiration of peritoneal fluid. Paracentesis is a relatively safe procedure and a valuable diagnostic tool in patients with ascites. Indications for paracentesis include new-onset ascites, respiratory distress or impairment secondary to massive ascites, and suspected bacterial peritonitis. Paracentesis with placement of an indwelling catheter has been used to manage abdominal compartment syndrome in critically ill pediatric patients, including extracorporeal membrane oxygenation patients.[5,6]

Paracentesis in a patient with ascites has no absolute contraindications. Patients who require paracentesis often have liver dysfunction with coagulopathy. Coagulopathy is not a contraindication, but correction of the coagulopathy may be needed before the procedure. To avoid introducing bacteria into the peritoneal cavity, paracentesis should not be performed through an area of infected skin.

Equipment
The following is a general list of supplies for performing a paracentesis:

• Chlorhexidine solution
• Sterile towels, gloves, and gauze sponges

- Local anesthetic with labeled syringe and needle
- Large-bore IV catheter or spinal needle (16–20 gauge)
- Syringe to aspirate sample (≥20 mL)
- Sterile specimen container
- Percutaneous catheter set (if drain to be left in place)

Technique

Place the patient in a supine position with the head of the bed elevated 30°. The bladder should be emptied. Verify by physical examination and ultrasonography the presence of ascites before the procedure, The preferred sites for paracentesis are in the midline 2 cm below the umbilicus through the avascular linea alba or, in patients with portal hypertension, a lateral approach to avoid the a vascularized linea alba and hemorrhagic complications. The lateral approach involves the left or right lower quadrant, a few centimeters above the inguinal ligament and lateral to the rectus abduminus muscle. Inspect the site with bedside real-time ultrasound to locate a target of ascites.

Prepare the site with chlorhexidine solution and drape with sterile towels. Infiltrate local anesthetic into the skin and subcutaneous tissues. Attach a syringe to the needle or IV catheter and advance it through the skin with caudal traction applied to the skin to create a "Z track." Advance the needle while applying suction to the syringe. When free flow of fluid is noted through the needle, hold the catheter or needle in place while a fluid sample is collected. Clamping a hemostat to the needle at the skin surface may help maintain the appropriate insertion depth. If using an IV catheter, as soon as fluid is obtained, advance the catheter over the needle into the peritoneal cavity, then remove the needle and attach the syringe to the catheter. Place the aspirated sample of peritoneal fluid in a sterile specimen container. Then, remove the needle or catheter, apply direct pressure, and place a sterile pressure dressing. For ongoing drainage, place a pigtail catheter using a modified Seldinger technique and secure it to a drainage device.

Complications

Complications from paracentesis can result from direct injury to intra-abdominal structures. Complications include persistent ascitic fluid leak, bladder and bowel perforation, bleeding, peritonitis, abdominal wall hematoma, and bleeding.

Pericardiocentesis

Pericardiocentesis is the percutaneous aspiration of fluid or air from the pericardial space. The absolute indication for pericardiocentesis is cardiac tamponade, but it may be needed for diagnostic purposes with pericardial effusion. Pericardiocentesis can be performed without imaging guidance, although using imaging guidance may lower the risk and increase the success rate of the procedure.

When performing pericardiocentesis for cardiac tamponade, there are no contraindications. The presence of aortic dissection is considered a major contraindication. For elective pericardiocentesis, coagulopathy is a contraindication, as is a loculated effusion not accessible by the subxiphoid approach. Operator inexperience may be considered a relative contraindication for elective pericardiocentesis.

Equipment

The following is a general list of supplies for performing pericardiocentesis:

• Chlorhexidine solution
• Sterile towels, gloves, and gauze sponges
• Labeled local anesthetic syringe and needle
• IV catheter, spinal needle, or introducer needle (16–20 gauge)
• Syringe to aspirate sample (≥20 mL)
• Sterile specimen container
• Percutaneous catheter set (if a drain to be left in place)

Technique

Place the patient in a supine position with the head elevated 30°. Confirm the presence of a pericardial effusion with echocardiography in all patients except those with suspected cardiac tamponade in cardiac arrest. Prepare the area around the xiphoid and the lower costal margin with chlorhexidine and drape with sterile towels. Infiltrate local anesthetic in the skin and subcutaneous tissue at the junction of the xiphoid process and the left costal margin. Insert the needle with a syringe attached below the junction of the xiphoid process and the left costal margin with a 30 to 45° angle and aim toward the left clavicle. Apply suction while advancing the needle. Stop the needle advancement as soon as fluid or air is aspirated. If blood is aspirated, careful evaluation is needed to determine the source of the blood—pericardial or intracardiac. Techniques for determining the origin of blood aspirated include echocardiography with agitated saline instilled via the needle, clotting of the blood, or the hematocrit level of the patient's blood versus the aspirated sample. Once pericardial origin of the fluid is certain, collect a sample and placed it in a sterile specimen container for further analysis. Perform drainage by needle aspiration; if ongoing drainage is needed, place a pigtail catheter using a modified Seldinger technique.

Complications

Cardiac puncture is not an uncommon complication of pericardiocentesis. This complication can range from minor injury with no clinical significance to a life-threatening injury requiring emergent repair. Other complications include coronary artery laceration, pneumothorax, hemothorax, hemoperitoneum, injury to bowel and diaphragm, and cardiac arrest.

Ventriculoperitoneal Shunt Tap

Ventriculoperitoneal (VP) shunting for hydrocephalus is a common procedure in pediatric patients. Since their introduction during the 1940s, shunts remain the mainstay of hydrocephalus treatment. The cerebrospinal fluid (CSF) is shunted from the lateral ventricles of the brain into the peritoneum via the shunt hardware, which consists of a ventricular (proximal) catheter, a valve mechanism, and a peritoneal (distal) catheter. Figure 4.1 shows a typical shunt system. The distal catheter can also be placed into pleural cavity, right atrium, or gall bladder.

Tapping or aspirating the shunt is performed for both diagnostic reasons (e.g., to evaluate for shunt infection or blockage) and therapeutic reasons (e.g., to alleviate high intracranial pressure or to inject medications such as chemotherapeutic agents or antibiotics).

The clinical diagnosis of a shunt malfunction can be challenging. The importance and role of a shunt tap is controversial in the diagnosis of shunt malfunction. When available, a neurosurgeon should perform this procedure. The intensivist should be able to perform the procedure in a life-threatening emergency, such as impending herniation.

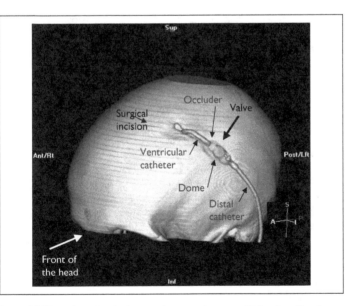

Figure 4.1 Three-dimensional reformatted computed tomographic imaging of head showing ventriculoperitoneal shunt components. (Courtesy of D. Doug Cochrane, MD, Professor of Pediatric Neurosurgery, British Columbia Children's Hospital) *Note to editors: I am trying to get a new figure that demonstrates the shunt on the right side of the head.- SS*

A VP shunt tap is not without risk, because a functioning noninfected shunt may become an infected shunt that needs revision. The risk of infection from a shunt tap is 2% to 5%.[7-9] It is important to exclude other common conditions and infections that may mimic shunt malfunction. Shunt infections are unlikely more than 3 months after placement.

There are few contraindications to a shunt tap. Absolute contraindications include infection over the entry site and severe coagulopathy. In addition, the lack of shunt imaging or information about the shunt type may cause unwanted problems. Potential complications include infection, bleeding, and CSF leak from the puncture site. The risk of introducing infection from a tap is low, but the consequences of a shunt infection may be dire. Sterile technique is crucial.

A small risk exists of bleeding from subcutaneous vessels at the entry site of the needle during the tap. Minimize the risk of bleeding by using a small needle and by checking for coagulation parameters before the procedure. A small needle also reduces the risk of CSF leak.

Equipment

A lumbar puncture kit suffices for the shunt tap with little additional equipment. The following is a list of supplies used for the procedure:

* Sterile gloves and mask
* Povidone–iodine, chlorhexidine, or 2% chlorhexidine gluconate
* Sterile drape
* Butterfly needles, 23 or 25 gauge
* Syringe, 3 to 5 mL
* Three-way stopcock
* CSF manometer
* Sterile gauze
* Wound dressing
* Specimen tubes for CSF collection

Technique

Except in the presence of immediately life-threatening situations (impending herniation), consult a neurosurgeon before tapping a VP shunt. Carefully review shunt imaging to locate the part of shunt hardware that can be tapped. There are a variety of shunt systems. Most shunt systems incorporate a reservoir, often a smooth, rounded bubble that can be palpated under the skin. In other systems, a part of the actual valve, usually a smooth domelike structure, may serve as the reservoir and can be tapped. The reservoir /valve hardware may be visible as a bump on the scalp in younger children. There are other shunt systems, such as shunts with slit valves, which may not have a reservoir to allow puncture.

Use of injectable local anesthesia is generally unnecessary, because infiltrating the skin and subcutaneous tissue with local anesthetic may be as painful as the shunt tap itself. Application of a topical local anesthetic cream before the procedure is useful in children when time permits.

Positioning the patient and maintaining his or her comfort during the procedure is important. The patient should be supine, with the head flat and oriented so the VP shunt reservoir is upright. The shunt hardware is usually placed on the right side of the patient, so the reservoir and the valve lie on the right side of the head. If hair overlies the reservoir, part and clean the hair away; shaving may disturb skin integrity, increasing the risk of infection. If shaving is necessary to identify the reservoir, use a hair trimmer rather than a razor.

Technique

Clean the skin thoroughly with an antiseptic solution in circles outward from the entry site at least three times and allow to dry. Place a sterile fenestrated drape over the reservoir/valve site. Insert a small (23 or 25 gauge) butterfly (scalp vein) needle perpendicular to the skin into the reservoir. When the reservoir is entered, a drop in resistance is felt. Advance slowly until the bevel of the needle is fully inside the reservoir.

Hold the needle securely in place and observe spontaneous flow as the CSF fills the tubing. If flow is poor, adjust the needle to achieve optimal positioning. Avoid removing the needle and reinserting, if possible, because of the increased risk of infection and patient discomfort. If flow remains slow, then aspirate gently with a 3- or 5-mL syringe. This starts the flow unless there is a proximal obstruction. If CSF is aspirated easily, the pressure in the ventricular system may be low. Stop aspirating if resistance is felt or it is difficult to aspirate, which may indicate obstruction. In addition, aspiration can result in the choroid plexus being drawn into the shunt tip, precipitating shunt blockage. Poor flow is correlated strongly with proximal shunt obstruction.[9,10]

When flow is obtained, attach a manometer to measure the opening pressure. If a manometer is not available, the tubing of the butterfly needle can be used as a fluid column and measured with a tape measure. It is measured vertically from the top of the CSF column to the level of the reservoir (entry site of the needle) or to the level of the tragus of the ear. Allow the CSF to drip slowly into the sample tubes through the end of the needle tubing or three-way stopcock. Collect 3 to 5 mL of the sample for analysis. Send the CSF sample for cell count, protein level, glucose level, Gram stain, and culture.

If the opening pressure is greater than 20 cm H_2O, more CSF may be drained to decrease the intracranial pressure. This temporizes the patient's condition until definitive treatment.

To assess distal shunt function, fill the manometer with sterile saline and occlude the proximal occluder if present. This action allows the fluid to run distally into the valve and the peritoneal catheter. Observe the fluid column as fluid flows into the shunt system distally. The presence of the occluder depends on the shunt valve type.

When sufficient information and CSF sample for routine analysis have been obtained, withdraw the needle from the reservoir and apply gentle pressure over the entry site with sterile gauze. Clean any the debris or blood. Apply a small adhesive bandage to the puncture site.

The findings of a shunt tap may be inconclusive. High opening CSF pressures (>20 cm H_2O) are associated with distal shunt obstruction in approximately 90% of cases,[11] whereas poor flow is a good indicator of proximal shunt obstruction.

References

1. Shiver S, Blaivas M, Lyon M. A prospective comparison of ultrasound-guided and blindly placed radial arterial catheters. *Acad Emerg Med.* 2006;13(12):1275–1279.
2. Ganesh A, Kaye R, Cahill AM, et al. Evaluation of ultrasound-guided radial artery cannulation in children. *Pediatr Crit Care Med.* 2009;10(1):45–48.
3. King MA, Garrison MM, Vavilala MS, Zimmerman JJ, Rivara FP. Complications associated with arterial catheterization in children. *Pediatr Crit Care Med.* 2008;9(4):367–371.
4. Froehlich CD, Rigby MR, Rosenberg ES, et al. Ultrasound-guided central venous catheter placement decreases complications and decreases placement attempts compared with the landmark technique in patients in a pediatric intensive care unit. *Crit Care Med.* 2009;37(3):1090–1096.
5. Sharpe RP, Pryor JP, Gandhi RR, Stafford PW, Nance ML. Abdominal compartment syndrome in the pediatric blunt trauma patient treated with paracentesis: report of two cases. *J Trauma.* 2002;53(2):380–382.
6. Prodhan P, Imamura M, Garcia X, et al. Abdominal compartment syndrome in newborns and children supported on extracorporeal membrane oxygenation. *ASAIO J.* 2012;58(2):143–147.
7. Noetzel MJ, Baker RP. Shunt fluid examination: risks and benefits in the evaluation of shunt malfunction and infection. *J Neurosurg.* 1984;61:328–332.
8. Kulkarni AV, Drake JM, Lamberti-Pasculli M. Cerebrospinal fluid shunt infection: a prospective study of risk factors. *J Neurosurg.* 2001;94:195–201.
9. Miller JP, Fulop SC, Dashti SR, Robinson S, Cohen AR. Rethinking the indications for the ventriculoperitoneal shunt tap. *J Neurosurg Pediatrics.* 2008;1(6):435–438.
10. Rocque BG, Lapsiwala S, Iskandar BJ. Ventricular shunt tap as a predictor of proximal shunt malfunction in children: a prospective study. *J Neurosurg Pediatrics.* 2008;1(6):439–443.
11. Shapiro AMJ, Lakey JRT, Ryan EA, et al. Islet transplantation in seven patients with type 1 diabetes mellitus using a glucocorticoid-free immunosuppressive regimen. *N Engl J Med.* 2000;343(4):230–238.

Chapter 5

Basic Pediatric Hemodynamic Monitoring

Jorge G. Sainz and Bradley P. Fuhrman

Historical Perspective

In critically ill children, applications of science and technology to physiological monitoring enable us to distinguish normal from abnormal physiology. Until fairly recently, only temperature, heart rate, blood pressure, and respiratory rate were used to follow the course of illness. Advanced invasive and noninvasive monitoring has only been possible for about 50 years. The developing of catheter over needle devices, the widespread use of the Seldinger technique, the evolution of the medical and nursing specialties of critical care, and the electronic revolution of the 1960s made possible the cardiorespiratory monitoring we use today.

The state-of-the-art monitoring tools currently in use and future technologies under development will continue to complement clinical care. It is unlikely, however, that monitoring devices will ever supplant the vigilant clinician at the bedside. Monitoring systems do not make clinical decisions; clinicians do. Hemodynamic parameters are often meaningless unless coordinated with physical findings and knowledge of disease processes. The same hemodynamic profile may have a very different meaning from one patient to another. For example, a patient with early septic shock and one with aortic insufficiency might both have normal systolic but low diastolic pressure. Fundamentally, cardiorespiratory monitoring targets the assessment of adequacy of oxygen uptake, delivery, and use.

Pulse Oximetry, Mixed Venous Oxygen Saturation Monitoring, and Near-Infrared Spectroscopy

Pulse Oximetry

Monitoring and optimizing oxygen delivery and tissue oxygenation are key therapeutic strategies to treat critically ill patients. Restoration and assurance of adequate tissue oxygenation are important targets of treatment. Frequent assessments of oxygen saturation, partial pressure of dissolved oxygen, regional oxygenation, and tissue oxygen extraction help clinicians follow the progression and resolution of critical illness.

Pulse oximetry is used in critical care units around the globe. Its technology is elegant and practical. Hemoglobin molecules are analyzed noninvasively by red and infrared absorption. Oxygenated and deoxygenated hemoglobin absorb light at different wavelengths. Pulsatile differences in absorption are attributed to arterial blood and allow for the estimation of arterial oxygenation saturation. This value does not provide much informa tion on tissue oxygenation, but it does define the state of oxygenation of arterial blood.

Pulse oximetry does have limitations. In the upper range, despite large changes in pO2, there is little difference in saturation because of the flatness of the oxyhemoglobin dissociation curve. At saturations less than 70%, accuracy is diminished. Carboxyhemoglobin and methemoglobin have absorption spectra similar to oxyhemoglobin.[1] Their presence may elevate apparent oxygen saturation falsely. At high concentrations, these abnormal hemoglobins, which do not deliver usable oxygen to tissues, may hide the true extent of oxygen deficiency by masquerading as oxyhemoglobin.[2]

Poor arterial pulsation, which occurs in low perfusion states or hypothermia, interferes with the accuracy of pulse oximetry. Motion of the monitored extremity may also interfere with accuracy.

Mixed and Central Venous Oxygen Saturation Monitoring

Regional tissue conditions, such as temperature, pH, and 2-3 DPG concentration, influence the download of oxygen molecules at the capillary level. Specific organs have different metabolic oxygen consumption rates depending on their specific oxygen demand indexes and critical illness stressors. Adequacy of tissue perfusion is also specific to each tissue. *Mixed venous blood* is a mixture of blood returning from all these tissues. It is sampled only imperfectly under most circumstances. The difference between arterial and venous oxygen saturations (mixed venous blood measured or sampled at a site in the pulmonary artery) is normally only about 25%, allowing a significant oxygen surplus to ensure adequate oxidative metabolism. Therefore, mixed venous oxygen saturation is helpful in determining the body's overall extraction of oxygen; however, it offers little clinical insight into organ-specific oxygen extraction and consumption or potential organ-specific deficit (Box 5.1). Moreover, it is an invasive measurement. Oximetric pulmonary artery catheters allow continuous monitoring of mixed venous saturation, but their use is increasingly uncommon. *Central venous oxygen saturation* is often used to estimate oxygen extraction and can be very useful for following trends, but it is even more dependent on the sampling location. Samples taken from the superior vena cava are typically much more desaturated than those taken from the

Box 5.1 Common Causes for Altered Venous Oxygen Saturation Levels

Abnormally Low Venous Oxygen Saturation
- Inadequate cardiac output
- Low hemoglobin level
- Arterial desaturation
- Increased metabolic rate without compensatory increased oxygen delivery

High Venous Oxygen Saturation
- Inability to extract oxygen (occasionally in late septic shock)
- Metabolic poisons (e.g., cyanide)
- Large systemic arteriovenous malformation (when overall cardiac output is sufficient to meet metabolic needs)

inferior vena cava, reflecting, in large part, the greater oxygen consumption of the brain compared with organs below the diaphragm, especially the kidneys (Box 5.2).

Near-Infrared Spectroscopy

The degree of oxygen extraction by individual organs is a useful and measurable marker for adequate oxidative metabolism. Near-infrared spectroscopy measures the transmission of near-infrared light through tissue—a phenomenon dependent on the oxygen-carrying states of both hemoglobin and the cytochrome aa_3. It appears to be of value for trending intracranial perfusion, and may prove useful for other tissues. It is not yet sufficiently quantifiable for individual measurements. In fact, in a study of cerebral oxygenation, one-third of cadavers were found to have near-infrared spectroscopy values greater than the lower limit of normal.[3]

Box 5.2 Oxygenation Values

Assorted normal values
- Systemic arterial oxygen saturation, 95% to 100%
- Mixed venous saturation, more than 70%
- Central venous saturation, 65% to 75%
- Oxygen extraction ratio, 25% to 35%
- P_aCO_2–$P_{ET}CO_2$, 2 to 5 mm Hg

Useful Calculations
- Oxygen delivery
  - $CO \times CaO_2$
  - (Heart rate × Stroke volume) × $[(SaO_2 \times Hgb(g) \times 1.36) + (PaO_2 \times 0.003)]$
- Oxygen consumption
  - VO_2 (Oxygen consumption) $\approx$ Cardiac output × Hb × $(SaO_2 - SvO_2)$

Hemodynamic Monitoring

Circulatory monitoring often requires that fluid-filled conduits be used to connect transducers (which convert pressure waves into electric voltage changes)
to vascular access catheters. If the fluid in these conduits applies additional
pressure to the transducer, that pressure is added to the vascular pressure and
included in the transducer output. To avoid this inaccuracy, transducers are
generally placed at a level horizontal to the left atrium and set to read "zero"
when opened to air (rather than 760 mm Hg, which approximates ambient
pressure). The same principal is used to position and "zero" fluid-filled tubing properly used to measure intracranial or abdominal pressure (Figure 5.1).

Monitoring

Central venous pressure (CVP) monitoring is indicated in pediatric patients if
there is concern that intravascular volume is insufficient to support adequate
cardiac output, that cardiac function may not be adequate to limit the volume
of blood in the veins, or if there is concern that excessive vascular volume has

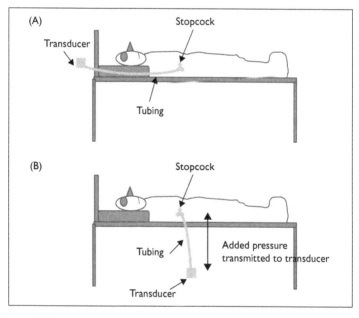

Figure 5.1 Vascular catheters are generally zeroed to atmosphere at the level of the left
atrium by opening a stopcock to air. (A) The transducer is usually positioned at that level on
the bed. (B) If the transducer were to fall off the bed, it would then sense the weight of the
fluid column in the tubing and add that to the measured vascular pressure.

overloaded the venous capacitance system. Central venous catheters are also often used to deliver vasoirritant medications, rapid fluid boluses (if indicated clinically), and hyperosmolar agents, and, if located properly, may be used to monitor central or mixed venous oxygen saturation. The rapid spread and availability of bedside ultrasound in the pediatric intensive care unit impacted positively the safety and success of obtaining vascular access in critically ill children.

CVP measures the back-pressure to venous return and the forward pressure to right ventricular filling in diastole. It offers a clinical perspective on right ventricular function. It is important to remember that right ventricular filling is influenced by multiple forces that act simultaneously. For example, an increase in positive end-expiratory pressure can decrease preload by decreasing diastolic right ventricular transmural pressure, thereby decreasing flow and venous return to the right heart.[4] However, at the same time, measured CVP may increase if airway pressures are transmitted to the vascular system (Figure 5.2).

Obviously, CVP must be interpreted in the context of airway pressure (or positive end-expiratory pressure). Elimination of positive end-expiratory pressure during measurement of CVP provides a first approximation of the

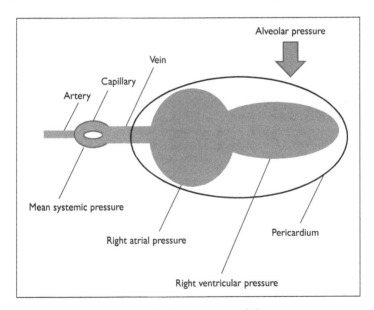

Figure 5.2 Mean systemic pressure (capillary mean pressure) drives venous return to the right heart. Right ventricular diastolic pressure opposes right ventricular filling. Alveolar pressure reduces functionally the compliance of the right ventricle by decreasing transmural ventricular filling pressure.

Table 5.1 Interpreting Central Venous Pressure (CVP)	
Low CVP	**High CVP**
Volume depletion	Volume overload
Dehydration	Cardiac dysfunction
Hemorrhage	Heart failure
Vasodilatation	Pulmonary hypertension
Hyperthermia	Tricuspid insufficiency
Sepsis	High airway pressure
Drug effect	transmitted to central veins
	High intra-abdominal pressure

right ventricular preload, but may cause secondary changes in pulmonary vascular resistance that defeat the purpose of the maneuver. (Measured in the femoral vein, CVP may be elevated by high intra-abdominal pressure and may provide a particularly poor estimate of right-heart filling.)

Clearly, a low measured CVP implies room for further volume expansion. An elevated CVP is more difficult to interpret. "Trending" the CVP tells a lot about responses to volume infusion and inotropic support (Table 5.1).

Arterial Pressure Monitoring

Continuous arterial pressure monitoring is usually undertaken in children who need frequent blood pressure monitoring, frequent blood sampling, a means to exchange or transfuse large volumes of blood, or therapy with vasoactive agents. Blood circulates through the arterial tree by virtue of tremendous force generated by the left ventricle. Blood pressure is a function of the blood flow rate and resistance of the arterial circulation, but it is also a function of arterial capacitance and blood volume. Pressure varies with the measurement site, as is the case with noninvasive measurements, being higher when measured in the lower extremities than in the upper. It reflects cardiovascular function directly, and ultimately impacts oxygen delivery and tissue oxygenation.

Although a valuable means of hemodynamic monitoring, arterial cannulation has risks and is subject to artifact (Figure 5.3). Accidental decannulation can lead to rapid and significant blood loss in children. Thrombosis of small and large vessels can occur. Cerebral embolism can result from vigorous flushing. Vascular insufficiency can occur, especially when collateral flow is inadequate (such as when the brachial artery is entered above its bifurcation into radial and ulnar vessels, or when the radial artery is cannulated at the wrist, and ulnar flow is inadequate). Risk of intra-arterial drug infusion, site infection, and limb ischemic necrosis must also be considered when performing arterial cannulation.

Continuous monitoring reveals changes in arterial pressure over the respiratory cycle. Spontaneous inspiration enhances right heart filling, thereby

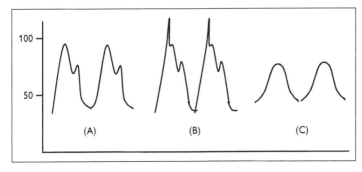

Figure 5.3 (A) appropriate high fidelity tracing. (B) resonance in the system (initial high spike in the tracing) overestimates systolic blood pressure. (C) overdamped (often by air or clot in the tubing or vessel) underestimates systolic blood pressure and overestimates diastolic pressure. In both (B) and (C), mean pressure is similar to (A) unless damping is very severe.

crowding the left ventricle and reducing left ventricular inflow (ventricular inter-dependence). It also reduces the pressure surrounding the heart, opposing left ventricular ejection. The net effect is a decrease in left ventricular ejection and arterial pressure during spontaneous inspiration. The reverse of these effects occurs during positive-pressure mechanical ventilation. Pericardial tamponade, which restricts total cardiac volume in diastole, exaggerates these findings over the respiratory cycle.

End-Tidal Carbon Dioxide Monitoring

Estimation of end-tidal carbon dioxide ($EtCO_2$) concentration at the bedside is another valuable tool in the critical care monitoring armamentarium. This measurement is easy to perform in mechanically ventilated patients and can also be used to estimate arterial partial pressure of carbon dioxide ($PaCO_2$) in spontaneously breathing patients. Carbon dioxide (CO_2) is produced in energy metabolism. It diffuses passively into the blood and is transported from the systemic capillary bed to the pulmonary capillaries, where it equilibrates with alveolar gas. During expiration, alveolar gas is delivered to the upper airway. CO_2 concentration is then estimated by side-stream sampling or direct passage of exhaled gas through an infrared sensor. At the end of expiration, in normal patients, all gas in the upper airway has left the alveolus earlier in that same breath. The absorption of infrared light as it passes through end-tidal gas is proportional to the concentration of CO_2 in alveolar air. The monitor then, estimates functionally the concentration of CO_2 in pulmonary capillary blood.

Normal Capnograph

A number of factors[5] may alter $EtCO_2$ abruptly during mechanical ventilation at fixed settings (Figure 5.4). By increasing cardiac output abruptly at fixed-minute ventilation, the rate at which CO_2 is delivered to alveolar gas is augmented. This is a transient effect, and delivery to the lungs returns to normal as equilibrium is restored, despite the persistently greater cardiac output. Rapid infusion of sodium bicarbonate increases the amount of CO_2 presented to the pulmonary circulation. A decrease in minute ventilation raises $EtCO_2$ by packing the same number of molecules of CO_2 into the smaller minute ventilation. An increase in metabolism at constant-minute ventilation packs more CO_2 into a fixed volume of minute ventilation. Similar logic applies to most of the other factors listed in Box 5.3.

One noteworthy cause of low $EtCO_2$ is the presence of a poorly perfused (high V_A/Q) lung segment. Such a segment generates little or no CO_2 despite being ventilated. The rest of the gas that mixes to form end-tidal air is at equilibrium with pulmonary capillary blood. When the underperfused segment's exhaled air mixes with the equilibrated exhaled air, it dilutes the CO_2 present functionally, lowering $EtCO_2$ to less than that of pulmonary capillary blood. This causes the capnograph to underestimate arterial $PaCO_2$. Pulmonary

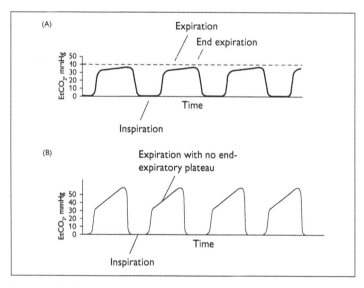

Figure 5.4 (A) Capnograph display. End-tidal partial pressure of carbon dioxide (pCO_2) is closely related to alveolar, pulmonary vein, and arterial pCO_2. (B) During severe bronchospasm, alveoli in different regions of the lung empty at different times and the end-expiratory plateau may not be reached before the next ventilator breath begins. Arterial pCO_2 may be significantly greater than end-tidal carbon dioxide.

Box 5.3 Factors Influencing End-Tidal Carbon Dioxide Transiently

Increased End-Tidal Carbon Dioxide (EtCO$_2$)
- Abruptly increased cardiac output
- Iatrogenic infusion of $NaHCO_3$
- Reperfusion state of regional circulation
- Hypoventilation
- Increased CO_2 production by increased metabolism

Decreased EtCO$_2$
- Hyperventilation
- Large alveolar dead space or high V_A/Q lung region
- Abruptly decreased in cardiac output
- Partially obstructive pulmonary circulation
- Obstruction and interruption of gas flow within the circuit analyzed

Absent EtCO$_2$
- Esophageal intubation, dislodgment of ETT
- Severe decrease in cardiac output
- Cardiac arrest

EtCO$_2$ Less Than PaCO$_2$
- Severe bronchospasm
- Pulmonary embolus/emboli

emboli lead to such poorly perfused lung segments and are associated commonly with EtCO$_2$ significantly lower than PaCO$_2$.

In patients with severe bronchospasm, gas from different alveoli reaches the sensor at different times, generating an EtCO$_2$ tracing with a delayed or absent plateau, and the measurement may underestimate arterial CO$_2$ significantly. The absence of a plateau may indicate a ventilator rate that does not allow adequate expiratory time (Figure 5.4).

Intra-abdominal Pressure Monitoring

A compartment syndrome develops when the pressure surrounding vessels approaches or exceeds vascular pressures. In the abdomen, a compartment syndrome is defined by an abdominal pressure of more than 12 mm Hg.[6] This can occur in the abdomen when it becomes tensely distended with fluid or air. An abdominal compartment syndrome is defined as an increase greater than normal pressure within the abdominal cavity that jeopardizes, if untreated, the vascular flow and viability of those organs contained within that space. It also impairs ventilation and glomerular filtration, as well as venous return from the lower extremities.

As the pressure within the abdominal cavity increases, blood flow to susceptible organs falls. Venous return via the inferior vena cava is impeded,

Box 5.4 Abdominal Compression Syndrome Grade

- Grade I, 12 to 15 mm Hg
- Grade II, 16 to 20 mm Hg
- Grade III, 21 to 25 mm Hg
- Grade IV, more than 25 mm Hg

reducing both cardiac output and mean arterial pressure. This impairs abdominal organ perfusion further, promoting a self-perpetuating cycle of organ edema, ischemia, additional ascites accumulation, and a massive inflammatory response.

The principles of intra-abdominal pressure monitoring are the same as described for vascular pressure monitoring. Pressures are measured in millimeters of mercury at end-expiration, in the supine position, and in the absence of muscle activity using a closed and continuous column of noncompressible fluid. The normal range for abdominal pressure in children is approximately 7 to 10 mm Hg,[7] and values related to the severity of an abdominal compartment syndrome are included in Box 5.4.

Pressure may be measured either directly or indirectly (Table 5.2). Using the direct technique, a needle or catheter is inserted into the abdomen. A transducer is set up and zeroed to monitor and record the pressure. This method, although invasive and not free of risk, allows for possible therapeutic removal of fluid. It also provides an opportunity to sample abdominal fluid for diagnostic purposes. However, this approach should be undertaken only after ultrasonography, because there may be scant fluid. The abdominal swelling may represent only visceral edema or a solid mass.

The indirect approach entails insertion of a Foley catheter to measure the pressures transmitted through the bladder wall. The bladder is first drained and then a small volume (1 mL/kg to a maximum of 25 mL) of saline is instilled to ensure fluid transmission of pressure.

Evidence suggests that physical examination alone is not as reliable and accurate as intravesicular abdominal pressure measurements to diagnose intra-abdominal hypertension, so an objective measurement should be performed when a suspicion of intra-abdominal hypertension is raised.

Table 5.2 Advantages (+) and Disadvantages (−) of Direct Versus Indirect Methods to Measure Abdominal Pressures

Method	Invasive	Therapeutic	Diagnostic
Direct	++	+++	+++
Indirect	+	0	+++

Key References

1. Watcha MF, Connor MT, Hing AV. Pulse oximetry in methemoglobinemia. *Am J Dis Child*. 1989;143:845–847.

2. Reynolds KJ, Palayiwa E, Moyle JT, Sykes MK; Hahn CE. The effect of dyshemoglobins on pulse oximetry: part I, theoretical approach and part II, experimental results using an in vitro test system. J Clin Monit. 1993;9:81–90.

3. Schwarz G, Litscher G, Kleinert R, Jobstmann R. Cerebral oximetry in dead subjects. *J Neurosurg Anesthesiol*. 1996;8:189–193.

4. Pinsky MR. Determinants of pulmonary arterial flow variation during respiration. *J Appl Physiol*. 1984;56:1237–45.

5. St John RE. Exhaled gas analysis: technical and clinical aspects of capnography and oxygen consumption. *Crit Care Nurs Clin North Am*. 1989;1:669–79.

6. Malbrain ML, Cheatham ML, Kirkpatrick A, et al. Results from the International Conference of Experts on Intra-abdominal Hypertension and Abdominal Compartment Syndrome: I. Definitions. *Intensive Care Med*. 2006;32(11):1722–1732.

7. Ejike JC, Bahjri K, Mathur M. What is the normal intra-abdominal pressure in critically ill children and how should we measure it? *Crit Care Med*. 2008;36:2157–2162.

Chapter 6

Respiratory Failure and Mechanical Ventilation

Jan Hau Lee and Ira M. Cheifetz

Respiratory failure with the need for mechanical ventilation is one of the most common indications for admission into the pediatric intensive care unit (PICU). Respiratory failure occurs when there is inadequate gas exchange resulting in hypoxemia and/or carbon dioxide (CO_2) retention. Although most commonly the result of primary lung injury (e.g., pneumonia, near drowning, inhalation injury, aspiration), respiratory failure can also be secondary to cardiac dysfunction, neurological abnormalities, blood product transfusions, sepsis, multiorgan system dysfunction, and many other clinical disorders.

To manage critically ill children optimally, pediatric intensivists must have a good working knowledge of both noninvasive and invasive respiratory support. In addition, they must understand the principles of common cardiorespiratory monitoring modalities and be able to interpret the results/values of these monitors. This chapter focuses on the fundamentals of noninvasive respiratory support, invasive mechanical ventilation, and respiratory monitoring modalities.

High-Flow Nasal Cannula

A high-flow nasal cannula (HFNC) provides flow that meets or exceeds a patient's spontaneous inspiratory demand. HFNC systems are available for use in infants, children, adolescents, and adults with flow rates ranging from 8 to 60 L/min. A key feature of all HFNC systems is the presence of an effective mechanism for heating and humidification (Figure 6.1).

Predominant mechanisms of efficacy with HFNC include

- Washout of nasopharyngeal dead space
- Matching of spontaneous inspiratory demands
- Generation of modest positive airway pressure
- Improved mucosal health with the applied heat and humidity

There is an increasing trend in the use of HFNC in infants and children as a respiratory support modality in viral bronchiolitis and during the postextubation period. Although HFNC is easy to apply and accepted more readily

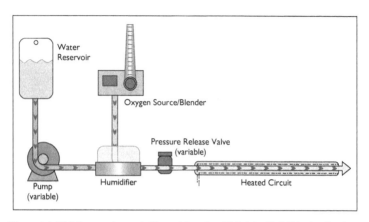

Figure 6.1 High flow nasal cannula (Figure 1 from Lee JH, Rehder KJ, Williford L, Cheifetz IM, Turner DA. Use of high flow nasal cannula in critically ill infants, children, and adults: a critical review of the literature. Intensive Care Med. 2013 Feb;39(2):247–257.)

by most patients, clinicians must be mindful of its ability to generate positive airway pressure that cannot be measured easily, leading to potential adverse effects, such as air leak and gas trapping.

Noninvasive Ventilation

Noninvasive ventilation (NIV) uses a mask or nasal prongs to provide positive pressure through the patient's nose and/or mouth. The main advantage of NIV is the avoidance of intubation and mechanical ventilation. This avoidance of intubation can potentially offer many "downstream" advantages, such as

- Decreasing the risk of nosocomial pneumonia
- Decreasing sedation requirements
- Allowing for mobility and, in some case, oral nutrition
- Potentially managing these children outside of the PICU (e.g., in a high-dependency, step-down unit)

The two main modes of NIV are continuous positive airway pressure (CPAP) and bilevel pressure support. Although CPAP provides for a single level of airway pressure throughout the respiratory cycle, bilevel pressure support allows for two different levels of airway pressure: inspiratory pressure for ventilatory support and expiratory pressure to maintain the lung recruited.

NIV can be considered in patients who meet the following criteria:

- Ability to protect the airway
- Adequate spontaneous breathing

- Cooperation with NIV application (e.g., the interface)
- Mild-to-moderate ventilation/oxygenation requirement
- Low risk of aspiration from abdominal distension
- No facial trauma/injuries

Despite the lack of definitive evidence, NIV is being used increasingly in children with respiratory distress from various etiologies. Taking into consideration the findings from adult studies of NIV, the clinician, when using NIV as a respiratory support modality, must be ready to escalate therapy to intubation and invasive respiratory support if the child does not improve after approximately 60 to 120 minutes of NIV support and to escalate immediately if the child experiences acute deterioration.

Conventional Mechanical Ventilation

The indications for intubation and mechanical ventilation are diverse and can be classified broadly into respiratory and nonrespiratory conditions. Respiratory diseases can lead to increased inspiratory workload, inability to maintain a patent airway, and ineffective gas exchange. Nonrespiratory conditions that may necessitate invasive ventilation include altered mental status resulting in an inability to protect the airway and severe shock states. Overall goals of mechanical ventilation are as follows:

1. To optimize gas exchange
2. To reduce the work of breathing
3. To ensure patient comfort
4. To minimize the risk for ventilator-induced lung injury (VILI)

Gas Exchange Goals

In severe acute lung injury, improved oxygenation is not correlated with improved clinical outcomes. The concept of accepting lower arterial oxygenation saturation is called *permissive hypoxemia*. Although the acceptable arterial oxygen saturation target remains controversial, ventilatory strategies should aim to provide adequate tissue and organ oxygenation while minimizing oxygen toxicity and VILI.

There are an increasing number of mechanical ventilation modes and ventilators currently being used in clinical practice. In general, conventional mechanical ventilation (CMV) can be classified into pressure-limited or volume-limited approaches. To date, no data exist to show that a particular conventional ventilator mode is superior to any other in terms of efficacy and safety. In this section, we focus on the general principles of mechanical ventilation concepts that are vital to ensure patient comfort and reduce morbidity and mortality.

Inspiratory Flow Pattern

The inspiratory flow pattern is perhaps the most important determinant of the choice of CMV mode for a particular patient. The two most commonly used flow patterns are variable decelerating flow and square-wave constant flow (Figure 6.2).

With a decelerating-flow pattern, the maximum flow is delivered near the start of inspiration, when large airway resistance is highest; flow then decreases during the remainder of inspiration. In a constant-flow (square-wave) pattern, the inspiratory flow rate is maintained the same throughout the inspiratory cycle. In contrast to constant flow, decelerating flow allows for lower peak inspiratory pressure (PIP) for a given tidal volume and inspiratory time with a higher mean airway pressure (MAP).

The choice of inspiratory flow pattern is based on the patient's underlying condition and more often on clinician/institution preference. In respiratory conditions of low compliance (such as acute respiratory distress syndrome [ARDS]; Table 6.1), the decelerating-flow pattern may be more appropriate because a lower PIP with an increased MAP is achievable, leading to better oxygenation and decreased risk for VILI. Variable decelerating flow is generally used in the pediatric setting to minimize PIP and optimize patient comfort in spontaneously breathing patients as flow is controlled by the patient (and the interaction between the patient and ventilator) and not by the clinician. Although practices may differ, we use decelerating flow routinely for all children admitted to our PICUs.

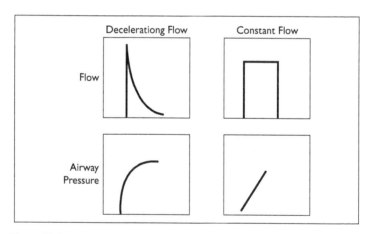

Figure 6.2 Decelerating-flow and constant-flow wave forms (Figure 1 from Ira M. Cheifetz. Invasive and Noninvasive Pediatric Mechanical Ventilation. Respiratory Care 2003; 48(4): 442–453.)

Table 6.1 Pediatric Acute Respiratory Distress Syndrome (PARDS) 2015 Consensus Definition

Age	Excludes patients with perinatal-related lung disease
Time of onset	Within 7 days of known clinical insult
Origin of edema	Respiratory failure not fully explained by cardiac failure or fluid overload
Chest imaging	New infiltrate(s) consistent with acute parenchymal disease
Invasive mechanical ventilation	Mild PARDS: $4 \leq OI < 8$, $5 \leq OSI < 7.5$
	Moderate PARDS: $8 \leq OI < 16$, $7.5 \leq OSI < 12.3$
	Severe PARDS: $OI \geq 16$, $OSI \geq 12.3$
Noninvasive mechanical ventilation	No severity stratification
	Full-facemask bilevel ventilation or CPAP ≥ 5 cm H_2O
	$PaO_2/FiO_2 \leq 300$
	$SaO_2/FiO_2 \leq 264$

CPAP, continuous positive airway pressure; FiO_2, fraction of inspired oxygen; OI, oxygenation index ($FiO_2 \times$ Mean airway pressure $\times 100/PaO_2$); OSI, oxygen saturation index ($FiO_2 \times$ Mean airway pressure $\times 100/SaO_2$ when $SaO_2 \leq 97\%$); PaO_2, arterial partial pressure of oxygen; SaO_2, arterial oxygen saturation

Special populations: Children with cyanotic heart disease and left ventricular dysfunction may be considered to have PARDS if they meet the criteria presented here *and* the acute deterioration in oxygenation is not explained by cardiac disease. Children with chronic lung disease may also be considered to have PARDS if they meet the criteria in the table. Classification of severity of PARDS is not applicable to children with cyanotic heart disease or children with chronic lung disease on baseline invasive ventilation.

Source: Modified from Pediatric Acute Lung Injury Consensus Conference Group. Pediatric acute respiratory distress syndrome definition. *Pediatr Crit Care Med*. 2015;16:428–439, Figure 2.

Patient–Ventilator Interaction

Optimization of patient–ventilator interaction is important

1. To ensure optimal patient comfort
2. To minimize the need for pharmacological sedation
3. To potentially reduce the duration of mechanical ventilation

Readily correctable patient–ventilator interaction abnormalities when identified correctly from an analysis of airway graphics (discussed in the next section) are

- Pulmonary overdistension
- Intrinsic positive end-expiratory pressure (PEEP)
- Patient–ventilator asynchrony

Positive End-Expiratory Pressure

The benefits of PEEP include

- Maintaining alveolar patency
- Restoring functional residual capacity
- Preventing alveolar collapse during expiration

PEEP is typically increased to a level that allows adequate oxygenation with an inspired fraction of oxygen of approximately 0.60 or less. A PEEP level of 10 to 15 cm H_2O, or even higher, may be required to achieve adequate oxygenation in certain clinical situations, such as severe ARDS. However, as PEEP levels exceed 12 to 15 cm H_2O in infants and children, the increase in mean intrathoracic pressure may affect cardiac output adversely, primarily by decreasing systemic venous return. In most cases, this can be addressed by intravascular volume loading and possibly inotropic support. In addition, significantly elevated PEEP levels may reduce the delta-P (i.e., distending pressure and tidal volume) that can be delivered while still maintaining the peak/plateau pressure (Pplat) to less than presumed toxic levels.

There is no recommended PEEP for each disease process. When an appropriate PEEP is applied to maintain the lungs at an ideal lung volume, further increases in PEEP should not be applied because there are no data to support improved outcome.

Low-Tidal-Volume Ventilation

Large tidal volumes can cause pulmonary overdistension and progressive secondary lung injury. The seminal study performed by the National Institutes of Health ARDS Network showed that adults with ARDS who were ventilated with a low tidal volume (6 mL/kg) had a 9% absolute decrease in mortality compared with adults who were ventilated with higher tidal volumes (12 mL/kg). Furthermore, when compared with the control group, Pplat was significantly lower in the low-tidal-volume group. It remains unclear whether lower tidal volume or lower Pplat is the key parameter. Thus, many clinicians would recommend limiting both for patients with acute lung injury: a tidal volume of 6 mL/kg and a Pplat less than 30 to 32 cm H_2O (discussed in subsequent paragraphs).

It must be noted that there is a lack of pediatric studies investigating the ideal tidal volume during invasive mechanical ventilation. Until such studies are performed, it seems reasonable to use a low-tidal-volume strategy in children with injured and, possibly, noninjured lungs. Recent observational data in pediatric populations demonstrated an inverse association between tidal volume (≤10 mL/kg) and improved outcome, but patients with higher tidal volumes and improved outcomes may represent a population with more normal lung compliance and, thus, a greater likelihood of a good outcome.

Another conclusion from studies of ARDS in adults is that the Pplat should be limited to less than approximately 30 to 32 cm H_2O to improve clinical outcome. The applicability of this observation to children requires further investigation. It is very possible that the "critical" limit for Pplat for infants and children may be less than 30 cm H_2O, and may vary with patient age and size.

By reducing minute ventilation, low-tidal-volume ventilation leads physiologically to hypercapnia. Most undesirable effects are reversible and minor when the pH is greater than approximately 7.20. Permissive hypercapnia, however, is not applicable to all patient groups. In general, this strategy should be avoided in patients with clinically significant intracranial pathology or pulmonary hypertension.

To ensure that a low tidal volume is applied accurately for a given patient, accurate tidal-volume determination is paramount. We propose that all infants and small children have a pneumotachometer placed at the end of the endotracheal tube to measure delivered tidal volumes reliably. This more accurate measurement (compared with tidal volumes measured at the ventilator expiratory valve or calculated as effective tidal volume using ventilator circuit compliance) may help minimize VILI in neonates and young children.

Troubleshooting

Any mechanically ventilated patient can deteriorate, resulting in hypoxia, CO_2 retention, and hemodynamic instability. A simple pneumonic—OPENED—can be used to troubleshoot acute problems that may arise during invasive ventilation:

O—*Obstruction*: kinked or blocked (e.g., with secretions) endotracheal tube (ETT) or blocked expiratory valve of the ventilator

P—*Pneumothorax/patient–ventilator dyssynchrony*

E—*Equipment failure*: faulty ventilator or circuits

N—*Nosocomial infection*

E—*Evolution of the underlying clinical process* (e.g., worsening respiratory disease)

D—*Dislodgment/disconnection*: dislodged ETT, circuit disconnection

If these acute factors are not present, other less common causes for clinical deterioration should be considered.

Extubation Readiness

Weaning is traditionally defined as the period of transition from full ventilatory support to complete spontaneous breathing, with the patient able to maintain effective gas exchange without mechanical support. In current practice, gradual weaning is less important than a routine assessment of extubation readiness. Assessment of extubation readiness should be part of the daily management plan of every intubated infant and child (Figure 6.3). Extubation readiness testing is a formal trial of spontaneous breathing to evaluate whether the patient is

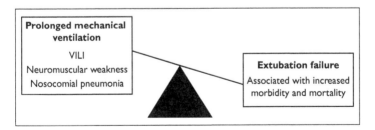

Figure 6.3 Balancing between prolonged mechanical ventilation and extubation failure. VILI, ventilator-induced lung injury.

ready to discontinue mechanical ventilation. Methods for extubation readiness testing include the use of variable pressure support and T-piece trials (with or without CPAP).

There are several objective extubation criteria in children; some are easier to perform than others, with some requiring fairly complex calculations. Criteria (Table 6.2) that have been applied in pediatrics include

- Spontaneous breathing trials
- Rapid shallow breathing index
- CROP, or compliance, respiratory frequency, oxygenation, and peak inspiratory pressure index
- Dead space-to-tidal volume ratio

Table 6.2 Pediatric Testing for Extubation Readiness

Predictive Indices	Formula/Components	Utility
Rapid shallow breathing index	f/V_T calculated during a spontaneous breathing trial (can be conducted either with a T-piece or pressure support)	Screening test with high sensitivity and low specificity. Should be considered early during the mechanical ventilation course. A pediatric rapid shallow breathing index of ≤8 breaths/mL/kg has been proposed previously as a threshold value.
CROP index	Dynamic compliance × Maximal negative inspiratory pressure × $[(P_aO_2/P_AO_2)/$Respiratory rate]	Conflicting results in studies and fairly complicated formula to use at the bedside.
Volumetric capnography	V_D/V_T	V_D/V_T >0.65 identifies patients at risk for extubation failure. To calculate volumetric capnography, an arterial blood gas measurement is required.
Leak test	Assessment for air leaking around ETT at a set inspiratory pressure (<20–25 cm H_2O)	Although the presence of an air leak is predictive of extubation readiness from an airway perspective, a negative test with all other parameters being optimal should not delay extubation unnecessarily.
NIF	Performed with a manometer attached to the ETT during inspiration	Used to assess strength of respiratory muscles. A NIF of at least −30 cm H_2O, although found to be predictive of extubation success, has not been validated and accepted as standard of care in children.

CROP, compliance, resistance, oxygenation, pressure; ETT, endotracheal tube; f, frequency of respiration; NIF, negative inspiratory force; P_aO_2, partial pressure of arterial oxygenation; P_AO_2, partial pressure of alveolar oxygenation; V_D, physiological dead space; V_T, tidal volume.

One of the more common cause of extubation failure in infants and children is upper airway obstruction. Although there are limitations and potential confounders (e.g., pre-extubation steroids), air leak testing is a relatively common practice within the PICU, but expert opinion and small, single-center studies propose that one should not delay extubation simply because a leak is absent, if all other conditions for extubation are favorable.

Unfortunately, there is no proven, single reliable method of assessing extubation readiness and predicting success of extubation. Until larger clinical trials are conducted in pediatrics, clinicians must use (1) their best judgment to determine whether the underlying need for intubation and mechanical ventilation in the first instance has been reversed or addressed appropriately and (2) available monitors and extubation assessment tools in deciding the optimal time for extubation.

Nontraditional Modes of Ventilation

In Table 6.3, we summarize the following nontraditional modes of ventilation: proportional assist ventilation, neutrally adjusted ventilator assist (commonly referred to as "NAVA"), airway pressure release ventilation (APRV), and adaptive support ventilation. At this point, current medical evidence does not demonstrate the superiority of any of these modes to any other, including conventional ventilator strategies.

Table 6.3 Nontraditional Modes of Ventilation				
Characteristics	PAV	NAVA	ASV	APRV
Key features	Spontaneous breathing mode, offers assistance to the patient in proportion to his or her effort	Electrical activity of the diaphragm provides the neural input to the ventilator, proper positioning of the electrical diaphragm catheter is key	Microprocessor-controlled algorithm that calculates the rate and tidal volume to optimize the patient's work of breathing	Patient may breathe spontaneously at any point during the respiratory cycle
Key ventilator settings by clinicians	Proportion of assistance to be provided to the patient	Trigger of the electrical activity of the diaphragm to start and end inspiratory cycle, amplification factor of this electrical activity (NAVA level)	Desired minute ventilation and degree of ventilator support	Four main parameters[a]: pressure$_{high}$ (P$_{high}$), pressure$_{low}$ (P$_{low}$), time$_{high}$ (T$_{high}$), time$_{low}$ (T$_{low}$)

(continued)

Table 6.3 Continued

Characteristics	PAV	NAVA	ASV	APRV
Advantages	Improve patient–ventilator interaction, improve sleep quality	Improve patient–ventilator synchrony, improve sleep quality	Reduce ventilation time in postoperative adult patients	Maintenance of spontaneous respiration with an "open lung" strategy, reduced need for sedation
Disadvantages	Limited application in children, presence of leak around ETT interferes with calculation of airway mechanics, requires ETT ≥6.0 mm in diameter	Requires accurate positioning of electrical diaphragm catheter		

APRV, airway pressure release ventilation; ASV, adaptive support ventilation; ETT, endotracheal tube; NAVA, neutrally adjusted ventilator assist; PAV, proportional assist ventilation.

[a] P_{high} is set well above the mean airway pressure (on conventional mechanical ventilation). T_{high} is usually set well above the usual inspiratory time for age. We propose that P_{low} be set at zero and T_{low} be set at an appropriately short time (usually 0.3–0.5 s) to ensure that the lung remains "open" throughout the ventilatory cycle.

High-Frequency Ventilation

The overarching strategy in the utility of high-frequency ventilation (HFV) is that of lung protection by using extremely low tidal volumes (i.e., tidal volume < dead space volume) to reduce the cyclic lung stretch that occurs during conventional ventilation, while maintaining the lung "open." There are three main modes of HFV, which are summarized in the following sections.

High-Frequency Oscillatory Ventilation

High-frequency oscillatory ventilation (HFOV) is the most commonly used mode of HFV. HFOV is often used when "toxic" CMV support is required to achieve the desired gas exchange goals. During the initial transition from CMV to HFOV, the general aim is to recruit lung (i.e., open lung strategy) with a relatively high MAP and then to decrease the MAP so the patient is ventilated on the expiratory limb of the flow–volume loop (Figure 6.4). Thus, the initial MAP is usually set about 4 to 6 cm H_2O more than that required during conventional ventilation. The ability to wean the fraction of inspired oxygen is an indicator of good lung recruitment.

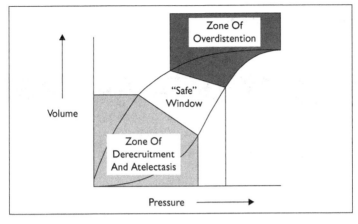

Figure 6.4 Hysteresis loop to show area of safe ventilation in high-frequency oscillatory ventilation (Figure 1 from John H. Arnold. High-frequency ventilation in the pediatric intensive care unit. Pediatric Critical Care Medicine 2000;1(2): 93–99.)

The initial amplitude is titrated clinically to a "wiggle" of the middle abdomen/upper thighs and then adjusted according to subsequent arterial blood gas (ABG) results, generally allowing for hypercapnia. Transcutaneous monitoring of gas exchange during HFV should be considered. Care must be taken to ensure that the amplitude is not more than three times the MAP, especially in younger patients. Finally, frequency is dependent on the age of the infant/child and the underlying condition. In general, a higher frequency is preferable compared with a lower frequency (with amplitude adjusted accordingly) to achieve the desired degree of ventilation.

High-Frequency Jet Ventilation

High-frequency jet ventilation (HFJV) is most commonly used in infants with severe respiratory failure. The principle behind HFJV is a high-frequency jet pulsation down the center of the airways with margination of CO_2 along the periphery of the airways. Unlike HFOV, in which exhalation is an active process, the continuous passive exhalation of the jet ventilation is a key feature of this mode.

Because HFJV clears CO_2 efficiently, this mode of ventilation is useful in certain clinical situations in which permissive hypercapnia may not be appropriate (e.g., significant pulmonary hypertension, combination of acute lung injury and traumatic brain injury, bronchospasm). However, the use of HFJV much beyond infancy has been limited by the power output of the jet ventilator.

High-Frequency Percussive Ventilation

The distinct advantage of high-frequency percussive ventilation is the ability to clear secretions from the lung. High-frequency percussive ventilation has been used most commonly in patients with burn injuries.

CHAPTER 6 Respiratory Failure and Ventilation

Adjunct Respiratory Therapies

Adjunct respiratory therapies are summarized in Table 6.4.

Table 6.4 Adjunct Respiratory Therapies in Severe Hypoxic Respiratory Failure

Adjunct Therapies	Pros	Cons
Inhaled nitric oxide	Improves oxygenation, reduces pulmonary vascular resistance (in those patients with pulmonary hypertension)	Not shown to improve survival, suggestion of increased risk of kidney injury in adults
Surfactant	Improves gas exchange and reduces length of stay in severe bronchiolitis	Lack of evidence for improved outcome in ARDS, potential adverse effects such as desaturation, bradycardia, and transient hypotension
Prone position	Improves V/Q matching and chest wall mechanics, improves survival in adults with severe ARDS	Risk of ETT obstruction, accidental catheter or tube dislodgment, ocular damage, and facial pressure ulcers
Corticosteroids	In adults, use within the first 2 weeks of established ARDS may reduce total days of mechanical ventilation and mortality	No conclusive studies in children
ECMO	Venovenous ECMO can be used to minimize oxygen toxicity and minimize VILI while achieving acceptable oxygenation and CO_2 clearance	Risk of complications (generally, bleeding and clotting) is real

ARDS, acute respiratory distress syndrome; CO_2, carbon dioxide; ECMO, extracorporeal membrane oxygenation; ETT, endotracheal tube; VILI, ventilator-induced lung injury; V/Q: ventilation–perfusion. iar to me.

Respiratory Monitoring

Careful bedside clinical examination forms the most important assessment and monitoring available to the intensivist. Examining for the presence of cyanosis, measuring the respiratory rate, and assessing the patient's work of breathing (presence of suprasternal, intercostal retractions; use of accessory muscles and paradoxical breathing) allow the clinician to monitor the progress of the critically ill child.

Continuous monitoring of the critically ill patient is the cornerstone of ICU cardiorespiratory care. Monitoring of blood oxygen saturation and CO_2 elimination complements the other components of respiratory monitoring, such as respiratory rate and physical examination findings.

Pulse Oximetry

Pulse oximetry is an indispensable tool in the ICU. This technology uses the principle of absorption of two different wavelengths between oxygenated and deoxygenated hemoglobin. Although the pulse oximeter is widely used, its limitations must be appreciated. Readings from the pulse oximetry can be inaccurate in the following situations:

• Presence of severe jaundice
• Dark skin pigmentation
• Significant movement artifact
• Impaired perfusion
• Low arterial oxygen saturation
• Elevated carboxyhemoglobin level

Blood Gas Monitoring

Blood gas monitoring is also indispensable and may be used for arterial, capillary, and venous blood. ABG analysis assists with an assessment of both oxygenation and ventilation whereas capillary blood gas and venous blood gas (VBG) analyses are useful to assess ventilation. Depending on the location of the central venous line tip, VBGs may be used to assess venous saturation as a surrogate for whole-body oxygen delivery/extraction. Peripheral VBGs should not be used. Blood gas values are not affected solely by gaseous exchange; they are also dependent on nonpulmonary factors such as perfusion and oxygen extraction, which may affect mixed venous oxygenation. In addition, there is natural variability in the measurements of arterial partial pressure of oxygen and arterial partial pressure of CO_2 ($PaCO_2$) in an individual patient. Thus, it is important that clinicians do not base their clinical decisions in general on isolated values, but instead base them on trends of these values.

Capnography

There are two categories of capnography: time-based capnography (also known as *end-tidal CO_2 monitoring*) and volumetric (or volume-based) capnography. Time-based capnography provides qualitative information on CO_2 waveforms as a function of time as well as a quantitative estimation of the partial pressure of CO_2. This is in contrast to volumetric capnography in which the exact net volume of CO_2 expired by the patient is measured (by a pneumotachometer/capnostat) and expressed as a volume measurement as a function of gas exhaled gas volume over time.

Several benefits of using continuous capnography in the pediatric critical care setting include the following:

• Confirmation of ETT placement
• Monitoring of the integrity of the ETT and ventilator circuit
• Assessment of pulmonary blood flow
• Assessment for extubation readiness

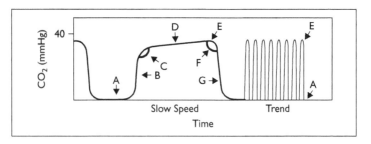

Figure 6.5 Volumetric capnography (Figure 2 from Ira M. Cheifetz and Timothy R. Myers. Should Every Mechanically Ventilated Patient Be Monitored With Capnography From Intubation to Extubation? Respiratory Care 2007; 52(4): 423–438.)

Capnography reveals an immediate disappearance of the CO_2 waveform when there is

- Apnea
- Severe airway obstruction
- Loss of cardiac output
- Severe interruption to pulmonary blood flow (e.g., severe pulmonary hypertension, pulmonary embolus)
- Interruption in the integrity of the ventilator circuit, including inadvertent extubation

Correct interpretation of the clinical waveforms of capnography is essential (Figure 6.5 and Figure 6.6). Abnormal pathologies can be inferred from alternations of the normal expired CO_2 waveform pattern. Because of normal anatomic/airway dead-space ventilation, there is always a small difference between $PaCO_2$ and partial pressure of $PaCO_2$ as measured at the level of the ETT (P_{ETCO2}), with P_{ETCO2} being slightly lower than P_aCO_2.

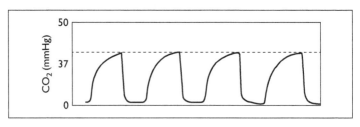

Figure 6.6 Time-based capnography in normal children and in bronchospasm (Figure 3 from Ira M. Cheifetz and Timothy R. Myers. Should Every Mechanically Ventilated Patient Be Monitored With Capnography From Intubation to Extubation? Respiratory Care 2007; 52(4): 423–438.)

In pathological processes in which alveolar dead space is increased, this difference is increased, with P_{ETCO_2} being much lower than $PaCO_2$. However, there may still be a reasonable correlation between these two values despite the gradient increasing with increasing dead space. Clinicians must be aware of the clinical condition of the patient and potential need for an ABG analysis to ensure that dead-space ventilation has not changed markedly.

Transcutaneous Gas Monitoring

By warming and vasodilating the skin, a transcutaneous CO_2 monitor is able to promote diffusion of gas from the capillary bed to the membrane of the monitor, resulting in a numerical display. We suggest the routine use of transcutaneous monitoring in ventilated patients in whom capnography is not possible (e.g., HFV).

Airway Graphics Analysis

Airway graphic analysis

- Assists the clinician in determining an optimal ventilator strategy for an individual patient
- Helps to optimize patient–ventilator interactions
- Minimizes the deleterious effects of mechanical ventilation

In the following sections, we discuss the three most common issues faced by clinicians in their care of mechanically ventilated patients in the PICU that can be informed by analysis of airway graphics.

Patient–Ventilator Asynchrony

The presence of patient–ventilatory asynchrony (Figure 6.7), if unrecognized, may lead to injudicious use of pharmacological sedation (and possibly neuromuscular blockade) and a resultant prolongation of the duration of mechanical ventilation. The two most important factors leading to asynchrony are (1) inadequate trigger sensitivity and (2) inadequate inspiratory flow.

Inadequate Trigger Sensitivity

Although now less common as a result of flow-triggering in most modern ventilators, an infant who is unable to trigger a mechanical breath will seem to be "fighting" with the ventilator and, thus, will be agitated. Instead of increasing sedative medications, improving trigger sensitivity allows better interaction between the patient and the ventilator.

Inadequate Inspiratory Flow

Flow asynchrony occurs when patients do not receive the inspiratory flow they desire during any point in the inspiratory cycle. Most commonly seen in a constant inspiratory flow mode, flow asynchrony can be managed by increasing the inspiratory flow (which may lead to an increased PIP) or changing to a variable, decelerating inspiratory flow mode. This latter option is generally preferred because it allows the inspiratory flow rate to

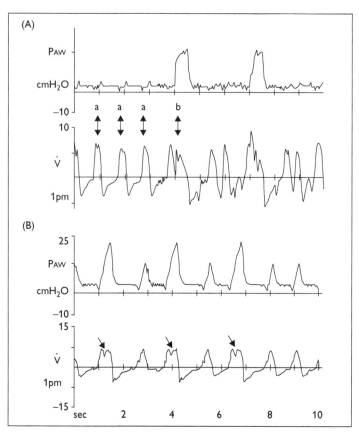

Figure 6.7 Patient–ventilator synchrony (Figure 4 from Ira M. Cheifetz. Invasive and Noninvasive Pediatric Mechanical Ventilation. Respiratory Care 2003; 48(4): 442–453.)

be better matched with the patient's spontaneous demand and pulmonary pathophysiology.

Pulmonary Overdistension

Overdistension of the lungs (Figure 6.8) can lead to volutrauma—a form of VILI—and increased pulmonary vascular resistance. Pulmonary overdistension can be noted readily by examining an upper inflection point on the pressure–volume curve. If present, peak airway pressure/tidal volume should be reduced as indicated clinically. It should be noted that excessive PEEP may also lead to overdistension. The goal is to use airway graphics to help achieve a more optimal lung volume.

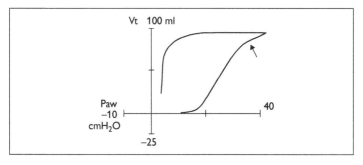

Figure 6.8 Overdistension (Figure 2 from Ira M. Cheifetz. Invasive and Noninvasive Pediatric Mechanical Ventilation. Respiratory Care 2003; 48(4): 442–453.)

Intrinsic PEEP

The presence of intrinsic PEEP can potentially lead to

- Air trapping
- Impaired gas exchange
- Trigger insensitivity
- Elevated mean intrathoracic pressure

By examining the flow-time graph, the presence of intrinsic PEEP can be identified (Figure 6.9). To ensure that inspiratory flow does not start before the

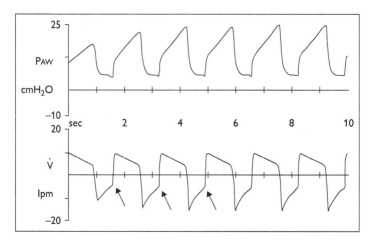

Figure 6.9 Intrinsic positive end-expiratory pressure (Figure 3 from Ira M. Cheifetz. Invasive and Noninvasive Pediatric Mechanical Ventilation. Respiratory Care 2003; 48(4): 442–453.)

prior breath returns to zero flow, the clinician should make sure of the presence of an adequate expiratory time.

Conclusion

Critical care clinicians need to be comfortable with the basic principles of noninvasive and invasive ventilation and respiratory monitoring to manage patients with respiratory distress/failure optimally. Low-tidal-volume ventilation is the only intervention to date that has been proved to change mortality (in adults with ARDS). Thus, the clinician should not be swayed to believe that any one mode of ventilation is superior to another. The clinician must use mechanical ventilation wisely, minimizing VILI at all times and keeping duration of mechanical ventilation as short as possible to serve each individual patient best. Respiratory monitoring tools should be used to achieve this ultimate aim in all mechanically ventilated infants and children.

Further Reading

Ventilation with lower tidal volumes as compared with traditional tidal volumes for acute lung injury and the acute respiratory distress syndrome: the Acute Respiratory Distress Syndrome Network. *N Engl J Med.* 2000;342(18):1301–1308.

Curley MA, Hibberd PL, Fineman LD, et al. Effect of prone positioning on clinical outcomes in children with acute lung injury: a randomized controlled trial. *JAMA.* 2005;294(2):229–237.

Arnold JH, Hanson JH, Toro-Figuero LO, Gutiérrez J, Berens RJ, Anglin DL. Prospective, randomized comparison of high-frequency oscillatory ventilation and conventional mechanical ventilation in pediatric respiratory failure. *Crit Care Med.* 1994;22(10):1530–1539.

Thomas NJ, Guardia CG, Moya FR, et al. A pilot, randomized, controlled clinical trial of lucinactant, a peptide-containing synthetic surfactant, in infants with acute hypoxemic respiratory failure. *Pediatr Crit Care Med.* 2012;13(6):646–653.

Antonelli M, Conti G, Moro ML, et al. Predictors of failure of noninvasive positive pressure ventilation in patients with acute hypoxemic respiratory failure: a multi-center study. *Intensive Care Med.* 2001;27(11):1718–1728.

Cheifetz IM. Invasive and noninvasive pediatric mechanical ventilation. *Respir Care.* 2003;48(4):442–453; discussion, 453–458.

Lee JH, Rehder KJ, Williford L, Cheifetz IM, Turner DA. Use of high flow nasal cannula in critically ill infants, children, and adults: a critical review of the literature. *Intensive Care Med.* 2012.

Mok YH, Lee JH, Rehder KJ, Turner DA. Adjunctive treatments in pediatric acute respiratory distress syndrome. *Expert Rev Respir Med.* 2014.

Randolph AG. Management of acute lung injury and acute respiratory distress syndrome in children. *Crit Care Med.* 2009;37(8):2448–2454.

Wratney AT, Cheifetz IM. Extubation criteria in infants and children. *Respir Care Clin North Am.* 2006;12(3):469–481.

Chapter 7

Cardiac Disease in Pediatric Intensive Care

Vamsi V. Yarlagadda and Ravi R. Thiagarajan

Children with congenital or acquired cardiac disease account for approximately 30% to 40% of admissions to pediatric intensive care units. The goal of this chapter is to provide a general overview of the evaluation and management of children with congenital and acquired heart disease requiring intensive care.

Cardiovascular Physiology

The main function of the cardiovascular system is to deliver oxygen and nutrients to tissues to maintain their metabolic function and to remove products of metabolic waste for excretion in other organs. Key concepts of cardiovascular performance include

- *Stroke volume (SV)*: the blood volume ejected from the ventricle with each beat and determined by myocardial preload, afterload, and contractility
- *Heart rate (HR)*: controlled by neural, baroreceptor, and chemoreceptor mechanisms
- *Cardiac output (CO)*: $CO = SV \times HR$. Although increases in HR cause increased CO, extreme tachycardia can decrease diastolic filling time and reduce SV and CO.
- *Systemic vascular resistance (SVR)*: determined by the contractile state of precapillary arterioles and larger arterioles, and regulated through a complex network of neural, hormonal, and local autoregulatory systems that influence vascular smooth muscle function
- *Blood pressure (BP)*: $BP = CO \times SVR$. BP represents an interaction of the heart with the vascular system (vascular tone). Although BP is commonly interpreted as CO, it is important to recognize that BP is also determined by SVR. *Therefore, BP may be normal in those with low CO but high SVR.*
- *Preload*: analogous to end diastolic volume (EDV) in the ventricle. Frank-Starling's law states that SV increases with increasing preload. In the presence of normal contractility, preload augmentation (e.g., via volume administration) increases SV and thus CO. "Recruitable stroke volume" is an increase in SV that can be achieved by increasing EDV. In clinical practice, EDV is difficult to measure, and we infer EDV by measuring ventricular

end diastolic pressure (EDP) using central venous pressure (CVP) for the right ventricle (RV), and left atrial (LA) pressure for the left ventricle (LV). The compliance of the myocardium determines EDP for any given EDV, and the relationship between EDP and SV is not linear. SV increases with increasing with EDP; but, at higher EDP, no further increase in SV occurs (Figure 7.1).

- *Afterload*: the tension and stress developed in the ventricular wall during ejection and the sum of all forces that resist blood ejection from the ventricle. Afterload, or ventricular wall stress, is determined by transmural pressure across the ventricular wall, thickness, and size of the ventricle as shown in Laplace's equation: $T = (P \times r)/2t$, where T is the circumferential wall stress, P is the transmural pressure, r is the ventricle radius, and t is the ventricular wall thickness. In the LV, for example, LV transmural pressure = LV intraluminal pressure (LVEDP) − LV extraluminal pressure (intrathoracic or pleural pressure). Starling's law states that force of muscle shortening is dependent on the load against which it shortens. Thus, with increasing

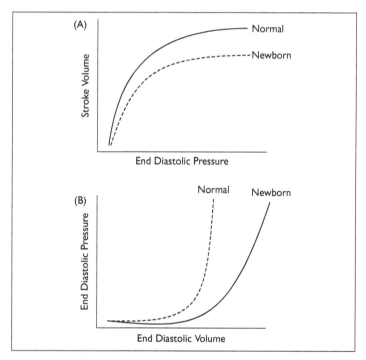

Figure 7.1 (A) Relationship of stroke volume and end diastolic pressure in mature and immature myocardium. (B) Myocardial compliance in mature and immature myocardium.

afterload, muscle shortening is decreased and slowed. In the presence of normal myocardial contractility, an increase in afterload is compensated by an increase in contractility. In patients with cardiac failure, the application of positive-pressure ventilation results in a more positive pleural pressure and thus a lower LV transmural pressure, resulting in decreased afterload. SVR, aortic and vascular inflow impedance, inertia properties of blood, and presence of outflow tract obstruction are also important determinants of afterload.

• *Contractility*: the ability of the myocardium to contract independently of other factors (preload and afterload) and determined by the health of the myocardium. The force and rapidity of contraction is related to the amount of free intracellular calcium available. Cyclic adenosine monophosphate plays an important role in myocardial contractility by increasing release and decreasing reuptake of calcium in the sarcoplasmic reticulum. Thus, agents that increase activity of adenyl cyclase and cyclic adenosine monophosphate act as inotropes.

Neonatal Myocardial Function

The neonatal myocardium is immature in structure, function, and innervation compared with the adult myocardium. Neonatal myocardial tissue contains fewer contractile elements, decreased sympathetic innervation, β-adrenergic receptor concentration, and immature sarcoplasmic reticulum with impaired release of cytosolic calcium for myocardial contractility. In addition, the myofibrils are arranged in a disorganized fashion. Thus, neonates may require larger doses of inotropic agents and are dependent on plasma levels of calcium to improve myocardial contractility. Decreased myocardial compliance impairs the ability to increase CO in response to volume loading (Figure 7.1). Therefore, HR is an important determinant of CO, and bradycardia in the neonate results in a low CO. Finally, the newborn myocardium is unable to increase force of contraction in response to increased afterload.

Cardiopulmonary Interactions

Interactions among the heart, lungs, and intrathoracic pressure are now recognized as important issues to consider in children with heart disease receiving mechanical ventilation in the intensive care unit (ICU). During normal inspiration, negative pleural pressure results in increased preload (systemic venous return) and increased CO. During mechanical ventilation, intrathoracic pressure becomes positive, resulting in decreased preload and CO. Shekerdemian et al. showed a 16% reduction in CO in children receiving positive-pressure ventilation.

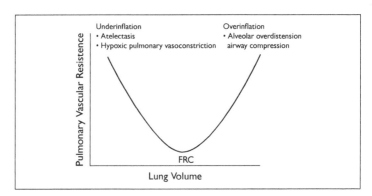

Figure 7.2 Lung inflation and pulmonary vascular resistance. FRC, functional residual capacity.

The RV pumps to the low-resistance pulmonary circulation and thus performs lower stroke work compared with the LV, which pumps to the high-resistance systemic circulation. Pulmonary vascular resistance (PVR) is lowest when lung inflation is at functional residual capacity (FRC) (Figure 7.2). Lung underinflation results in atelectasis and hypoxic pulmonary vasoconstriction, and hyperinflation results in alveolar distension and compression of the pulmonary capillaries. Both conditions lead to increased PVR. Thus, maintaining FRC while using low mean airway pressure (MAP) during mechanical ventilation is important.

Evaluation of Cardiac Disease in Children

Cardiovascular dysfunction may occur as a result of primary heart disease or as part of other systemic diseases (e.g., septic shock). Presenting features vary with severity of heart disease. Cyanosis (deoxyhemoglobin >5 g/dL), murmur, arrhythmia, failure to thrive, congestive heart failure, and pulmonary edema are usual manifestations of heart disease in children.

Evaluation of children with heart disease requires a through history and physical examination and assessment with chest X-ray (CXR) and electrocardiogram (ECG). Echocardiography (ECHO) is an important diagnostic tool and can provide information on cardiac function and anatomy. Investigations such as cardiac catheterization, computed tomography, and magnetic resonance imaging (MRI) can provide specialized information on function and structure, and may be required in some patients.

Central venous catheters can be used to monitor CVP, and intra-arterial catheters can provide continuous assessment of BP. The utility and risks of placing invasive catheters must always be considered before placing them.

In children undergoing cardiac surgery, additional intracardiac vascular catheters can provide information on right atrial (RA) and LA pressures, and pulmonary artery (PA) pressures. A number of measurements such as CO, SVR, and PVR can be calculated from these values and can help with diagnosis and management. Normal values for intracardiac pressures and saturation, and formulas to calculate various hemodynamic parameters, typically obtained with intravascular catheters in the ICU or catheterization laboratory, are shown in Figure 7.3 and Table 7.1. Adequacy of CO and tissue oxygen delivery function can also be assessed using mixed venous oxygen saturation (measured in the PA in the absence of intracardiac shunts), blood oxygen saturation in the superior vena cava (SVC), and serum lactate levels.

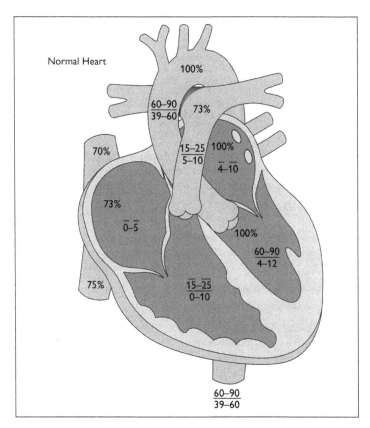

Figure 7.3 Normal values for intracardiac pressures and blood oxygen saturation.

Table 7.1 Formulas for Calculating Hemodynamic Parameters

Parameter	Formula	Normal Range
CI (Fick principle)	$VO_2/(CaO_2 - CvO_2) \times BSA$	Infant, 160–180 mL/min/m²; child, 100–130 mL/min/m²
CaO₂	$CaO_2 = (1.34 \times Hb \times SaO_2) + (PaO_2 \times 0.003)$	
Systemic vascular resistance index	$79.9 \times (MAP - CVP)/CI$	800–1600 dyne-s/cm⁵/m²
Pulmonary vascular resistance index	$79.9 \times (MPAP - LAP)/CI$	80–240 dynes-s/cm⁵/m²
Oxygen delivery	$CI \times CaO_2$	570–670 mL/min/m²
Pulmonary: systemic blood flow ratio ($Q_p:Q_s$)	$(SaO_{2\,AORTA} - SaO_{2\,SVC})/ (SaO_{2\,PV} - SaO_{2\,PA})$	1

BSA, body surface area; CaO₂, arterial oxygen content; CI, cardiac index; CvO₂, mixedvenous oxygen content; CVP, central venous pressure; Hb, hemoglobin concentration (g/dL); LAP, left atrial pressure; MAP, mean arterial pressure; MPAP, mean pulmonary artery pressure; PaO₂, partial pressure of oxygen in arterial blood; PA, pulmonary artery; PV, pulmonary vein; Q_p, pulmonary blood flow; Q_s, systemic blood flow; SaO₂, oxygen saturation; SVC, superior vena cava; VO₂, oxygen consumption.

Congenital Heart Disease

Congenital heart defects (CHDs) are the most common forms of birth defects, affecting 1% of births per year, and are the leading causes of birth defects associated mortality in infants. A third of children born with CHDs become critically ill and require surgical management during the first year of life.

Types of CHDs

A clinical classification of CHD types based on the presence of cyanosis and pulmonary blood flow is shown in Table 7.2. Some forms of CHDs (e.g., corrected transposition of the great vessels) are not covered in this classification.

Hemodynamic Consequences of CHDs

Effects on hemodynamics vary by the type CHD

Left–to-right shunt: A left-to-right shunt can occur at the ventricle, atrium, or great vessels and results in increased pulmonary blood and pulmonary congestion. The magnitude of the shunt depends on the size of the lesion, SVR, PVR, and ventricular compliance. The shunt can be quantified during cardiac catheterization as a ratio of pulmonary blood flow (Q_p) to systemic blood flow (Q_p/Q_s; normal value = 1).

Outflow obstruction: Obstruction to the pulmonary or aortic outflow tract results in increased pressure proximal to the obstruction. In children, the ventricles respond to the increase workload with hypertrophy. In

Table 7.2 Classification of Congenital Heart Disease

Acyanotic	Cyanotic
Increased pulmonary blood flow	Increased pulmonary blood flow
A. Septal defects	d-Transposition of great arteries
Atrial septal defects	Truncus arteriosus
Ventricular septal defects	Total anomalous pulmonary venous return
Atrioventricular canal defects	Hypoplastic left heart syndrome
B. Great vessel communications	
Patent ductus arteriosus	
Aortopulmonary window	
Normal pulmonary blood flow	Decreased pulmonary blood flow
Aortic stenosis	Tetralogy of Fallot
Coarctation of aorta	Tricuspid atresia with pulmonary stenosis
Pulmonary stenosis	Ebstein's anomaly
	Critical pulmonary stenosis

the neonate, however, obstruction usually causes ventricular dilation and dysfunction. Signs and symptoms of outflow obstruction depend on the severity of the outflow obstruction, which can be quantitated by measuring a pressure gradient across the obstruction either by ECHO or cardiac catheterization.

Mixing of pulmonary venous return and systemic venous blood: In patients with single-ventricle lesions, venous mixing usually occurs at the atrial level. The single ventricle's output is distributed to the systemic and pulmonary circulation. The presence or absence of pulmonary or systemic outflow obstruction and/or magnitude of SVR and PVR determines $Q_p:Q_s$.

Evaluation of CHDs

Age at presentation and symptomatology vary by type and severity of CHD. The history and physical examination should be conducted with a plan to determine the severity of the CHD, and to help assess the need and timing of intervention. Physical examination should include review of vital signs, four-limb BP measurement, pulse oximetry, and auscultation for murmurs.

Evaluation should include review of ECG and CXR. ECHO is commonly used to confirm diagnosis and evaluate cardiac anatomic details for intervention. Cardiac catheterization can provide important hemodynamic information to assess severity and need for intervention. In many cases, cardiac catheterization is therapeutic and can be used to treat or to help stabilize hemodynamics, so surgical management of the CHD can occur at a later and more optimal time. Newer modalities of imaging such as MRI can help obtain information on anatomy and physiology important for the management of some forms of CHDs. Finally, assessments should be conducted for abnormalities in other organ systems, which occur in 29% of children with CHDs and include skeletal, gastrointestinal, and respiratory tract abnormalities. Noncardiac mal-formations often complicate management of CHDs and require involvement of other specialist services.

Special Consideration in Evaluation of a Newborn with Suspected CHD

Prenatal diagnosis of CHDs is now more common and has facilitated plan-ning delivery and postnatal management. In the absence of prenatal diagno-sis, four-limb BP, pre- and postductal peripheral oxygen saturation (SaO_2), and hyperoxia testing can help diagnose CHDs. The systolic BP gradient between the upper and lower limbs (>10 mm Hg) suggests coarctation of the aorta. Differential cyanosis suggested by higher preductal (right hand) more than postductal (legs) SaO_2 is seen in patients with ductal-dependent left heart obstruction (e.g., critical aortic stenosis) and persistent pulmo-nary hypertension (PH) of a newborn. A consensus statement from the American Academy of Pediatrics on using pulse oximetry as a screening tool to detect CHDs is now available. A postductal SaO_2 level less than 95% 24 hours after birth may need evaluation to rule out CHDs. Hyperoxia test-ing may be required to differentiate cyanosis resulting from a lung disease from cyanotic CHDs. A preductal arterial partial pressure of oxygen less than 150 mm Hg measured from a blood gas drawn from the right radial artery while breathing 100% oxygen suggests the presence of cyanotic con-genital heart disease.

Preoperative Management of Newborn Infants with Suspected or Confirmed CHDs

Neonates with ductal-dependent CHDs presenting with shock after clo-sure of the PDA require resuscitation with prostaglandin (PGE_1; usual dose, 0.01–0.1 µg/kg/min) to establish patency of the PDA, volume expansion, and inotrope support, and mechanical ventilation. Apnea and respiratory depres-sion are known side effects of PGE_1, thus some neonates without shock started on PGE_1 may require control of the airway and mechanical ventilation for apnea or respiratory insufficiency.

Some neonates may require emergency cardiac catheterization for inter-ventions to improve hemodynamic stability further (e.g., balloon atrial septos-tomy in d-transposition of the great arteries to improve mixing at the atrial level) or to provide definitive treatment (e.g., balloon pulmonary valvuloplasty in critical pulmonary stenosis). In patients with common mixing lesions, ensur-ing adequate systemic perfusion requires management of pulmonary blood flow by balancing PVR and SVR.

Surgical Intervention for CHDs

Neonates with ductal-dependent CHDs require operative management dur-ing the neonatal period. Surgical interventions are usually undertaken when hemodynamic stability and end-organ recovery have occurred. For older children with CHDs, timing and type of intervention depend on the lesion, symptoms, hemodynamic consequences of the CHD, and local practice patterns.

Many surgical procedures for CHDs require the use of cardiopulmonary bypass (CPB). Recent advances in CPB techniques have allowed the conduct of complex cardiac surgical procedures during the newborn period, even in premature newborns. Total body hypothermia is commonly used during CPB. Some procedures are conducted with circulatory arrest under deep hypothermic conditions (body temperature, 18–22°C). Myocardial protection during cardiac surgery is usually achieved with cardioplegia solutions injected into the aortic root or directly into the coronary artery. Heparin is used to provide anticoagulation during CPB and is typically reversed with protamine sulfate. CPB elicits a systemic inflammatory response that results in increased capillary permeability and interstitial edema, and is most pronounced in neonates. CPB causes dysfunction of other organs, including lungs, kidney, and brain, that may complicate postoperative care.

Postoperative Management of Children with CHDs

Postoperative care of children and adults with CHDs requires a coordinated effort of a team of multidisciplinary caregivers including medical, surgical, nursing, allied health care professionals, and family members. Postoperative care starts with the transfer of information from the operating room team to the ICU providers. Information on intraoperative course and results of intraoperative imaging should be obtained from the operating room team. Postoperative assessment should include physical examination, review of hemodynamic data, laboratory data, ECG, and CXR. Evaluation of the postoperative patient should be focused on diagnosing residual heart defects, assessing CO, presence of bleeding, and status of end-organ function.

Postoperative cardiovascular management should aim to optimize CO and tissue oxygen delivery by ensuring adequate preload, myocardial contractility, and afterload; ensuring sinus rhythm; and reducing oxygen consumption (Box 7.1). A postoperative course deviating from the expected course for type and physiology of CHD should be evaluated promptly for the presence of residual heart defects that may impair recovery.

Weaning from mechanical ventilation and extubation should be considered when hemodynamic stability and hemostasis have been achieved. Other postoperative considerations include adequate pain control, nutrition, and care of the patient's family.

Common challenges in postoperative care of children undergoing CHD surgery include the following:

1. *Postoperative low cardiac output syndrome* (*LCOS*): Several studies have shown that CO falls 6 to 12 hours after surgery for CHDs, and more commonly so in infants. The etiology of postoperative LCOS is multifactorial

Box 7.1 Management of Postoperative low cardiac output syndrome

1. Rule out residual or uncorrected structural defects
   - Physical examination
   - Echocardiography and/or cardiac catheterization
2. Ensure adequate preload
   - Volume expansion to maintain atrial filling pressures
3. Support myocardial contractility
   - Inotropes (dopamine or epinephrine)
4. Reduce afterload
   - Vasodilators or inodilators
   - Positive pressure ventilation
5. Manage rhythm
   - Treatment of arrhythmia
   - Atrioventricular sequential pacing for heart block
6. Reduce oxygen consumption
   - Mild hypothermia
   - Mechanical ventilation
   - Pain management, sedation, and neuromuscular blockade
7. Provide mechanical ventilation
   - Maintenance of functional residual capacity to lower pulmonary vascular resistance
8. Monitor for recovery
   - Monitoring of mixed venous oxygen saturation or serum lactate levels
9. Provide mechanical circulatory support
   - Consideration of extracorporeal membrane oxygenation for failure of conventional medical therapies

and includes inflammatory response to CPB and myocardial injury from the procedure. Clinical manifestations include tachycardia, decreased skin perfusion, decreased urine output, hypotension, tachypnea, decreased mixed venous oxygen saturation, increased atrial filling pressures, and lactic acidosis. Prompt recognition and management of LCOS is imperative in optimizing outcomes for children undergoing cardiac surgery. The principles of management of LCOS are outlined in Box 7.1. Prophylactic use of milrinone after cardiac surgery has been shown to decrease the incidence of LCOS. Residual heart defects should be ruled out in patients with LCOS. Patients who do not respond to medical interventions may need mechanical circulatory support, usually with extracorporeal membrane oxygenation (ECMO).

2. *LCOS resulting from restrictive right ventricle*: In neonates and young infants undergoing cardiac surgical procedures that involve reconstruction of the RV outflow tract (e.g., Tetralogy of Fallot, pulmonary atresia, truncus arteriosus), diastolic dysfunction of a noncompliant or hypertrophied

RV can result in LCOS. Possible causes of diastolic dysfunction include preoperative RV hypertrophy or myocardial injury from right ventriculotomy. Elevated RV EDP results in increased RA pressures and systemic venous hypertension. Although RV systolic function is generally preserved, elevated RV EDP impacts LV compliance and function adversely through changes in the configuration of the interventricular septum and ventricular interdependence. Manifestation of restrictive RV physiology includes LCOS with increased RA pressure, tachycardia, hypotension, decreased pulse pressure, oliguria, and metabolic acidosis. Systemic venous hypertension results in hepatic congestion, increased chest drain losses, pleural effusion, and ascites. In patients with restrictive RV physiology, demonstration of antegrade blood flow into the PA during atrial systole using Doppler ECHO suggests the diagnosis. Although antegrade flow into the PA during atrial systole is abnormal, it contributes to CO (30%). Antegrade diastolic flow is impaired during the inspiratory phase of positive-pressure mechanical ventilation, and the use of excessive MAP during mechanical ventilation may be detrimental. Management includes maintenance of RV preload, prompt management of arrhythmias, and administration of vasoactive support, sedation, and paralysis. The mechanical ventilation strategy should use the lowest MAP that maintains FRC, and early extubation when possible is beneficial. Restrictive RV physiology is made worse by residual left-to-right shunt or RV outflow obstruction, and these should be investigated. In most instances, RV diastolic function will improve, and recovery is expected. Creating a fenestration in the atrial septum can lower elevated RA pressure and maintain LV preload.

3. *Postoperative pulmonary hypertensive crisis*: PH (PA systolic pressure, >35 mm Hg, PA mean pressure, >25 mm Hg; or PA pressure, >50% systemic pressure) often complicates postoperative management of CHDs. Postoperative PH is often seen in lesions with large left-to-right shunts (VSD, complete atrioventricular canal defects, truncus arteriosus, large PDA, and aortopulmonary window), and left-sided obstructive lesions (total anomalous venous return and mitral stenosis). Systemic inflammation following CPB contributes to the transient elevation of PVR and PH. Acute PH crisis is characterized by an acute elevation of PVR resulting in increased RV pressure, RV dysfunction, and decreased CO. The increased RV pressure can shift the interventricular septum into the LV, altering LV compliance and reducing CO. Acute distension of hypertensive pulmonary arterioles can compress small airways and result in difficulty with ventilation. The usual triggers for PH crisis include pain, noxious stimuli, hypoventilation, and atelectasis. Management includes narcotics (to reduce sympathetic stimulation) neuromuscular blockade, increased FiO_2, moderate hyperventilation and alkalosis, and inhaled nitric oxide.

4. *Postoperative cardiac arrhythmia*: Arrhythmias can lead to a significant morbidity after CHD repair and occur in 15% to 48% of postoperative patients. Arrhythmias are common in patients with residual volume or

pressure overload and after ventricular incisions. Consultation from a cardiac electrophysiologist should be sought, if possible, for the diagnosis and management of cardiac arrhythmias. Discerning the type of arrhythmia is an important step and requires information on HR (tachycardia or bradycardia), regularity, presence of p waves and their ratio and relationship to the QRS complex, and QRS morphology (in comparison with baseline ECG). Determining whether the QRS complex is narrow can help differentiate tachycardia originating from the atrioventricular node junction versus from the atrium. Wide complex tachycardia should always be assumed to be ventricular tachycardia unless proved otherwise. Alternatively, wide complex tachycardia can be a form of supraventricular tachycardia with aberrant conduction. A 12-lead ECG can help determine the type of tachycardia. In some cases, atrial wire studies using temporary pacing wires in postoperative patients may help better understand the mechanism of tachycardia. Management in stable patients may require electrolyte replacement, gentle weaning of inotropes when possible, mild hypothermia (35°C), sedation and muscle relaxation, antiarrhythmic medication, and temporary pacing. Reentrant atrial tachycardia may be amenable to intravenous adenosine administration or overdrive pacing. Patients who are unstable hemodynamically or pulseless require cardiopulmonary resuscitation and electrical cardioversion or defibrillation. Postoperative heart block is a known complication in the surgical repair of CHDs and may require atrioventricular sequential pacing. Waiting approximately 10 days for recovery of AV node function may be required to avoid unnecessary placement of a permanent pacemaker.

Single-Ventricle CHDs

Patients with single-ventricle CHDs have absence or hypoplasia of one of the two ventricles. The single ventricle receives both the systemic and pulmonary venous return and ejects into both outflow tracts. Initial management depends on the presence and severity of obstruction of the systemic or pulmonary outflow tract as outlined in Table 7.3. Staged single-ventricle palliation aims to separate the pulmonary and systemic venous circulation typically in three stages (Figure 7.4).

Stage 1 Palliation: Norwood Operation
Stage 1 is used for the single ventricle with systemic outflow tract obstruction (e.g., HLHS) and consists of systemic outflow tract reconstruction (Damus-Kaye-Stansel anastomosis and reconstruction of the aortic arch), atrial septectomy, PDA ligation, and construction of a source of pulmonary blood flow with either a Blalock-Taussig shunt (systemic [usually innominate or subclavian

Table 7.3 Management of Postoperative Patients after Stage 1 Palliation

Scenario	Physiology/Etiology	Management
SaO_2 = 85% SvO_2 = normal Normotensive	$Q_p = Q_s$ Balanced flow	Usual management
SaO_2 >90% Hypotension	$Q_p > Q_s$ ↑SVR ↓PVR	Afterload reduction Inotrope support Avoidance of hyperventilation Sedation and paralysis
	Aortic arch obstruction	Catheter or surgical intervention
Acute ↓SaO_2 Hypotension Acute ↓$ETCO_2$	BT shunt thrombosis	Heparinize Ventilate with 100% FiO_2 Catheter or surgical shunt intervention ECMO to stabilize patient if needed
SaO_2 = 75%–85% Hypotension SvO_2 low	Low cardiac output	Inotrope support Afterload reduction Sedation paralysis VO_2 decrease
	Aortic arch obstruction AVVR	Catheter or surgical intervention

AVVR, atrioventricular valve regurgitation; BT, Blalock-Taussig; ECMO, extracorporeal membrane oxygenation; $ETCO_2$, end tidal carbon dioxide; FiO_2, fraction of inspired oxygen; PVR, pulmonary vascular resistance; Q_p, pulmonary blood flow; Q_s, systemic blood flow; SaO_2, arterial oxygen saturation; SvO_2, venous oxygen saturation; SVR, systemic vascular resistance; VO_2, oxygen consumption.

artery] to PA) or a right ventricle-to-PA conduit (Figure 7.4). The systemic and pulmonary circulations are in parallel, and CO is distributed to both. The balance of SVR and PVR determines Q_p:Qs. Because pulmonary and systemic venous returns mix in the atrium, PA and systemic SaO_2 are equal. If one assumes normal lung function (pulmonary vein SaO_2, 100%) and adequate cardiac output (SVC SaO_2, 70%) then a peripheral SaO_2 of 85% indicates balanced circulation with Q_p:Q_s of 1:1. Systemic SaO_2 thus reflects the balance of Q_p:Q_s. Those with higher SaO_2 have higher Q_p compared with Q_s and may present with symptoms of low CO.

Postoperative management aims to balance Q_p:Q_s. This is achieved by decreasing SVR using afterload reduction. Hyperventilation and use of high FiO_2 may decrease PVR and should be avoided. Support of myocardial contractility with inotropes is often required. In patients with systemic-to-pulmonary artery shunts, blood flow from the aorta to the pulmonary artery in diastole can result in systemic steal and coronary ischemia. This phenomenon is not

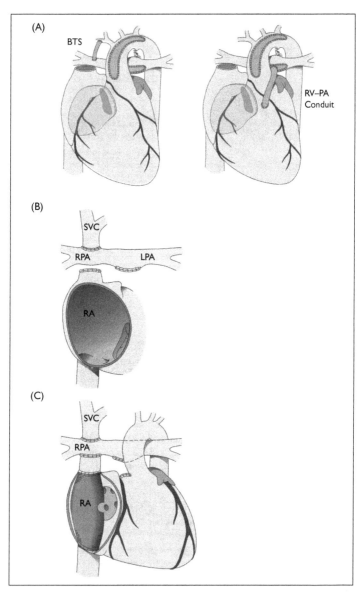

Figure 7.4 Operative details of the three stages of single-ventricle palliation. (A) Norwood operation. (B) Bidirectional Glenn operation. (C) Lateral tunnel. BTS, Blalock-Taussig shunt; LPA, left pulmonary artery; PA, pulmonary artery; RA, right atrium; RPA, right pulmonary artery; RV, right ventricle; SVC, superior vena cava.

Table 7.4 Palliation of Single-Ventricle Congenital Heart Defects	
Stage	**Age**
Stage 1	*Newborn*
No outflow tract obstruction	PA band
Outflow tract obstruction	
A. Pulmonary obstruction	
PDA dependent	Systemic-to-PA shunt
Non-PDA dependent	No intervention until cyanosis and then systemic-to-PA shunt
B. Systemic obstruction	Stage 1 palliation (Norwood)
Stage 2	*3–6 months*
	Superior cavopulmonary connection (bidirectional Glenn)
Stage 3	*18–24 months*
	Total cavopulmonary connection (Fontan)
	Lateral tunnel Fontan
	Extracardiac Fontan

PA, pulmonary artery; PDA, patent ductus arteriosis .

seen in patients receiving RV-to-PA conduits, which has led to their widespread adoption.

An approach to managing patients after stage 1 palliation is shown in Table 7.4. In patients with systemic-to-pulmonary artery shunts, acute desaturation, hypoxemia, loss of shunt murmur, and sudden decrease in end-tidal carbon dioxide should raise the suspicion of shunt thrombosis. These patients may progress to cardiac arrest and need resuscitation with ECMO before intervention for shunt recanalization.

Stage 2 Palliation: Bidirectional Glenn Operation

The venous return from the upper body is directed via the SVC into the PA (Figure 7.4). After this operation, pulmonary blood flow is dependent on cerebral blood flow. Therefore, factors that increase cerebral blood flow (hypercarbia and acidosis) can increase pulmonary blood flow and SaO_2. However, these factors may also increase PVR. This operation results in decreased volume load to the single ventricle and improved myocardial performance. Persistent hypoxemia after the operation warrants evaluation in the cardiac catheterization laboratory to diagnose anatomic obstruction of the new venous return pathway and to look for venous collaterals that drain blood away from the SVC. Systemic hypertension is common after the operation, resulting from either improved myocardial performance or as a response to increased cerebral venous pressure, and may require management with antihypertensives.

Stage 3 Palliation: Total Cavopulmonary Connection (Fontan Operation)

This is the final step in the separation of the pulmonary and systemic circulation in a single-ventricle CHD. It is achieved by directing the venous return from the inferior vena cava (IVC) into the PA. Current operative strategies to achieve this include creating a lateral tunnel along the free wall of the RA directing IVC flow into the PA or using an extracardiac conduit outside the right atrium to direct IVC flow into the PA. A fenestration in the Fontan tunnel allows shunting of blood from the Fontan baffle into the LA and allows decompression of high systemic venous pressures often seen during the early postoperative period. This maintains LV preload at the expense of lower SaO_2. The fenestration can be closed at a later time in the cardiac catheterization laboratory.

Several physiological considerations are important during postoperative management after the Fontan operation. CO is dependent on pulmonary blood flow and blood shunted from the venous circulation across the fenestration into the systemic atrium. Pulmonary blood flow and therefore CO may also be decreased by anatomic obstruction of the PA or increased PVR. In some cases, occlusion of the Fontan fenestration can cause low CO because of reduced filling of the systemic atrium. These patients have low CO with high SaO_2. Finally, use of high levels of MAP during mechanical ventilation can impair systemic venous return, reduce pulmonary blood flow, and decrease CO.

Thus, after undergoing the Fontan operation, patients often require judicious intravascular volume expansion, mechanical ventilation with low MAP for gas exchange, prompt correction of metabolic acidosis, afterload reduction, and pacing for atrioventricular dysynchrony. Early extubation from mechanical ventilation should be considered when possible. Table 7.5 describes causes and management of LCOS in the Fontan circulation. Persistent pleural effusions, arrhythmias, and hypoxemia may complicate the postoperative course and may require cardiac catheterization for hemodynamic assessment and management.

Acquired Heart Disease

Acquired heart disease includes primary myocardial disease (e.g., cardiomyopathies, acute myocarditis, infectious endocarditis, acute rheumatic fever) and cardiac involvement in other systemic diseases (e.g., sepsis, metabolic disease, Duchenne muscular dystrophy, Friedreich's ataxia, systemic lupus erythematosus). Evaluation and management of children with acquired heart disease is similar to those with CHDs. Congestive heart failure or acute cardiogenic shock is often the predominant feature at presentation, and evaluation and management are aimed at managing cardiovascular dysfunction.

Table 7.5 Considerations for Management of Fontan Circulation

Scenario	CVP	LAP	SBP	SaO₂	Management
Ideal circulation	10–15 mm Hg	4–6 mm Hg	80–90 mm Hg	85%–95%	Manage as usual
Hypovolemia	Low	Low	Low	85%–95%	Expand volume
Increased PVR PA obstruction	High	Low	Low	Low	Reduce PVR Ventilate Correct acidosis Administer inhaled nitric oxide Perform catheterization or surgery
Fenestration occlusion	High	Low	Low	High	Open fenestration
Ventricular dysfunction AVVR AV dissociation	High	High	Low	Expected range	Maintain preload Provide inotrope support Reduce afterload Pace Provide mechanical circulatory support Take down Fontan
Tamponade			Very low		Relieve Tamponade

AV, atrioventricular; AVVR, atrioventricular valve regurgitation; CVP, central venous pressure (Fontan pressure); LAP, left atrial pressure; PA, pulmonary artery; PVR, pulmonary vascular resistance; SaO₂, arterial oxygen saturation; SBP, systolic blood pressure.

Viral Myocarditis

Myocarditis is an inflammatory process affecting the myocardium and is associated with a wide spectrum of clinical presentations and etiological agents including infectious and noninfectious agents. Common causes of viral myocarditis include Coxsackie B, ECHO, and adenoviruses. Clinical presentation of myocarditis varies from asymptomatic to cardiogenic shock. History is typically nonspecific; however, a history of a viral syndrome before the onset of CHF may be present. Myocarditis tends to affect infants and adolescents. Chest pain, tachycardia out of proportion to fever, and signs of CHF may be present. ECG findings include nonspecific ST-T wave changes, ventricular or atrial ectopy, and conduction defects. Cardiomegaly and pulmonary edema are often seen on CXR. ECHO shows decreased cardiac function with normal cardiac anatomy. Serum creatine phosphokinase and cardiac troponin I levels are elevated in pediatric myocarditis and can aid in diagnosis. Definitive diagnosis of viral myocarditis is made with an endomyocardial biopsy showing lymphocytic infiltration and myocytolysis. Polymerase chain reaction examination of myocardial biopsy specimen has helped improve the identification of viral genomes in the myocardial cell. Delayed enhancement sequences using gadolinium contrast cardiac MRI can diagnose myocardial inflammation and is used increasingly to provide noninvasive diagnosis of myocarditis.

Management of patients with myocarditis is largely supportive, with pharmacological therapy aimed at optimizing CO and systemic oxygen delivery. Patients with myocarditis should be monitored and managed in the ICU. Preload, afterload, and myocardial contractility should be optimized. Volume administration needs to be judicious and given slowly, with monitoring of CVP if available. Vasoactive agents are the primary means of augmenting BP and CO. Administration of intravenous immunoglobulin (2 g/kg) may improve ventricular function and 1-year survival. Benefits from the use of other immunosuppressive agents (prednisone, cyclosporine, azathioprine) have not been demonstrated clearly in children. Ventricular tachycardia may occur, could be life threatening, and should be treated promptly. Many children recover cardiac function and survive to hospital discharge. Some (estimated, 12%–40%) develop dilated cardiomyopathy and some require cardiac transplantation at initial presentation.

Patients with acute fulminant myocarditis often present in cardiogenic shock and may require emergent airway management, inotrope support, and mechanical circulatory support. ECMO is often required for cardiovascular support in these patients, especially in those with ventricular arrhythmias, severe lactic acidosis, and end-organ dysfunction at presentation.

Summary

Cardiac disease is a common reason for ICU admission in children. Diagnosis and treatment of congenital and acquired cardiac diseases require knowledge of cardiac anatomy, physiology, medical, and surgical options for optimal management. Treatment options for heart disease in children are expanding and require a multidisciplinary team-based approach.

Further Reading

Andropoulos DB, Chang AC. Pediatric cardiovascular intensive care. In: Allen HD, Driscoll DJ, Shaddy RE, Feltes TF, eds. Moss and Adams' Heart Disease in Infants, Children, and Adolescents. 8th ed. Philadelphia: Lippincott Williams & Wilkins; 2013;483–529.

Marino BS, Bird GL, Wernovsky G. Diagnosis and management of the newborn with suspected congenital heart disease. Clin Perinatol. 2001;28(1):91–136.

Redington AN. Cardiopulmonary and right–left heart interactions. In: Allen HD, Driscoll DJ, Shaddy RE, Feltes TF, eds. *Moss and Adams' Heart Disease in Infants, Children and Adolescents*. 8th ed. Philadelphia: Lippincott Williams & Wilkins; 2013:546–551.

Shekerdemian LS, Bush A, Lincoln C, Shore DF, Petros AJ, Redington AN. Cardiopulmonary interactions in healthy children and children after simple cardiac surgery: the effects of positive and negative pressure ventilation. *Heart*. 1997;78(6):587–593.

Teele SA, Allan CK, Laussen PC, Newburger JW, Gauvreau K, Thiagarajan RR. Management and outcomes in pediatric patients presenting with acute fulminant myocarditis. *J Pediatr*. 2011;158(4):638–643.

Wessel DL. Managing low cardiac output syndrome after congenital heart surgery. *Crit Care Med*. 2001;29(10)(suppl):S220–S230.

Chapter 8

Pediatric Shock

Recognition and Management

Diana Pang and Joseph A. Carcillo

Shock is a state of *acute energy failure* in which there is not enough adenosine triphosphate (ATP) production to support cellular respiration. Cellular respiration begins with metabolism of glucose to acetyl coenzyme A, entry into the Krebs cycle, electron transport, oxidative phosphorylation, and production of carbon dioxide, water, and ATP. Shock and dysoxia usually occur concomitantly, and inadequate oxygen (O_2) delivery is a key component of shock (Figure 8.1). Clinical signs of shock are presented in Box 8.1.

Types of Shock

The key factors in the recognition and treatment of shock vary by its etiology (Table 8.1). The seven most common types of shock are as follows:

1. *Hypovolemic*: inadequate intravascular volume
   a. Blood loss (trauma, hemorrhage, vessel injury or rupture)
   b. Fluid loss (emesis, diarrhea, polyuria)
2. *Anemic/hemorrhagic*: low hemoglobin concentration and/or active bleeding
   a. Blood loss
   b. Decreased production of red blood cells
   c. Increased destruction of red blood cells
3. *Cardiogenic*: low cardiac output (CI <2.0 L/min/m²) resulting from cardiac dysfunction
   a. Structural abnormalities (e.g., ductal-dependent congenital cardiac lesions)
   b. Congestive heart failure
   c. Cardiomyopathy, myocarditis
4. *Vasoplegic* (aka *distributive*): low vascular tone
   a. Neurogenic (e.g., spinal cord injury)
   b. Anaphylactic
      i. Immunoglobulin E-mediated reactions to foods, drugs, insect bites
      ii. Complement-mediated reactions to blood products
5. *Septic*: encompassing characteristics of hypovolemic, cardiogenic, and distributive shock; includes toxin and cytokine-mediated endothelial dysfunction and loss of vascular tone

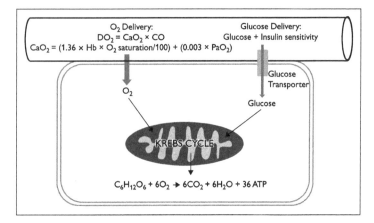

Figure 8.1 Cellular respiration occurs in the mitochondria, where glucose and oxygen (O_2) yield carbon dioxide, water, and adenosine triphosphate (ATP). O_2 delivery depends on the arterial content of O_2 and cardiac output. O_2 molecules diffuse into the cell and mitochondria. Glucose enters the cell via the glucose transporter.

ATP, adenosine triphosphate; $C_6H_{12}O_6$ – hexose (simple sugars, e.g., glucose, fructose); CaO_2 – arterial oxygen content blood; CO – cardiac output; CO_2 – carbon dioxide; DO_2 – oxygen delivery; H_2O – water; Hb – hemoglobin; O_2 – Oxygen; PaO_2 – arterial partial pressure of oxygen

Box 8.1 Clinical Signs of Shock at Early and Late Stages

Early

- Ill appearance
- Tachycardia to more than the 98th percentile for age (unless hypothermic)
- Tachypnea for age
- Capillary refill more than 2 seconds or flash capillary refill
- Abnormal pulse pressure
  - Narrow pulse pressure, suggesting cardiac failure
  - Wide pulse pressure, suggesting septic or vasodilatory shock

Late

- Hypotension
- Anion gap metabolic acidosis, more than 16 mEq/L
- Elevated lactate, more than 2 mmol/L

Table 8.1 Summary of Shock States, Recognition, and Management

Shock/Dysoxia State	Recognition	Management
Hypovolemic	Capillary refill >2 s High shock index	Fluid resuscitation
Anemic	Pallor Capillary refill >2 s High shock index	Blood transfusion If anemia is from decreased production or increased destruction, must be given in small aliquots over several hours.
Cardiogenic (ischemic)	Capillary refill >2 sec High shock index $AVDO_2$ >5% SVO_2 <70% Lactate >2 mmol/L AG >16 mEq/L	Inotropes Inodilators
Vasoplegic (distributive)	Flash capillary refill High shock index	If neurogenic: fluid resuscitation If anaphylactic: IM or SQ epinephrine, fluid resuscitation, histamine blockers, steroids
Septic	Capillary refill >2 s or flash capillary refill High shock index Suspicion of infection	Antibiotics Fluid resuscitation Inotropes, inodilators, and/or inovasopressors
Metabolic	Hypo- or hyperglycemia in the setting of any of the previously listed shock states Lactate >2 mmol/L AG >16 mEq/L	If hypoglycemic: dextrose infusion If hyperglycemia: dextrose and insulin infusion
Cellular dysoxia	$AVDO_2$ <3% SVO_2 >70% Lactate >2 mmol/L AG >16 mEq/L	Dextrose infusion Citrate Levocarnitine Coenzyme Q10

AG, anion gap; $AVDO_2$, arterio-venous oxygen content difference; IM, intramuscular; SQ, subcutaneous; SVO_2 central venous oxygen saturation.

6. *Metabolic*: inadequate glucose substrate to fuel the Krebs cycle and produce ATP, which leads to anion gap acidosis resulting from organic acid
   intermediates produced by catabolism of protein and fat
   a. Hypoglycemia
   b. Hyperglycemia with extreme insulin resistance or absence of insulin

7. *Cellular dysoxia*: when mitochondrial dysfunction prevents ATP production despite adequate O_2 and glucose delivery
   a. Metabolic crises in children with metabolic syndromes (e.g., medium-chain acyl-coenzyme A dehydrogenase deficiency, methylmalonic acidemia)
   b. Cyanide poisoning

Management: Goal-Directed Therapy

Implementation of therapies that reverse derangements before ATP deficiency occurs can *prevent* shock. Resuscitation to clinical goals is the first priority in *treatment* of shock (Box 8.2, Table 8.2, Figure 8.2).

1. Clinical goals
   a. Appropriate mental status for age and development
   b. Urine output more than 1 mL/kg/h
   c. Signs of adequate CO and normal peripheral vascular tone
      i. Capillary refill time less than 2 seconds
      ii. Easily palpable distal pulses
      iii. Concordance between peripheral and core temperatures (37.0–38.0°C)
      iv. Normal arterial pressure tracing (Figure 8.3)
         1. Increased steepness of upstroke with better cardiac contractility
         2. Summation of the reflection wave with higher systemic vascular resistance
         3. Absent respiratory variation in systolic blood pressure with better preload.
         Note: Hypotension is a very late sign of shock. As a result of significant vasoconstriction in response to hypovolemia, hypotension is not seen until 30% to 50% of blood volume is lost (Figure 8.4). Earlier signs of shock must be recognized and treated (tachycardia, elevated shock index [heart rate/systolic blood pressure]).

2. Hemodynamic and O_2 utilization goals
   a. Normal heart rate (HR) for age
   b. Normal perfusion pressure for age (dependent on mean arterial pressure [MAP]; Box 8.2)
      i. Effective fluid resuscitation
         1. ↑ MAP – CVP: ↑ perfusion pressure
         2. ↓ HR and ↑ SBP: ↓ shock index
      ii. Excessive or ineffective fluid resuscitation
         1. ↓ MAP and ↑ CVP: ↓ perfusion pressure
         2. ↑ HR and ↓ SBP: ↑ shock index

Box 8.2 Resuscitation Goals

The overall goal of resuscitation is to normalize clinical, hemodynamic, and biochemical derangements.

Clinical
- Nontoxic appearance
- Normal respiratory rate for age
- Equal core and peripheral temperatures
- Capillary refill less than 2 seconds
- Urine output more than 1 mL/kg/h

Hemodynamic and Oxygen Use
- Normal heart rate for age
- Normal perfusion pressure for age (Mean arterial pressure [MAP] – Central venous pressure [CVP])
  - Term newborn, more than 55 mm Hg
  - Infant, more than 60 mm Hg
  - Toddler, more than 65 mm Hg
  - School age child, more than 65 mm Hg
  - Adolescent, more than 65 mm Hg
- SVO_2 saturation, more than 70%
- Improved Cardiac Index (CI)
  - CI more than 2.0 L/min/m^2 for cardiogenic shock
  - CI 3.3–6.0 L/min/m^2 for septic shock
- Arterial-venous oxygen content difference 3% to 5%
- Mean pulmonmary artery occlusion pressure 5–10 mm Hg
- Mean left atrial pressure 5–10 mm Hg

Biochemical
- Anion gap less than 16 mEq/L
- Lactate less than 2.0 mmol/L
- Normoglycemia

Table 8.2 Fluid Resuscitation

Fluid Therapy	Dosage	Comments
Isotonic crystalloid (e.g., 0.9% NaCl)	20–40 mL/kg	More or less may be needed. Dose to meet resuscitation goals.
Colloid (e.g., 5% albumin)	20–40 mL/kg	Start with smaller doses in children at risk of myocardial dysfunction (5–10 mL/kg).
		In all patients, monitor for signs of heart failure/fluid overload:
		Hepatomegaly
		Rales
		Wet cough
		Tachypnea
Packed red blood cells	10 mL/kg	In chronic anemia with cardiac failure, a smaller volume should be administered slowly.

Fluid resuscitation can be with isotonic crystalloid, colloid, or red cells. Patients must be monitored for signs of fluid overload and heart failure during fluid resuscitation.

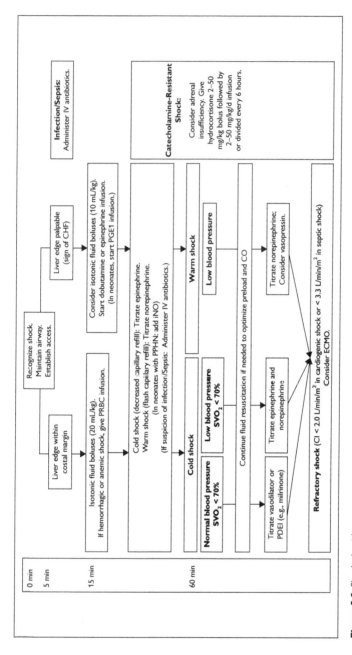

Figure 8.2 Shock algorithm.

CHF – congestive heart failure; CI – cardiac index; CO – cardiac output; ECMO – extracorporeal membrane oxygenation; iNO – inhaled nitric oxide; IV – intravenous; PDEI – phosphodiesterase inhibitor; PGE1 – prostaglandin E1; PPHN – persistant pulmonary hypertension of the newborn; PRBC – packed red blood cell; SVO2 – central venous oxygen saturation

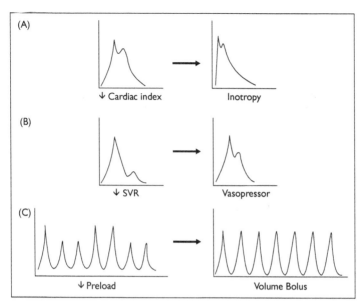

Figure 8.3 (A) Decreased upstroke is a sign of decreased cardiac contractility. Inotropes will increase the upstroke. (B) Separation of the reflection wave from the arterial wave is a sign of decreased systemic vascular resistance (SVR). Vasopressors will lead to summation of the two waveforms. (C) Respiratory variation of arterial systolic blood pressure is a sign of decreased preload. Fluid resuscitation will abrogate the variation.

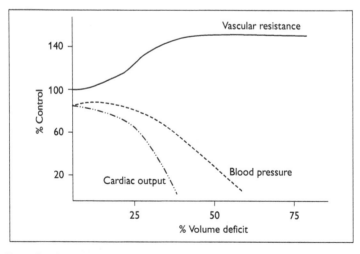

Figure 8.4 Systemic vasoconstriction can maintain blood pressure despite 25% hypovolemia and reduced cardiac output.

c. Mixed venous O_2 saturation (SVO_2) more than 70%, measured from SVC

d. CI more than 2.0 L/min/m² in cardiogenic shock or 3.3 to 6.0 L/min/ m² in septic shock

Although the most accurate measurements are derived from thermodilution techniques using pulmonary artery catheters, noninvasive estimates can be obtained with portable Doppler ultrasonography or electric cardiometry.

3. Biochemical goals

a. Lactate less than 2.0 mmol/L. Elevated lactate is one sign of anaerobic metabolism. *Note:* Lactate is also increased in conditions without shock (e.g., metabolic disorders, lymphoproliferative disorders, liver failure).

b. Anion gap (AG) less than 16. Increased AG can be the result of anaerobic metabolism (ischemic shock) or organic acidemia (metabolic shock and cellular dysoxia). *Note:* Non-AG acidosis following fluid resuscitation with 0.9% NaCl is the result of strong ions Na^+ and Cl^-, not energy failure or shock.

Therapies

Specific therapies to treat shock are as follows.

1. *Fluid therapy.* Fluid therapy is the hallmark of hypovolemic shock resuscitation (Table 8.2). If signs of fluid overload or heart failure develop while shock persists, fluid resuscitation should be stopped and vasoactive agents should be started.

a. Isotonic crystalloid (e.g., 0.9% NaCl, Ringer's lactate) or colloid (e.g., 5% albumin)

Dose: 20 to 40 mL/kg infused rapidly via a manual pressure bag or electronic rapid infusion system. Infusion through a large-bore (18–20 gauge) intravenous catheter or intraosseous needle ensures the fastest resuscitation.

Note: For neonates and children with cardiac failure (e.g., from cardiomyopathy or congenital heart disease), aggressive fluid resuscitation may lead to decreased cardiac output and cardiovascular collapse. Therefore, volumes of 5 to 10 mL/kg should be given judiciously with continuous clinical and hemodynamic monitoring.

b. Blood products: Packed red blood cells (PRBC) should be given for anemic/hemorrhagic shock.

Dose: 10 mL/kg will increase Hb concentration by 2 to 3 g/dL (depending on the Hb concentration of the transfused cells).

Note: When transfusing children with hypervolemia or cardiac dysfunction, consider administering a diuretic during or after the transfusion to prevent adverse sequelae of fluid overload. In contrast, patients with hemorrhagic shock are *hypovolemic* and therefore do not need diuresis.

2. Catecholamines (Table 8.3)
   a. Dobutamine: synthetic racemic catecholamine with dose-dependent β1 and α2 adrenergic effects; most effective in congestive heart failure
      i. Low dose (2.5–5 µg/kg/min): β1 agonist effects predominate → inotropy and chronotropy
      ii. High dose (>10 µg/kg/min): increasing α2 agonist effects → inhibition of norepinephrine release → ↓ vascular tone → hypotension
   b. Epinephrine: Endogenous catecholamine increases contractility during stress and shock with dose-dependent β1, β2, α1, and α2 effects.
      i. Low dose (0.05 µg/kg/min): β1 agonist → inotropy and chronotropy
      ii. High dose (0.3 µg/kg/min): α1 agonist → ↑ vascular tone → ↑ afterload
      Note: Patients with heart failure and increased systemic vascular resistance may be harmed by high doses unless epinephrine is administered concomitantly with a vasodilator or inodilator.
   c. Dopamine
      i. Endogenous catecholamine with both inotropic and vasopressor qualities, as well as effects on the dopamine D1 receptor (renal vasodilation) and dose-dependent β1 and α1 effects. Dopamine mediates its adrenergic effects through the release of norepinephrine from the sympathetic vesicles.
         1. Low dose (3–10 µg/kg/min): β1 agonist → inotropy
         2. High dose (>10 µg/kg/min): α1 agonist → ↑ vascular tone
         Note: Dopamine may be less effective in neonates or children who have exhausted their catecholamine reserves.
   d. Norepinephrine: endogenous catecholamine with both inotropic and vasopressor qualities, stimulating β1, α1, and α2 receptors. Even at low doses (0.01–0.05 µg/kg/min), norepinephrine has vasopressor qualities that predominate over inotropic effects.

3. Inodilators
   a. Phosphodiesterase inhibitors (PDEIs)
      i. Type III PDEIs (milrinone, amrinone, enoximone, pentoxifylline): Bind competitively to cyclic adenosine monophosphate (cAMP) and prevent hydrolysis of cAMP by phosphodiesterase 3.
      Effects: Lusitropy (improve diastolic function, ventricular relaxation), inotropy, and vasodilation. By inhibiting hydrolysis of cAMP, milrinone effectively increases β1 and β2 effects of high-dose epinephrine (inotropy and vasodilation, respectively) when α1 effects (vasoconstriction) predominate.
      Toxicity: In the setting of renal insufficiency, clearance of milrinone by the kidneys is decreased, and hypotension and tachyarrhythmias can occur. In this case, discontinue milrinone and consider norepinephrine to counteract vasodilation-mediated hypotension.

Table 8.3 Commonly Used Medications to Treat Shock

Medication	Effect	Dosage	Comments
Catecholamines			
Dobutamine	Low dose: inotrope (β1 agonist) High dose: afterload reduction (α2 agonist)	2.5–5 μg/kg/min	
Epinephrine	Low dose: inotrope (β1 agonist) High dose: vasopressor (α1 agonist)	0.05–1 μg/kg/min	Potent inotropic catecholamine
Dopamine	Low dose: inotrope (β1 agonist) High dose: vasopressor (α1 agonist) Vasodilator (D1 receptor) for renal arteries	2–20 μg/kg/min	Age-specific insensitivity (less effective in newborns)
Norepinephrine	Inotrope and vasopressor (β1, α1, α2 agonist)	0.05–1 μg/kg/min	Potent vasopressor; absent β2 effect distinguishes it from epinephrine
Inodilator			
Milrinone	Inotrope, lusitrope, vasodilator (type III PDEI)	0.2–0.75 μg/kg/min	Metabolized predominantly by the kidney
Vasopressor			
Vasopressin	Vasopressor (V1 agonist) without inotrope activity	0.0002–0.002 U/kg/min	
Vasodilators			
Nitroprusside	Systemic arterial vasodilator (cGMP-mediated)	0.3–1 μg/kg/min	Monitor cyanide and isothiocyanate metabolites
Inhaled nitric oxide	Pulmonary vasodilator (cGMP-mediated)	5–20 ppm	For neonates with PPHN
Prostaglandin E1	Prevents PDA closure	0.05–0.1 μg/kg/min	Should be started in all newborns with shock because 50% of neonatal shock occurs in newborns with ductal-dependent congenital heart disease
Steroid			
Hydrocortisone	Glucocorticoid and mineralocorticoid effects	Bolus dose: 2–50 mg/kg; infusion: 2–50 mg/kg/day	

cGMP, cyclic guanosine monophosphate; PDA, patent ductus areteriosus; PDEI, phosphodiesterase inhibitor; PPHN, persistant pulmonary hypertension of the newborn.

ii. Type V PDEIs (sildenafil, dipyrimadole): Potentiate pulmonary vaso-dilator effects of inhaled nitric oxide (iNO).

b. Isoproterenol: Synthetic derivative of norepinephrine that has strong $\beta 1$ and $\beta 2$ effects. Can be used for treatment of pulmonary hyperten-sive crises with right ventricle failure, severe bradycardia, heart block, and refractory status asthmaticus.

Note: Use with caution. Should not be used in the setting of myocardial ischemia. Even in patients without existing myocardial ischemia, effects on increased HR and lower SVR can lead to subendocardial ischemia (increase in myocardial O2 demand not met by concomitant increased myocardial O2 delivery).

c. Levosimendan: Calcium-sensitizing agent that improves contractility in adult heart failure and refractory septic shock. Causes vasodilation of pulmonary arterial beds.

4. Vasopressors
   a. Phenylephrine: Pure $\alpha 1$ agonist. In addition to treating hypotension resulting from decreased systemic vascular tone, phenylephrine can be used for reversal of Tetralogy of Fallot spells unresponsive to conven-tional therapies. In that case, systemic arterial vasoconstriction leads to left-to-right shunting and perfusion of the lungs.
   b. Vasopressin: V1 receptor agonist that leads to systemic vasoconstric-tion. Useful in catecholamine-resistant shock.
      Note: Can reduce cardiac output in children with poor cardiac function by increasing afterload.
   c. Angiotensin: Mediates vasoconstriction via the phospholipase C path-way and increases aldosterone secretion.

5. Vasodilators
   a. Nitrosovasodilators
      i. Nitroprusside: systemic and pulmonary vasodilator. Stimulates NO production → arteriolar vasodilation → decreased afterload → improved CO. Useful in cardiogenic shock associated with high systemic vascular resistance.
      Note: Risk of cyanide toxicity with use of nitroprusside, especially in the setting of renal insufficiency (Nitroprusside + O_2-Hb → NO + MetHb + CN^-). If concern of cyanide toxicity, stop nitroprusside and consider administration of Na thiosulfate.
      ii. Nitroglycerin: Dose-dependent coronary artery, pulmonary venous, systemic arterial vasodilator
   b. α-Adrenergic antagonists
      i. Phentolamine: Can be used in combination with epinephrine or norepinephrine to offset their α-agonist effects.
      ii. Phenoxybenzamine: Can be used to reverse hypertension in pheo-chromocytoma and provides afterload reduction in neonates with single-ventricle physiology.

6. Prostaglandin E1: Prevents closure of the patent ductus arteriosus. Should be started in all newborns with shock because 50% of neonatal shock occurs in newborns with ductal-dependent congenital heart disease. An echocardiogram should be performed as soon as possible to identify any cardiac lesions.

7. Hydrocortisone: Adrenal insufficiency should be considered in catecholamine-resistant shock. Hydrocortisone, not methylprednisolone or dexamethasone, should be used for shock because it has both gluco-corticoid and mineralocorticoid effects. Risks of centrally and peripherally mediated adrenal insufficiency include chronic illness treated with long-term steroids, congenital central nervous system (CNS) anomalies, acquired CNS injury, and Waterhouse-Friderichsen syndrome. Patients present with persistent hypotension despite adequate volume resuscitation and infusions of epinephrine and/or norepinephrine. A low, random cortisol level (e.g., <18 µg/dL) in a stressed patient is consistent with adrenal insufficiency. (During acute shock, cortisol levels can reach 150 to 300 µg/dL.)

8. Other medical therapies
   a. Dextrose (+ insulin if needed): to deliver adequate glucose substrate and increase ATP production.
   b. Mitochondrial substrates may be useful in patients with inborn errors of metabolism.
      i. Levocarnitine
      ii. Coenzyme Q10
      iii. Citrate
   c. Tri-iodothyronine: Hypothyroidism should be suspected in children with shock who require epinephrine and/or norepinephrine, have tri-somy 21, a CNS illness, or a pan-hypopituitary state.

9. Extracorporeal mechanical support: In patients who remain in ischemic shock despite use of the discussed therapies, extracorporeal mechanical support can attain a 50% survival in children and 80% in neonates.
   a. Extracorporeal membrane oxygenation (ECMO)
      i. Indications for consideration of venoarterial ECMO
         1. Severe shock resulting from primary cardiac failure
         2. CI less than 2.0 L/min/m² despite appropriate fluid, inotrope, and vasodilator management
         3. Greater than 1 µg/kg/min epinephrine
      ii. Indications for consideration of venovenous ECMO
         1. Shock resulting from primary respiratory failure resulting in cardiac dysfunction
         2. Oxygenation index more than 40
   b. Left ventricular assist device and intra-aortic balloon pump may be used in larger children and adolescents.

Summary

Shock is a common, time-sensitive cause of death in critically ill children and thus requires early recognition and goal-directed treatment to attain the best outcomes. Therapies should be directed to timely reversal of anemia, hypoxia, ischemia, and glycopenia. Initially, fluids and inotropes should be used to reverse shock and return to normal cardiac output, blood pressure, and SVO_2 >70%. Vasopressors, vasodilators, hydrocortisone, tri-iodothyronine, and extracorporeal mechanical support may also be required to accomplish this goal.

Further Reading

Brierley J, Carcillo JA, Choong K, et al. Clinical practice parameters for hemodynamic support of pediatric and neonatal septic shock: 2007 update from the American College of Critical Care Medicine. Crit Care Med. 2009;37(2):666–688.

Dalton HJ, Siewers RD, Fuhrman BP, et al. Extracorporeal membrane oxygenation for cardiac rescue in children with severe myocardial dysfunction. Crit Care Med. 1993;21(7):1020–1028.

Dolbec K, Mick NW. Congenital heart disease. Emerg Med Clin North Am. 2011;29(4):811–827, vii.

Weiss SL, Selak MA, Tuluc F, et al. Mitochondrial dysfunction in peripheral blood mononuclear cells in pediatric septic shock. Pediatr Crit Care Med. 2015;16(1):e4–e12.

Chapter 9

Neurocritical Care

Steven L. Shein and Robert S. B. Clark

Brain injury is the most common proximate cause of death in pediatric intensive care units (PICUs). For children who survive critical illness, long-standing brain damage and residual brain dysfunction can impact quality of life significantly. Therefore, minimizing neurological injury to improve patient outcomes is a priority of neurocritical care. This may be accomplished by implementing specific targeted therapies, avoiding pathophysiological conditions that exacerbate neurological injury, and using a multidisciplinary team that focuses on contemporary care of children with neurological injury and disease.

Overarching Principles

Anatomic Considerations

The brain accounts for approximately 80% of the contents of the cranial vault. Cerebrospinal fluid (CSF) and cerebral blood volume (CBV) each account for approximately 10%. Because the cranial vault is generally rigid, the expansion of any of these compartments (or the presence of a mass lesion) necessitates contraction of another compartment (capacitance) to prevent an increase in intracranial pressure (ICP)—referred to as the *Munro-Kellie doctrine*. The primary reservoir reacting to acute changes in CBV or mass lesions is the CSF, facilitated by displacement into the spinal cord subarachnoid space and/ or absorption in arachnoid villi. CSF is then replaced at an average rate of 18 mL/h. The secondary reservoir, after CSF capacitance is exhausted, is CBV. Because CBV proportional to cerebral blood flow (CBF), this occurs at the expense of CBF and may result in ischemia. When both CSF and CBV capacitance are exhausted, further increases in ICP may lead eventually to herniation of brain structures into adjacent intracranial compartments and one or more of the following herniation syndromes:

• *Central*: Increased ICP in both cerebral hemispheres causes the diencephalon to herniate underneath the tentorium, causing brainstem compression. Level of arousal decreases progressively and symptoms evolve through the *diencephalic stage* (hypertonicity, small and reactive pupils, decorticate posturing, Cheyne-Stokes respirations), *midbrain–upper pons stage* (midposition pupils with variable reactivity, decerebrate posturing, hyperventilation), *lower pons–medullary stage* (nearly absent motor function [lower extremities may withdraw to plantar stimulation], midposition and fixed pupils, failure of oculovestibulo/cephalic reflexes, ataxic respirations), and *medullary stage* (generalized flaccidity, fixed pupils, apnea, eventual brain death).

* *Subfalcine/cingulate*: Increased ICP in one cerebral hemisphere causes herniation of the cingulate gyrus underneath the falx cerebri, causing paresis of the contralateral lower extremity.
* *Uncal*: A lateral mass pushes the uncus of the temporal lobe and the hippocampus over the edge of the tentorium, compressing the brainstem unilaterally and causing ipsilateral third-nerve palsy (mydriasis with absent or sluggish response to light, ptosis, and inferior/lateral deviation of the eye) and hemiparesis (can be ipsi- or contralateral). As herniation progresses, consciousness becomes depressed, pupils become unresponsive to light, decorticate/decerebrate posturing develops, and cardiorespiratory instability ensues.
* *Cerebellar/tonsillar*: Increased pressure in the posterior fossa may lead to herniation of the cerebellar tonsils through the foramen magnum, causing brainstem dysfunction such as apnea and cardiovascular instability. Upper brainstem function (e.g., pupillary light reflexes) may be preserved, although lower cranial nerve palsies may be present. Loss of consciousness is from reticular activating system compression.
* *Upward*: In a patient with supratentorial decompression (surgical or ventricular drain), contents of the posterior fossa may herniate upward into the diencephalic region.

Physiological Considerations

Coupling of CBF and Cerebral Metabolism
The cerebrovascular bed is tightly regulated such that adequate CBF is delivered to meet metabolic demands. In general, CBF is coupled linearly with cerebral metabolic rate for oxygen and cerebral metabolic rate for glucose (Figure 9.1). Thus, CBF is coupled directly with level of consciousness and is also increased during other situations of heightened metabolism, including fever and seizures, both relevant to PICU patients.

Important features related to the coupling of CBF and CBV include the following:

* Normal CBF in an awake adult human is ~50 mL/100 g brain/min.
* The ischemic threshold in humans is considered to be less than 20 mL/100 g brain/min.
* If CBF and metabolism are coupled, therapeutic maneuvers that would reduce CBV include sedation, narcotics (if level of discomfort or intolerance of procedures is increasing metabolism), and lowering body temperature.

Blood Pressure Autoregulation
Within a physiological range of mean arterial pressure (MAP), CBF is constant (Figure 9.2). When autoregulation is intact, increased cerebral perfusion pressure (CPP) leads to cerebral arterial and arteriolar vasoconstriction (thus decreasing CBV); and, vice versa, decreased CPP leads to vasodilation (thus

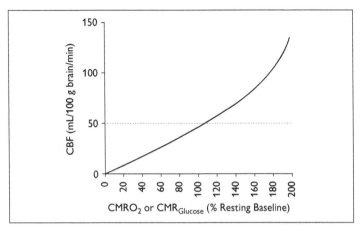

Figure 9.1 Coupling of cerebral blood flow (CBF) and metabolism. $CMR_{Glucose}$, cerebral metabolic rate for glucose; $CMRO_2$, cerebral metabolic rate for oxygen.

increasing CBV). Given that CBF is proportional to the blood vessel radius to the fourth power, changes in blood vessel diameter change inversely with CPP to maintain constant CBF.

- CPP = MAP – ICP (or MAP - central venous pressure (CVP) if CVP is >ICP)
- Poiseuille's law: $Q = (\pi \Delta Pr^4)/(8\eta l)$, where Q is CBF, P is CPP, r is radius, η is viscosity, and l is length

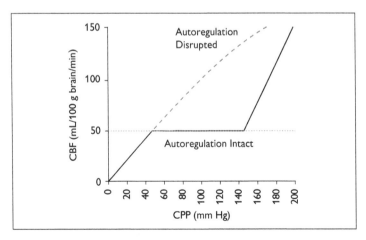

Figure 9.2 Cerebral perfusion pressure (CPP)–cerebral blood flow (CBF) autoregulation.

- Normal autoregulatory range in healthy adults for MAP is ~60 to 160 mm Hg (CPP, ~50–150 mm Hg)
- If autoregulation is intact, therapeutic maneuvers that would reduce CBV include increasing CPP (P) and reducing blood viscosity (η) via hyperosmolar agents such as mannitol and hypertonic saline.

Limited pediatric data indicate that the upper limit of autoregulation likely correlates with age, similar to the age dependency of systolic blood pressure, whereas the lower limit may be surprisingly similar to adult levels (e.g., MAP ~60 mm Hg in one study of anesthetized children age 6 months–14 years). The autoregulatory range can be "reset" with chronic hypertension. With impaired or disrupted autoregulation, as observed with severe brain injury, most notably traumatic brain injury (TBI) and hypoxic–ischemic encephalopathy (HIE), CBF (and consequently CBV) changes proportionally with CPP (Figure 9.2).

Carbon Dioxide Reactivity and CBF Response to Hypoxemia

When carbon dioxide (CO_2) reactivity is intact, CBF rises and falls linearly with $PaCO_2$ (Figure 9.3). This is thought to be related to rapid diffusion of CO_2 from the blood into brain tissue with subsequent changes in tissue pH and corresponding vasodilation (as pH decreases) or vasoconstriction (as pH increases).

CBF remains relatively constant throughout the range of physiological PaO_2, with the exception of conditions of hypoxemia (Figure 9.3). When PaO_2 drops to less than 60 mm Hg, CBF increases profoundly. Of note, with extreme instances of hypocarbia, as seen in extreme hyperventilation, local

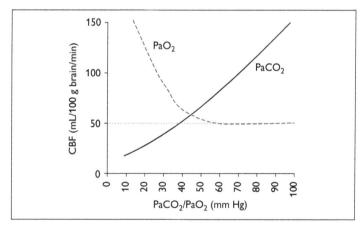

Figure 9.3 $PaCO_2$– and PaO_2–cerebral blood flow (CBF) relationships.

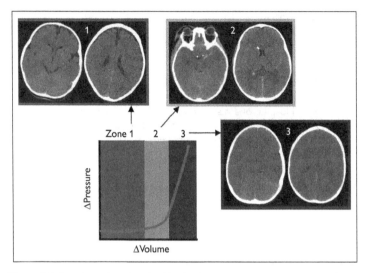

Figure 9.4 Compliance-based cerebral blood volume–intracranial pressure relationships.

brain tissue hypoxia counteracts CO_2-induced vasoconstriction (in normal brain) via numerous mediators (including H^+, adenosine, and so on).

- Normal CO_2 reactivity results in a 2% to 3% change in CBF for every 1 mm Hg change in $PaCO_2$.
- If CO_2 reactivity is intact, increased ventilation reduces CBV.
- If the patient is hypoxemic, increasing PaO_2 more than 60 mm Hg reduces CBV.

Intracranial Compliance

In normal brain, physiological changes in CBV related to changes in CBF are off-set by opposite changes in CSF volume, resulting in constant ICP (Figure 9.4). In other words, in normal brain, intracranial compliance is equal to zero (no change in ICP for a given change in CBV, Zone 1, Figure 9.4). In pathological conditions, the compliance curve shifts to the right, where physiological changes in CBV—as seen with incremental changes in CBF—result in a corresponding change in ICP (Zone 2, Figure 9.4). In extreme cases (Zone 3, Figure 9.4), even small changes in CBV can result in dramatic changes in ICP.

- Compliance = ΔPressure/ΔVolume
- Clinical conditions for compliance-based CBV–ICP relationships
  - Zone 1: Normal brain
  - Zone 2: Moderate global or focal edema, moderate mass lesion (includes stroke), hydrocephalus, malignant hypertension
  - Zone 3: Massive global edema, large mass lesion, central venous obstruction

- Therapeutic maneuvers to shift the compliance curve to the left include reducing CBV (discussed earlier), external CSF drainage, removal of mass lesions, and surgical decompression.

Clinical Management

At Children's Hospital of Pittsburgh of UPMC, we have established a care model composed of a multidisciplinary team that focuses on contemporary care of children with neurological injury and disease. Early consultation and involvement of relevant subspecialty services (e.g., neurology, neurological surgery) is essential.

Approach to the Child with Altered Mental Status

Initial Stabilization

Altered mental status is a common indication for admission to a PICU. Initial management should focus on stabilization of the airway, breathing, and circulation to ensure adequate gas exchange and oxygen delivery. Endotracheal intubation, fluid resuscitation, and vasoactive medications may be required. Factors that may prompt intubation include absence of airway protective reflexes (e.g., cough, gag), severe coma (i.e., Glasgow Coma Scale [GCS] score ≤8 points), and significant hypoxemia and/or hypercarbia. Specific etiologies should be treated when diagnosed or highly suspected based on history (e.g., TBI, ischemia, status epilepticus, meningitis, toxic exposure, hypoglycemia). Naloxone administration should be strongly considered if opiate ingestion is a possibility, and other antidotes provided as indicated.

Physical Examination

Overall level of consciousness is commonly classified using the GCS score (Table 9.1), which has been shown to be associated with outcome after TBI, but has not been validated in other types of brain injury. Cranial nerve (CN) examination may help localize neurological injuries. Symmetric pupils may be large (tectal lesions), midposition (midbrain lesions), small (diencephalic lesions, metabolic disorders), or pinpoint (pontine lesions). Pupil asymmetry can be seen with neurological injury and represents a harbinger of many herniation syndromes (discussed earlier). An abnormally large pupil (mydriasis) is best appreciated in bright light. Dysfunction of CN III (e.g., uncal herniation, posterior communicating artery aneurysm) may cause mydriasis. An abnormally small pupil (miosis) is best appreciated in dim light and may be the result of dysfunction of the sympathetic fibers (Horner's syndrome; e.g., carotid artery dissection or brachial plexus injury). Conjugate gaze can be deviated laterally (seizures, ipsilateral pons/cortex injury) or downward (midbrain compression). Dysconjugate gaze can be secondary to extraocular muscle weakness, CN III palsy (ipsilateral lateral/inferior deviation), CN IV palsy (ipsilateral superior deviation), or CN VI palsy (associated with intracranial hypertension in diffuse injury). With the oculocephalic reflex ("dolls eyes")

Table 9.1 Glasgow Coma Scale Score for Children and Infants

Component	Child	Infant	Score, pt
Eye opening	Spontaneous	Spontaneous	4
	To speech	To speech	3
	To pain only	To pain only	2
	No response	No response	1
Best verbal response	Oriented, appropriate	Coos, babbles	5
	Confused	Irritable cries	4
	Inappropriate words	Cries to pain	3
	Incomprehensible sounds	Moans to pain	2
	No response	No response	1
Best motor response	Obeys commands	Moves spontaneously and purposefully	6
	Localizes painful stimuli	Withdraws to touch	5
	Withdraws in response to pain	Withdraws in response to pain	4
	Flexion in response to pain	Abnormal flexion posture to pain	3
	Extension in response to pain	Abnormal extension posture to pain	2
	No response	No response	1

The Glasgow Coma Scale score is the sum of all three components.

maneuver, eyes will either deviate contralaterally (normal: eyes remain fixed on visual target) or remain fixed in the neutral position (abnormal brainstem function: eyes move with the head). With the oculovestibular reflex ("cold caloric") maneuver, eyes may not move at all (abnormal brainstem function), may deviate ipsilaterally only (abnormal cortical function) or may deviate slowly ipsilaterally with a fast return to a neutral position (normal). Other pertinent cranial nerve examinations include corneal reflexes (CN V and VII) and cough/gag reflex (CN IX and X).

Diagnostic Studies

Diagnostic tests that are appropriate for comatose children include blood glucose, chemistry panel, ammonia, blood gas, liver function tests (LFTs), complete blood count (CBC), lactate, pyruvate, toxicology screen, and cultures/titers for infection. Other laboratory tests to consider include metabolic tests (amino acids, organic acids, and so on), autoimmune tests, and thyroid function tests. Lumbar puncture (LP) may be indicated but should be delayed if signs of intracranial hypertension are present; if LP is delayed, it is important to begin presumptive therapies (for infection) in the interim. Neuroimaging before an LP may be, but is not always, informative. Head computed tomographic (CT) scanning is often indicated to evaluate for signs of increased ICP, trauma, infection, or mass effect. Magnetic resonance imaging (MRI) may be warranted, especially if stroke is a possible diagnosis. An electroencephalogram (EEG) is valuable if convulsive or nonconvulsive seizures are suspected.

Prevention of Secondary Injury

In many acute neurological injuries (e.g., TBI, stroke), primary injury often results in irreversible tissue damage. In addition, other regions may be vulnerable to further or "secondary" injury. Prevention and treatment of secondary injury represents one of the primary roles of the critical care physician. Although some aspects of care are disease specific (see appropriate section), prevention and/or immediate treatment of the following pathophysiological conditions should be strongly considered in all neurologically injured patients:

* Hypoglycemia
* Hypotension
* Hypoxia
* Seizures
* Hyponatremia
* Hyperthermia

Monitoring

ICP Monitoring

Invasive ICP monitoring is widely, but not uniformly, used in neurocritical care for select indications. ICP can be measured with a catheter placed into the ventricle (external ventricular drain [EVD]) or into the brain parenchyma. EVDs allow for treatment of intracranial hypertension via CSF drainage, although CSF diversion precludes concurrent ICP measurement whereas parenchymal monitors measure ICP continuously, which is associated with increased detection of ICP crises. Measurement of ICP is used most commonly in severe TBI, but has also been reported in other conditions (Figure 9.5).

EEG and Other Neuromonitoring

EEG is a widely accepted bedside neuromonitor. EEG is used most commonly to diagnose seizures. It can help guide antiepileptic drug (AED) therapy and is necessary when targeting burst-suppression. In addition to its use in status epilepticus, continuous EEG monitoring is gaining acceptance for use in patients with HIE, such as after prolonged cardiac arrest, TBI, and hepatic encephalopathy.

Emerging neuromonitoring techniques include assessment of brain oxygenation including the use of noninvasive near-infrared spectroscopy and invasive parenchymal brain-tissue oxygen sensors (PbO_2 monitor), and microdialysis to measure metabolic by-products invasively.

Neuroimaging

CT scans are the most widely used imaging technique for acute intracranial processes. CT scans are inexpensive, readily available, and fast, but are limited by radiation exposure, insensitivity to acute ischemic lesions, and relatively poor

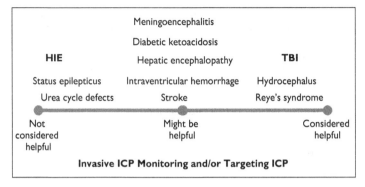

Figure 9.5 Select neurocritical care indications for invasive ICP monitoring and/or using ICP as a therapeutic target. HIE, hypoxic–ischemic encephalopathy; ICP, intracranial pressure; TBI, traumatic brain injury.

imaging of posterior fossa pathology. Noncontrast CT scanning is used typically to identify acute traumatic lesions and to diagnose intracranial hemorrhage, which appears bright. Contrast CT scanning can detect blood–brain barrier dysfunction and excess vascularity, and is used more commonly in the diagnosis of tumors, infections, and inflammatory lesions. MRI provides increased sensitivity for many lesions, but is more expensive and time-consuming. A large number of MRI sequences beyond T1 (CSF = dark) and T2 (CSF = white) are available. Acute ischemic lesions (bright on diffusion-weighted images, dark on ADC maps) can be detected within minutes of onset. MRI can also detect tumors, edema (bright on both diffusion-weighted images and apparent diffusion coefficient maps), infections, demyelinating lesions, and vascular lesions. Magnetic resonance angiography and magnetic resonance venography detect vascular occlusions, aneurysms, and dissections. CT angiography is also useful in these circumstances, although invasive angiography may be indicated if imaging-based angiography is negative or inconclusive.

Other modalities for imaging cranial vault contents exist. Ultrasound via an open fontanelle can assess ventricular size and intraventricular hemorrhage, but is less sensitive for ischemic injury, intraparenchymal hemorrhage, subdural hematomas, and epidural hematomas. Doppler ultrasound does not require an open fontanelle and measures blood flow velocity, typically in the middle cerebral artery. Velocity is a surrogate of CBF that depends on assumptions of blood vessel diameter.

Common Conditions Requiring Neurocritical Care

Traumatic Brain Injury
- Classification and presentation
  - TBI is classified most commonly by mechanism (blunt, penetrating, abusive, and so on) or severity. A patient with a postresuscitation GCS

score of 8 points or less is classified as having severe TBI; a patient with a postresuscitation GCS score of 9 to 11 points is classified as having moderate TBI. Children usually present with altered mental status, although TBI should also be considered in any child with seizures, cardiorespiratory compromise, or cardiac arrest, especially in infants (abusive head trauma). Similarly, children who present with altered mental status after a traumatic injury may have another cause, as well, for their altered sensorium, such as seizures or ingestion.

- Management
  - Guidelines for the management of pediatric severe TBI were originally published in 2003 and updated in 2012. Early collaboration and frequent communication with neurosurgical and trauma surgery services is imperative.
  - *Initial stabilization*: Resuscitation of a child after severe TBI should focus on preventing hypotension, hypoxia, and hypercarbia. Endotracheal intubation is recommended for any child with a GCS score of 8 points or less, or any child requiring urgent surgical intervention. Rapid sequence intubation should be used, although modified to include bag-mask ventilation during induction to limit hypoxia and hypercarbia. In addition, strict cervical (C)-spine precautions should be followed during intubation. Lidocaine attenuates intracranial hypertension from endotracheal suctioning, leading some practitioners to use it during intubation of a child with suspected intracranial hypertension. Hypotension should be treated aggressively with isotonic fluid resuscitation (and blood products for hemorrhage or coagulopathy) and vasopressors if needed.
  - *Laboratory studies*: On presentation: CBC, coagulation profile, electrolytes, osmolality (Osm), blood gas, LFTs, amylase, lipase, type and screen. During ICU admission: follow electrolytes (especially sodium), serum Osm, blood gas, CBC and coagulation profile.
  - *Imaging*: On presentation: head CT scan and C-spine X-rays should be obtained on any child in whom TBI is suspected. During ICU admission: Indications for a repeat CT scan include new findings on neurological examination (including worsened coma) or unexplained intracranial hypertension. MRI may give valuable long-term prognostic data, but has not been evaluated thoroughly for acute management of TBI. Angiography may be needed to assess for traumatic aneurysms and dissections, and damage to central veins and venous sinuses.
  - *PICU*: Secondary injuries (discussed earlier) should be prevented. Prophylactic hyperventilation ($PaCO_2$ <30 mm Hg) should be prevented. Antiseizure prophylaxis with fosphenytoin or levetiracetam or continuous EEG should be considered, especially when using neuromuscular blockade. Extremes in fluid balance should be avoided. Hyponatremia exacerbates cerebral edema and lowers seizure threshold and should be avoided using isosmolar fluids. Children with TBI are at particular risk of hyponatremia (syndrome of inappropriate

antidiuretic hormone [low urine output] or cerebral salt wasting [high urine output]) and hypernatremia (diabetes insipidus [high urine output]). Dextrose containing intravenous fluids are generally avoided for the first 48 hours after injury (unless hypoglycemia occurs). Early enteral nutrition is supported. Systemic steroids are contraindicated.

- Special considerations: treatment of intracranial hypertension
  - Indications for ICP monitoring: (1) GCS score of 8 points or less after resuscitation, (2) rapidly declining level of consciousness, (3) mass lesion with shift, and (4) moderate TBI (GCS score, 9–11 points) without ability to follow neurological examination (surgical procedure planned, non-neurological requirement for neuromuscular blockade).
  - Intracranial hypertension, typically defined as an ICP of 20 mm Hg or more, is associated with death and unfavorable outcome after TBI. ICP typically peaks 48 to 72 hours after injury. Intracranial hypertension crises are diagnosed most accurately using an ICP monitor, but should also be suspected in children with anisocoria, bradycardia/hypertension (Cushing's response), apnea, or decorticate/decerebrate posturing. Suggested treatment based on published guidelines and our practice and experience at the Children's Hospital of Pittsburgh of UPMC is summarized in Box 9.1.
  - Weaning therapies for ICP after a period of more than 24 hours without intracranial hypertension is a reasonable practice.

Hypoxic–Ischemic Encephalopathy
- Classification and presentation
  - Acute HIE is most frequently secondary to cardiac arrest. Cardiac arrest in children is usually a consequence of asphyxia (in contrast to cardiac etiology in adults). Etiologies of asphyxial cardiac arrest include drowning, respiratory failure from pneumonia, asthma or airway obstruction, and CNS depression (from toxic ingestion, trauma, tumor, hydrocephalus, or metabolic process), and other causes such as trauma or sepsis. Cardiac etiologies of cardiac arrest include congenital heart disease, dysrrhythmias (e.g., long QT syndrome), myocarditis, or cardiomyopathy. Common presenting symptoms include coma, seizures, and multisystem organ failure (in cases of prolonged cardiac arrest). Although certain regions are more vulnerable to hypoxia–ischemia (including the hippocampus, cerebellum, basal ganglia, and brainstem), prolonged hypoxia–ischemia can cause global brain injury. Pathophysiological mechanisms include excitotoxicity, activation of cell death pathways (e.g., apoptosis, necrosis), oxidative stress, mitochondrial damage, and inflammation.
- Management
  - Acute resuscitation of a child with ongoing arrest is covered in another chapter. The American Heart Association (AHA) published guidelines for management of children after CA in 2015.

Box 9.1 Treatment Considerations for Intracranial Hypertension

General Management
- Placement of head of bed at 30°
- Optimization of sedation/analgesia
- Consideration of neuromuscular blockade
- $PaCO_2$ target, 35 mm Hg
- Adequate central perfusion pressure: more than 40 mm Hg for infants and toddlers, more than 50–60 mm Hg for children, more than 60 mm Hg for adolescents
- Intermittent or continuous cerebrospinal fluid (CSF) drainage (we use continuous CSF drainage with the reservoir at 10 cm above midbrain)
- Prevention and/or treatment of seizures

Intracranial Pressure of 20 mm Hg or More for More Than 5 Minutes
- First-tier therapies
  - CSF drainage if using an EVD with intermittent drainage
  - Bolus of analgesic or sedative (avoid hypotension!)
  - Hyperosmolar therapies
    - Mannitol bolus 0.25 to 1.0 g/kg (monitor for hypovolemia)
    - Saline 3% (1–5-mL/kg bolus and/or infusion starting at 0.5–1 mL/kg/h titrated to control intracranial pressure (ICP). Monitor serum Na^+ closely; typical therapeutic range, 140 < Na^+ < 155. Monitor closely for rebound intracranial hypertension during weaning of therapy.
  - Moderate hyperventilation: $PaCO_2$ less than 32 mm Hg (monitoring for cerebral ischemia recommended)
- Second-tier therapies and management of refractory ICP
  - Repeat imaging, surgical intervention if indicated
  - Limited period of profound hyperventilation (monitoring for cerebral ischemia recommended; hyperventilate aggressively for clinical signs of herniation)
  - Moderate hypothermia (32–34°C)
  - Barbiturate coma (titrated to burst-suppression; vasopressors likely needed to maintain central perfusion pressure)
  - Trial of induced systemic hypertension (may increase ICP if autoregulation not intact)
  - Decompressive craniectomy

Based on published guidelines and the practice and experience at the Children's Hospital of Pittsburgh of UPMC.

- *Initial stabilization*: Resuscitation of a child at risk for HIE is similar to management of the patient with TBI and should focus on preventing secondary injury. Endotracheal intubation is recommended for any child who remains in a coma after cardiopulmonary resuscitation. Hypotension should be treated aggressively with goal-directed (especially in the instance of cardiac etiology of arrest) isotonic fluid resuscitation and vasopressors if needed.

- *Laboratory studies*: Initial laboratory studies include blood gas, CBC, chemistry panel, LFTs, toxicology screen, coagulation studies, troponin, lactate, and central venous oxygen saturation. Parameters of organ function are commonly deranged and should be followed serially.
- *Imaging*: A head CT scan may identify causes of cardiopulmonary arrest (e.g., trauma, intracerebral hemorrhage, tumor) and provide evidence of injury severity (e.g., cerebral edema). Plain X-rays (e.g., chest, abdomen), electrocardiography, and echocardiography should also be strongly considered to assess for non-CNS causes of arrest and resultant organ dysfunction. MRI may provide valuable prognostic data.
- *PICU*: After CA, establishment of normal parameters of cardiopulmonary function are paramount. Fluid resuscitation and vasoactive medication administration are often required during the post-CA period and should be titrated to adequate CPP. Normocarbia is an appropriate target, as both hypocarbia and hypercarbia are associated with unfavorable outcome following pediatric cardiac arrest. Hypoxemia should be avoided. Normoxemia (SaO_2, 94%–99%) is an appropriate goal because hyperoxemia after cardiac arrest is associated with unfavorable outcome in adults (although this is controversial in children). EEG is often warranted to evaluate for nonclinical seizures and should be considered especially if neuromuscular blocking agents are used. Electrographic seizures can be seen in nearly half of children after cardiac arrest, and AED therapy should be strongly considered. Thorough assessment for the cause of the cardiac arrest should be undertaken and possible etiologies treated (e.g., antibiotics for possible infection). Hyponatremia, hypoglycemia, and fever should be prevented and/or treated. Early enteral nutrition is often limited by systemic ischemia and gut injury. Treatment of intracranial hypertension and ICP monitoring are generally not used in patients after cardiac arrest (exceptions include those with CNS etiologies such as TBI, tumor, or intracerebral hemorrhage)
- Special considerations: therapeutic hypothermia (TH)
  - Moderate TH of 32 to 34°C has been used to improve neurological outcome in adults following out-of-hospital ventricular fibrillation/ventricular tachycardia arrest and in asphyxiated neonates at risk for HIE. More recent data from both children and adults suggest that controlled normothermia is equally effective following an out-of-hospital cardiac arrest. Based on these data and the current AHA recommendations, either controlled normothermia (36–37.5°C) or hypothermia (32–34°C) is a reasonable option following cardiac arrest. The AHA recommends that elevated body temperatures should be actively prevented for at least 5 days following a cardiac arrest.
  - Exclusion criteria for TH include coagulopathy, bleeding, and hemodynamic instability.
  - If used, TH should be initiated rapidly. External cooling (e.g., ice packs, fans, cooling blankets) and internal cooling (e.g., infusion of cold saline,

lavage with cold fluids, cooling of gas in the mechanical ventilator circuit, specialized blood cooling catheters) may be used.
- It is reasonable to continue TH for 12 to 72 hours and rewarming should be done slowly (≤1°C every 4–6 hours). Rewarming may precipitate hypovolemia, hyperkalemia, and seizures.
- Reported complications of TH include coagulopathy, electrolyte abnormalities, dysrhythmmias, and infection.

Status Epilepticus
- Classification and presentation
  - Status epilepticus (SE) was defined in recently published guidelines as 5 minutes or more of continuous seizure activity or recurrent seizure activity without a return to neurological baseline. Refractory SE (RSE) is defined loosely as SE that does not respond to standard treatment regimens. A child with SE may present with active clinical seizures or decreased level of consciousness as a result of the postictal state, adverse effects of AEDs, nonconvulsive SE (NCSE), or any combination thereof. Mortality rates in children with SE are approximately 3% to 9%, and range up to 32% in RSE. Outcome is worse with prolonged seizures, so rapid and aggressive therapeutic interventions appear logical. Initial diagnostic studies should focus on common causes of SE that may be amenable to treatment, including CNS infections, TBI, posterior reversible encephalopathy syndrome, and metabolic derangements (e.g., hypoglycemia, hyponatremia). However, febrile SE is the most common etiology.
- Management
  - *Initial stabilization*: Children with SE are at high risk of respiratory failure resulting from airway obstruction and decreased respiratory drive. Supplemental oxygen is often required to prevent hypoxemia, and endotracheal intubation may be required until seizures are controlled. Prolonged mechanical ventilation is usually associated with RSE or secondary to another pathological process. Children with SE are also at risk of cardiovascular dysfunction, often related to undesirable effects of AED administration, although it may also be related to the underlying condition or, in extreme cases, neurogenic pulmonary edema. Hypotension should be corrected aggressively. Correction of electrolyte disturbances is important. Intravenous fluids containing dextrose (unless the patient is on a ketogenic diet) and normal saline are typically indicated (lower serum sodium lowers seizure threshold). Treatment with appropriate antimicrobial agents (e.g., vancomycin, ceftriaxone, acyclovir) is warranted pending culture results if infection is suspected.
  - *Laboratory studies*: Blood glucose, chemistry panel, toxicology screen, AED levels (if applicable), and infectious workup (e.g., CBC, C-reactive protein, blood culture). Further tests (e.g., LFTs, inborn error of metabolism labs) may be indicated as well. LP may be warranted, but should

be delayed if intracranial hypertension is suspected, and deferred until the airway is secured and seizures have been controlled.

- *Imaging*: A noncontrast head CT scan can evaluate for signs of trauma or hemorrhage. Also consider a study with contrast to evaluate for signs of infection. MRI is often valuable for uncovering an etiology; however, it should be deferred until seizures have been controlled.
- *EEG*: EEG is essential for management of SE. Continuous EEG (cEEG) is recommended for patients "not waking up after clinically obvious seizures cease" to evaluate for NCSE. NCSE is detected in ~40% of critically ill children by cEEG, including those who had clinical seizures before diagnosis. However, it is not known whether aggressive treatment of NCSE improves outcome.
- *PICU*: AEDs should be administered and titrated aggressively in children with SE. Benzodiazepines are the first-line agents recommended in expert guidelines published in 2012. Intravenous administration is generally preferred, although some benzodiazepines may be administered by other routes (e.g., intramuscular, rectal, buccal, nasal). Midazolam (consider 0.1 mg/kg) and lorazepam (consider 0.1 mg/kg) are commonly used agents; diazepam may be associated with decreased efficacy and increased respiratory depression. Addition of a second agent when seizures persist despite two doses of benzodiazepines is reasonable; agents to consider include phenytoin/fosphenytoin (consider 15–20 mg PE/kg), phenobarbital (consider 15–20 mg/kg), valproate sodium (consider 20 mg/kg) and levetiracetam (consider 20 mg/kg). Pyridoxine should be considered in neonates and young children. Children with RSE often require continuously administered AEDs, such as midazolam (consider starting at 0.1–0.2 mg/kg/h) or pentobarbital (consider loading with 2–5 mg/kg and starting infusion at 1 mg/kg/h) with rapid titration. Continuous AED infusion often requires cardiorespiratory support and warrants cEEG. Seizures that persist despite AED infusions may require alternate therapies, such as ketamine, inhaled anesthetics, hypothermia, initiation of the ketogenic diet, or neurosurgical intervention. It is reasonable to begin to decrease therapeutic intensity after seizures have been controlled adequately for more than 24 hours, although this should be decided in conjunction with the neurology team.

Meningitis/Encephalitis

- Classification/presentation
  - Symptoms of meningoencepahlitis include fever, lethargy, irritability, confusion, seizures, vomiting, headache, photophobia, rash, and neck stiffness. Noninfectious etiologies of encephalopathy (e.g., autoimmune syndromes, toxins [sedatives, anticholinergics, salicylates, organophosphates, heavy metals, and so on], hypoglycemia, DKA, inborn error of metabolism, hyponatremia, hepatic failure, uremia,

vasculitides, Reye's syndrome) should be considered. Common infectious causes of meningoencephalitis include bacteria (neonates: Group B *Streptococcus, Escherichia coli, S. pneumonia, L. monocytogenes*; infants/children: *S. pneumonia, N. meningitidis, H. influenzae* type B; tuberculosis), viruses (e.g., herpes viruses [HSV, VZV, CMV, EBV, HHV6], enterovirus, arboviruses), fungi, and parasites.

- Management
  - *Initial stabilization*: Children with profound CNS depression resulting from suspected meningoencephalitis may require endotracheal intubation related to airway obstruction, hypoventilation/apnea, and/or inability to protect their airway. Children with bacterial meningitis may present with septic shock and should be treated accordingly.
  - *Laboratory studies*: Blood glucose (hypoglycemia not uncommon), chemistry panel (hyponatremia and syndrome of inappropriate antidiuretic hormone not uncommon), CBC, coagulation studies, blood cultures and viral studies are routine. Consider C-reactive protein and other labs as indicated.
  - *CSF*: An LP should be performed in all patients with possible meningoencephalitis when the procedure can be performed safely. An opening pressure should be measured and recorded. Complications include cerebral herniation and spinal epidural hematoma. Contraindications include signs of intracranial hypertension (e.g., coma, decerebrate or decorticate posturing, abnormal pupils, bradycardia), coagulopathy, purpura, cardiorespiratory instability, and active seizures. Early empiric antimicrobial therapy and delay of LP until resolution of contraindications should be strongly considered. Common CSF studies include cell counts, protein, glucose, gram stain, culture, and polymerase chain reaction for specific organisms. Classic findings in CSF include marked leukocytosis (predominantly neutrophils), increased protein and decreased glucose with bacterial meningitis; moderate leukocytosis (predominantly lymphocytes), mildly increased protein and normal glucose with viral meningitis; and moderate leukocytosis (predominantly lymphocytes), markedly increased protein and decreased glucose with tuberculous meningitis.
  - *Imaging*: Head CT scan to evaluate for signs of intracranial hypertension and/or a mass lesion should be considered before LP, especially if signs of intracranial hypertension are present, although a "normal" head CT scan does not rule out intracranial hypertension. MRI of the brain can be helpful in the diagnosis of meningoencephalitis and other encephalopathies.
  - *EEG*: An EEG is valuable because approximately one-third of patients with meningoencephalitis have seizures.
  - *PICU*: Rapid administration (preferably pre-PICU admission) of antimicrobials is paramount in a patient with suspected meningoencephalitis. Recommended regimens include ampicillin and cefotaxime or gentamicin for neonates, and vancomycin and ceftriaxone for infants, children, and

adolescents. Acyclovir is recommended for all patients with suspected encephalitis, and doxycycline should be administered if rickettsial/ehrlichial disease is suspected. Consultation with an infectious disease specialist is recommended. Although the available evidence is inconsistent, dexamethasone may decrease postmeningitis hearing loss but does not appear to impact survival. Dexamethasone should be considered in children older than 6 weeks to 3 months of age. Hydrocortisone may be valuable for vasopressor-resistant shock in children with fulminant meningococcemia. Inconsistent evidence also implies that glycerol (hyperosmolar therapy) may decrease postmeningitis hearing loss, but this practice is not included in the most recent NICE (United Kingdom) or Infectious Diseases Society of America (United States) guidelines.

- Special considerations: targeting ICP
  - Despite intracranial hypertension being common in patients with meningoencephalitis (diagnosed by measurement of opening pressure or suspected clinically), invasive ICP monitoring and ICP-directed treatment is not standard and is not commonly practiced. The only consensus indication for EVD placement is when meningitis results in obstructive hydrocephalus.
  - Empiric administration of hyperosmolar agents such as mannitol and/or hypertonic saline to children admitted to the PICU with meningoencephalitis and coma is rational, but not substantiated in the literature. If this approach is chosen, checking serum Na^+ (targeting 140 > Na+ > 155 mEq/L) and Osm (targeting <320 mOsm/kg) frequently is appropriate. Arterial and central venous pressure monitoring helps to avoid hypotension associated with osmotic dieresis, and Foley catheter placement prevents bladder rupture. Therapies can be tapered after mental status improves and response to antimicrobial treatment has been confirmed.

Stroke and Cerebrovascular Accidents

- Classification and presentation
  - Strokes are relatively uncommon in children (~2.5 per 100,000 children-years) but commonly require admission to a PICU. Approximately 55% of pediatric strokes are ischemic and most others are hemorrhagic. Cerebral venous sinus thromboses (CVSTs) are an additional cause of stroke. Children with stroke may present with acute, focal neurological deficits, but may also present with seizures or altered mental status/coma. Approximately half of all children with stroke have one or more identifiable risk factors. Common risk factors include congenital or acquired heart disease (ischemic or CVST), sickle cell disease (ischemic or hemorrhagic), polycythemia or anemia (CVST), trauma (ischemia or hemorrhagic), dehydration (CVST), infection (all types), and hypercoagulable–prothrombotic states (ischemic or CVST). Hemorrhagic stroke is often secondary to rupture of a vascular

abnormality (e.g., arteriovenous malformation or aneurysm) or hemorrhage into a tumor.

- Management
  - Guidelines for the management of acute stroke in children, published by the AHA, American College of Chest Physicians (ACCP), and the Royal College of Physicians, are available. Emergent neurology consultation is important.
  - *Initial stabilization*: Adequate oxygenation, ventilation, and systemic perfusion are essential, but specific resuscitation requirements vary widely among children with stroke. Close monitoring of any child with an acute stroke is warranted to identify deterioration quickly. This may require admission to a PICU even if the child does not require intensive care-level support at the time. Based on adult stroke guidelines, initial IVFs should be isotonic and without dextrose.
  - *Laboratory studies*: Evaluation should include CBC, chemistry panel, coagulation studies, hypercoagulable panel, infectious workup, and other studies to identify stroke risk factors.
  - *Imaging*: Urgent neuroimaging is vital. Some centers use head CT scanning as the initial test, but brain MRI is superior for diagnosis of an acute embolic stroke. Virtual angiography (magnetic resonance angiography/ magnetic resonance venography or CT angiography/CT venography) is recommended in all children with a stroke. Traditional angiography may be necessary if radiological studies are inconclusive and/or endovascular therapy is warranted. Echocardiography to identify intracardiac shunt is also standard.
  - *PICU*: Avoidance of secondary insults may limit damage to the penumbra (the susceptible area surrounding the infarcted brain tissue). Ventilatory support may be required in patients with a GCS score of less than 8 points. Decompressive craniectomy and/or ICP monitoring may be indicated in particularly malignant cases with mass effect and coma. Blood pressure management varies based on whether the stroke includes hemorrhage. A blood pressure floor to prevent any degree of hypotension and to optimize perfusion to the penumbra is recommended for ischemic stroke without hemorrhagic conversion, whereas a blood pressure ceiling is recommended for patients with hemorrhagic stroke and intraventricular hemorrhage resulting from rupture of an arteriovenous malformation or aneurysm.
- Special considerations: AHA, ACCP, and PCP guidelines
  - Although some recommendations vary among groups, all three recommend the following: (1) exchange transfusion to HbS less than 30% in a child with sickle cell disease and (2) no usage of tissue plasminogen activator for ischemic stroke outside of a research protocol. All three groups recommend anticoagulation in ischemic stroke with aspirin (Royal College of Physicians and ACCP), unfractionated heparin (ACCP and AHA), or low-molecular weight heparin (ACCP and AHA).

All three groups recommend anticoagulation in cases of extracranial arterial dissection (unfractionated or low-molecular weight heparin), unless there is intracranial hemorrhage. All three groups recommend anticoagulation for CSVT without intracranial hemorrhage (unfractionated or low-molecular weight heparin). Anticoagulation for CSVT with intracranial hemorrhage is recommended by the AHA and may be considered per the ACCP guidelines. The AHA and ACCP also recommend considering thrombolytic therapy in select cases of CSVT.

Hydrocephalus/Shunt Malfunction
- Classification/presentation
  - Acute hydrocephalus commonly presents with coma or other signs of intracranial hypertension. Macrocephaly may also be the presenting symptom, especially in infants. Hydrocephalus is categorized as obstructive (as a result of obstructed flow in a ventricle or an interventricular channel) or nonobstructive (resulting from inadequate resorption of CSF at the arachnoid villi). Causes may be congenital (e.g., prenatal CNS infection, Chiari malformation, aqueductal stenosis) or acquired (e.g., postintraventricular hemorrhage, acute infection/inflammation). Long-standing cerebral atrophy also may be associated with increased CSF (hydrocephalus *ex vacuo*).
- Management
  - *Initial stabilization*: Emergent neurosurgical consultation should be obtained in conjunction with initial stabilization.
  - *Laboratory studies*: Screening for other etiologies of altered mental status (e.g., CBC, chemistry panel) should be considered. LP is contraindicated in children with obstructive hydrocephalus. Obtaining a CSF sample from the shunt reservoir may be necessary to rule out ventriculitis in the absence of obvious shunt obstruction.
  - *Imaging*: Increased ventricle size on head CT scan (or on ultrasound in neonates) is the hallmark of hydrocephalus. Obstructive hydrocephalus causes ventricular dilation only proximal to the obstruction, whereas all ventricles are dilated in nonobstructive hydrocephalus. MRI is useful for delineating the cause of newly diagnosed hydrocephalus. In children with an existing ventricular drain, plain films provide information to assess catheter continuity.
  - *PICU*: Medical therapies such as hyperosmolar agents and hyperventilation may temporize intracranial hypertension and delay herniation, but are minimally effective treatments for hydrocephalus. Definitive treatment is surgical and warrants urgent neurosurgical consultation. Third ventriculostomy can treat obstructive hydrocephalus. A ventricular shunt treats obstructive or nonobstructive hydrocephalus. Complications of ventricular shunts include infection and mechanical fracture/obstruction and are most common within 6 months of placement.

Further Reading

Abend NS, Dlugos DJ. Treatment of refractory status epilepticus: literature review and a proposed protocol. *Pediatr Neurol*. 2008;38(6):377–390.

Au AK; Carcillo JA; Clark RS; Bell MJ. Brain injuries and neurological system failure are the most common proximate causes of death in children admitted to a pediatric intensive care unit. *Pediatr Crit Care Med*. 2011;12(5):566–571.

Brophy GM; Bell R; Claassen J, et al. Guidelines for the evaluation and management of status epilepticus. *Neurocrit Care*. 2012;17(1):3–23.

Fink EL, Clark RSB, Kochanek PM. Hypoxic–ischemic encephalopathy: pathobiology and therapy of the post-resuscitation syndrome in children. In: Furhman BP, Zimmerman JJ, eds. *Pediatric Critical Care*. 4th ed. Philadelphia, PA: Elsevier; 2011:971–992.

Kochanek PM; Carney N; Adelson PD, et al. Guidelines for the acute medical management of severe traumatic brain injury in infants, children, and adolescents: second edition. *Pediatr Crit Care Med*. 2012;13(suppl 1):S1–S82.

Kravljanac R; Jovic N; Djuric M; Jankovic B; Pekmezovic T. Outcome of status epilepticus in children treated in the intensive care unit: a study of 302 cases. *Epilepsia*. 2011;52(2):358–363.

Moler FW; Silverstein FS; Holubkov R; et al. Therapeutic hypothermia after out-of-hospital cardiac arrest in children. *N Engl J Med*. 2015;372:1898–1908.

Monagle P; Chan AK; Goldenberg NA; et al. Antithrombotic therapy in neonates and children: antithrombotic therapy and prevention of thrombosis, 9th ed: American College of Chest Physicians evidence-based clinical practice guidelines. *Chest*. 2012;141(2)(suppl): e737S–e801S.

Neumar RW; Nolan JP; Adrie C; et al. Post-cardiac arrest syndrome: epidemiology, pathophysiology, treatment, and prognostication: a consensus statement from the International Liaison Committee on Resuscitation. *Circulation*. 2008;118(23):2452–2483.

Pineda JA; Leonard JR; Mazotas IG; et al. Effect of implementation of a paediatric neurocritical care programme on outcomes after severe traumatic brain injury: a retrospective cohort study. *Lancet Neurol*. 2013;12(1):45–52.

Roach ES; Golomb MR; Adams R; et al. Management of stroke in infants and children: a scientific statement from a Special Writing Group of the American Heart Association Stroke Council and the Council on Cardiovascular Disease in the Young. *Stroke*. 2008;39(9):2644–2691.

Shoykhet M, Clark RSB. Structure, function, and development in the nervous system. In: Furhman BP, Zimmerman JJ, eds. *Pediatric Critical Care*. 4th ed. Philadelphia, PA: Elsevier; 2011:783–804.

Tunkel AR, Glaser CA; Bloch KC; et al. The management of encephalitis: clinical practice guidelines by the Infectious Diseases Society of America. *Clin Infect Dis*. 2008;47(3):303–327.

Visintin C, Mugglestone MA; Fields EJ; et al. Management of bacterial meningitis and meningococcal septicaemia in children and young people: summary of NICE guidance. *BMJ*. 2010;340:c3209.

Wainwright MS, Pediatric neurologic assessment and monitoring, In: Furhman BP, Zimmerman JJ, eds. *Pediatric Critical Care*. 4th ed. Philadelphia, PA: Elsevier; 2011:759–782.

Chapter 10

Sedation and Analgesia

Iskra I. Ivanova and Lynn D. Martin

Neonates, infants, and children undergoing intensive care are subjected to a number of noxious procedures and mechanical ventilation. Providing safe, effective sedation and analgesia in the pediatric intensive care unit (ICU) is an important part of everyday care activities. An understanding of the basic principles of sedation and the pharmacology of the most commonly used sedative and analgesic drugs is of paramount importance to the pediatric provider. The goals of sedation in the pediatric patient are

- Allay anxiety
- Obtain the child's cooperation
- Achieve immobilization
- Decrease awareness
- Alleviate discomfort and pain
- Keep the child safe

There are four levels of sedation defined by the American Society of Anesthesiologists (ASA) and they are provided in Table 10.1.

Table 10.1 Continuum of Depth of Sedation				
Domain	Minimal Sedation	Moderate Sedation	Deep Sedation	General Anesthesia
Responsiveness	Normal response to verbal stimulation	Purposeful response to verbal/tactile stimulation	Purposeful response to repeated/painful stimulation	Not able to be aroused, even with painful stimulus
Airway	Not affected	No intervention required	Intervention may be required	Intervention often required
Spontaneous ventilation	Not affected	Adequate	May be adequate	Frequently inadequate
Cardiovascular function	Not affected	Usually maintained	Usually maintained	May be impaired

Adapted with permission from American Society of Anesthesiologists. Practice guidelines for sedation and analgesia by non-anesthesiologists. *Anesthesiology*. 2002;96(4):1004–1017.

General Guidelines

Presedation Assessment

Sedation must be patient oriented and tailored to a specific goal while ensuring the child's safety. The presedation evaluation guidelines of the ASA involve three components

1. Medical history
2. Physical examination
3. Risk assessment: ASA physical status classification system (Table 10.2)

Particular caution is required for patients with an ASA physical status of 3 or more, who are at increased risk of sedation-related adverse events.

Fasting

For nonurgent procedural sedation, the patient should fast for a sufficient time to allow for gastric emptying, according to the ASA preprocedure fasting guidelines (Table 10.3):

Monitoring

Appropriate equipment for airway management and resuscitation of the pediatric patient should be available and checked before each sedation procedure. Especially relevant to critical care providers, in an emergency situation, the American Academy of Pediatrics and the American Academy of Pediatric Dentistry joint update recommended a checklist—SOAPME—to be followed:

- **S** (Suction)
- **O** (Oxygen)
- **A** (Airway)
- **P** (Pharmacy)
- **M** (Monitors)
- **E** (Equipment)

Table 10.2 American Society of Anesthesiologists (ASA) Physical Status (PS) Classification System	
Classification	**Description**
ASA PS 1	Normal healthy patient
ASA PS 2	Patient with mild systemic disease
ASA PS 3	Patient with severe systemic disease
ASA PS 4	Patient with severe systemic disease with constant threat to life
ASA PS 5	Moribund patient not expected to survive without the procedure
ASA PS 6	Brain-dead patient with organs harvested for donor purposes

Table 10.3 American Society of Anesthesiologists Preprocedure Fasting Guidelines

Time, h	Food or Liquid Allowed
2	Clear liquids
4	Breast milk
6	Infant formula, nonhuman milk, light meal

During pediatric sedation, data to be recorded at appropriate intervals before, during, and after the procedure include (1) pulse oximetry, (2) response to verbal commands if practical, (3) exhaled carbon dioxide (CO_2) monitoring, (4) blood pressure and heart rate, and (5) electrocardiography.

Sedatives and Hypnotics

See Table 10.4 for sedative and opiate medications and dosing, and Table 10.5 for benzodiazepine and opiate antagonists.

Table 10.4 Choice of Sedative Agents

Drug	Bolus Dose, IV	Duration of Action	Infusion Dose	Comments
Benzodiazepines				
Diazepam	0.05–0.3 mg/kg	15–30 minutes for seizures, 4–6 hours for sedation; duration limited by redistribution, but has long tissue half-life	NA	PO, 0.04–0.3 mg/kg
Lorazepam	0.05–0.1 mg/kg	Up to 8 h	NA	PO, same
Midazolam	0.03–0.1 mg/kg	20–30 min	0.05–0.1 mg/kg/h	PO, 0.5–1 mg/kg Nasal, 0.1–0.2 mg/kg
Opiates				
Alfentanil	10–20 µg/kg	<15 min	NA	Repeat 5–10 µg/kg

(continued)

Table 10.4 Continued

Drug	Bolus Dose, IV	Duration of Action	Infusion Dose	Comments
Fentanyl	1–5 µg/kg	30–60 min	5–20 µg/kg/h	Nasal, 1.5–2.0 µg/kg
Remifentanil	0.25–1 µg/kg	3–10 min	0.05–2 µg/kg/min	Consider potential for opioid-induced hyperalgesia
Sufentanil	0.1–1 µg/kg	Typically 5 min (dose dependent)	0.1–3 µg/kg/h	
Morphine	0.03–0.1 mg/kg	3–5 h	10–30 µg/kg/h	
Hydromorphone	0.01–0.02 mg/kg	4–5 h	0.006 mg/kg/h	
Methadone	0.05–0.1 mg/kg	6–8 h, but increases to 24–48 h with repeated doses	NA	*Not* for short-term sedation, generally used to treat iatrogenic withdrawal syndrome, can prolong QT interval, monitor QTc regularly in prolonged use
Other classes				
Etomidate	0.1–0.3 mg/kg	2–3 min (0.15 mg/kg) 4–10 min (0.3 mg/kg) (dose dependent)	NA	Infusion not recommended, causes transient adrenal insufficiency
Dexmedetomidine	0.3–1 µg/kg	60–120 min (dose dependent)	0.3–0.7 µg/kg/h	Nasal, 0.5–1 µg/kg
Ketamine	0.5–2 mg/kg	5–10 min IV 12–25 min IM	5–20 µg/kg/min	IM, 3–6 mg/kg
Propofol	1–2 mg/kg	3–15 min (dose dependent)	See Table 10.6	

IM, intramuscular; IV, intravenous; NA, not applicable; PO, per os.

Doses cited are IV unless otherwise specified.

Adapted from Gregory GA, Andropoulos DB. *Gregory's Pediatric Anesthesia*. 5th ed. Wiley-Blackwell, Oxford; 2012.

Table 10.5 Benzodiazepine and Opiate Antagonists

Drug	Bolus Dose	Infusion Dose	Comments
Flumazenil	5–10 µg/kg	NA	Repeat as needed
Naloxone	1–10 µg/kg	0.25–1 µg/kg/h	

NA, not applicable.

Doses cited are intravenous unless otherwise specified.

Adapted from Gregory GA, Andropoulos DB. *Gregory's Pediatric Anesthesia.* 5th ed. Wiley-Blackwell, Oxford; 2012.

Propofol

Propofol is currently the most commonly used intravenous (IV) anesthetic and preferred agent for induction and maintenance of anesthesia. Propofol enhances gating of the gamma-aminobutyric acid (GABA^A) receptor by GABA, the principal inhibitory neurotransmitter, and depresses excitatory synaptic transmission presynaptically.

Pharmacokinetics

Pharmacokinetics varies with age, which explains dosing differences among infants, children, and adults.

Pharmacodynamics

Propofol has little effect on cerebral blood flow (CBF) and intracranial pressure (ICP) when normocarbia is present, making it a good choice in the pediatric neurosurgical ICU.

Propofol depresses ventilation by decreasing sensitivity to CO_2. At therapeutic concentrations, the effect of propofol on cardiac contractility is insignificant. The main vascular effect on propofol is to lower vascular tone, probably because of both sympathetic nervous system inhibition and direct effect on the peripheral vasculature.

Propofol Infusion Syndrome

In the setting of a prolonged propofol infusion, severe toxic effects have occurred, likely caused by the uncoupling effect of propofol on the respiratory chain in the mitochondria. The clinical presentation includes lactic acidosis, rhabdomyolysis, and cardiovascular collapse. When propofol sedation is deemed beneficial, it is recommended to give less than 4 mg/kg/h for 48 hours or less.

Dosing

Propofol is widely available as 1% lipid carrier emulsion. The usual anesthesia induction dose is less than 1 month, 4 mg/kg; 1 month to 3 years, 5–6 mg/kg; 3–8 years, 3–5 mg/kg; more than 8 years, 3 mg/kg. Lower doses would be used for sedation settings. Loss of consciousness lasts for 5 to 10 minutes after a single injection; sedation is maintained with an infusion (measured in mg/kg/hr) as referenced in Table 10.6.

Table 10.6 Dosing Scheme for Propofol Continuous Infusion for Infants and Children by Age and Duration of Infusion

Age	Duration of Infusion, mg/kg/h			
	≤10 min	10–30 min	30–100 min	>100 min
<3 mo	25	20–15	10–5	2.5
3–6 mo	20	15–10	5	2.5
6–12 mo	15	10–5	5	2.5
1–3 y	12	9–6	6	6
Adult	10	8–6	6	4

Adapted from Steur RJ, Perez RSGM, De Lange JJ. Dosage scheme for propofol in children under 3 years of age. *Pediatr Anesth.* 2004;14:462–467.

Etomidate

Etomidate acts by interacting with the GABA^A receptor.

Pharmacokinetics

Etomidate is highly protein bound. In patients with kidney and liver failure and decreased protein binding, the sensitivity to the drug is increased. Etomidate is metabolized in the liver by the cytochrome P450 system to inactive metabolites. Clearance is decreased in cirrhotic patients.

Pharmacodynamics

Etomidate decreases ICP and has no significant effect on CBF. Etomidate depresses ventilation by decreasing sensitivity to CO_2, has minimal effect on heart rate and contractility, and vascular tone is impaired only slightly. Because of its excellent hemodynamic stability profile, etomidate is agent of choice for induction of anesthesia when hemodynamic control is important.

Etomidate impairs adrenal function. It blocks 11-β-hydroxylase, thus inhibiting conversion of cholesterol to cortisol. After an induction dose of etomidate, adrenal suppression lasts for 24 hours. This may have clinical significance in critically ill patients, who may already have compromised adrenal function.

Dosing

The induction dose is 0.3 to 0.6 mg/kg; consider lower doses of 0.2 to 0.3 mg/kg in children with compromised cardiovascular function. Continuous infusion of the drug is not recommended because of effects on adrenal steroid synthesis.

Dexmedetomidine

Dexmedetomidine is a selective α-2-adrenergic agent. It causes sedation without respiratory depression by acting on subcortical areas. It also provides analgesia by stimulating α-2-adrenoreceptors in the central and peripheral nervous systems.

Pharmacokinetics

Dexmedetomidine undergoes rapid redistribution (distribution half-life of 6 minutes) and has an elimination half-life of 2 hours. Dexmedetomidine is highly protein bound and undergoes nearly complete biotransformation in the liver to inactive metabolites that are excreted in the urine.

Pharmacodynamics

Dexmedetomidine reduces CBF and the cerebral metabolic rateproportionally. The CO_2 reactivity of the cerebral vasculature is unaffected.

Common cardiovascular effects are bradycardia and transient hypotension, usually responsive to slowing the infusion rate, or a fluid bolus. Transient hypertension has been observed and is associated with an initial peripheral vasoconstriction effect of dexmedetomidine before its central nervous system (CNS)-mediated vasodilatory effect. Reduce the dose in patients with impaired liver or renal function.

Dosing

The dexmedetomidine pharmacokinetic profile allows titration by infusion, with a relatively quick onset and offset of action. Because of its nonopioid mechanism of analgesia and lack of respiratory depression, dexmedetomidine is favored in the ICU setting to provide anxiolysis after surgical procedures, and sedation for mechanical ventilation. A loading dose of 0.5 to 1 µg/kg over 10 to 20 minutes is followed by a maintenance infusion of 0.2 to 0.7 µg/kg/h, titrated to a preferred sedation scale. The intranasal dose for procedural sedation is 0.5 to 1 µg/kg. As with all sedatives, physical dependence can occur with prolonged use. Clonidine has been used to prevent or treat withdrawal symptoms after prolonged (approximately >1 week) continuous administration.

Ketamine

Ketamine is a noncompetitive *N*-methyl-D-aspartate (NMDA) receptor antagonist. It inhibits presynaptic release of glutamate and potentiates GABA^A. Ketamine has opioid and muscarinic effects, and hypnotic, analgesic, and antihyperalgesic properties. Emergence after ketamine administration may be associated with a state of confusion (less frequently in children) that may be prevented by adjunct drugs such as benzodiazepines (BZDs).

Pharmacokinetics

Ketamine is metabolized by cytochrome P450 to norketamine, which has about 30% of the activity of ketamine. Norketamine (half-life, 4–6 hours) is responsible for some of the effects of ketamine. Drug redistribution occurs rapidly (initial distribution half-life, <15 minutes) and, after a single 1 mg/kg IV injection, the effect lasts 6 to 10 minutes.

Pharmacodynamics

Ketamine increases CBF and cerebral metabolic rate. When normocarbia is maintained, ICP does not increase. Ketamine does not depress ventilation, and the CO_2 response is intact. Tidal volume and respiratory rate are unchanged, with moderate bronchodilation. Airway reflexes are preserved, leading to relative airway protection. Ketamine increases arterial blood pressure, myocardial contractile force, and cardiac output, and sympathetic activity is preserved through the endogenous release of catecholamine stores. Critically ill patients may have limited endogenous catecholamine stores; in this setting, ketamine's direct myocardial depressive effects can produce hemodynamic instability.

Subanesthetic doses of ketamine are potentially antihyperalgesic—an anti-N-methyl-D-aspartate effect. Ketamine has opioid-sparing effects and limits opioid-induced hyperalgesia when used early during the time course of nociceptive stimulation.

Dosing

The usual dose of ketamine is 1 to 2 mg/kg IV for intubation and 0.5 to 1 mg/kg IV for minor procedures, 3 to 6 mg/kg IM; maintenance at 5 to 20 µg/kg/min.

Benzodiazepines

Benzodiazepines (BZDs) interact with the $GABA^A$ receptor, increasing its affinity for GABA. BZDs have hypnotic, sedative, anticonvulsant, anxiolytic, and antegrade amnestic properties.

Pharmacokinetics

Duration of action depends mainly on the affinity to the receptor. Midazolam and lorazepam have an affinity to the receptor 20 times greater than diazepam, hence the duration of action: diazepam, 2 hours; midazolam, 2 to 4 hours; and lorazepam, 24 to 72 hours. BZD metabolism takes place in the liver. Diazepam and midazolam have active metabolites that may accumulate when renal failure is present. BZD elimination depends mainly on hepatic function; in liver failure, clearance is reduced markedly.

Pharmacodynamics

BZDs are commonly used, preferred agents for procedural sedation in children. BZDs have a minimal effect on CBF and ICP, making them suitable for sedation in the neurosurgical ICU.

BZDs depress ventilation by decreasing sensitivity to CO_2, along with mild cardiovascular depression with minimal reduction in blood pressure secondary to a decrease in vascular resistance (in otherwise hemodynamically stable patients). Tolerance and tachyphylaxis can occur with longer infusions (>3 days). BZD withdrawal syndrome is associated with high-dose or long-term infusions (>7 days). Therefore, slow weaning of the drug is recommended if possible, via intermittent IV or per os (PO or oral) dosing of a BZD with a sufficiently long half-life (e.g., lorazepam, diazepam). Monitor for signs of withdrawal (tremor, diaphoresis, jitteriness, yawning/sneezing, uncoordinated/repetitive movements, loose stools, vomiting/gagging, fever) and consider using the pediatric-specific standardized assessment of withdrawal (e.g., using the Withdrawal Assessment Tool [WAT]).

Dosing

Midazolam 0.3 to 0.5 mg/kg PO (onset time 20–30 minutes) in children is useful for providing sedation for minor, nonpainful procedures. Midazolam can be used intranasally (0.1–0.2 mg/kg); however, this is not well tolerated by children because of its bitter aftertaste. For procedural sedation, dosing is 0.1 to 0.15 mg/kg IV. An infusion dose at 0.03 to 0.3 mg/kg/h is adjusted based on the clinical condition of the patient and desired sedation score.

Lorazepam: 0.05 to 0.1 mg/kg IV/PO
Diazepam: 0.05 to 0.3 mg/kg IV, 0.04 to 0.3 mg/kg PO

Flumazenil – Benzodiazepine Antagonist

Flumazenil is a specific BZD antagonist that blocks effects on the GABA inhibition pathway in the CNS. Flumazenil reverses all the effects of the BZDs. Its rapid elimination (half-life, 0.7–1.3 hours) makes continuous infusion of the drug necessary to maintain therapeutic efficacy. The dose is a 5 to 10 µg/kg IV bolus, repeating as necessary. Adverse effects include nausea, vomiting, anxiety, seizures, and cardiac arrhythmias.

Analgesics

Opioids

Opioids interact with specific opioid receptors (μ, δ, κ), with major sites of action being the spinal cord, the medulla, and the periaqueductal gray matter. Opioids have no significant effect on cerebral hemodynamics, provided CO_2 is kept normal. Opioids may depress ventilation and decrease functional residual capacity. Opioids have mild depressant effects on myocardial contractility and vascular tone. The incidence of respiratory depression, nausea/vomiting, pruritus, and urinary retention is similar for all opioids. As with BZDs, tolerance and tachyphylaxis can occur with longer infusions (>5 days). Opiate withdrawal syndrome is associated with high-dose or long-term infusions (>7 days). Therefore, slow weaning of the drug is recommended if possible, via intermittent IV or PO dosing of an opiate with a sufficiently long half-life (e.g., morphine, hydromorphone, methadone), and signs of withdrawal should be monitored.

Morphine

Morphine is primarily (60%) metabolized in the liver. In patients with decreased liver function, dosing must be adjusted. Although less than 10% of morphine is transformed to its active metabolite, morphine-6-glucuronide, the latter is two to eight times as potent as morphine. In renal failure, morphine and its metabolite elimination are impaired. Infants are very sensitive to the respiratory depressant effect of morphine as a result of reduced clearance and prolonged elimination half-life. In neonates and infants younger than 3 months, a continuous infusion at 0.01 to 0.03 mg/kg/h is the preferred mode of administration. Dosing is a 0.05 to 0.1 mg/kg IV bolus titrated to a desired effect.

Hydromorphone

Hydromorphone is a morphine derivative and is approximately five times as potent when given intravenously. Although individual patients may report differences in analgesia and side effects between morphine and hydromorphone, randomized controlled trials have found few differences in the frequency of side effects. Hydromorphone metabolites can accumulate in patients with renal impairment but do not seem to be associated with the respiratory depressant effects seen with morphine metabolites. Dosing is a 0.01 to 0.02 mg/kg IV bolus and an infusion of 0.006 mg/kg/h.

Fentanyl

Fentanyl has a long half-life (6–8 hours), slow intercompartmental clearance, and rapid increase in context-sensitive decrement times with increased duration of administration. This is a relevant consideration particularly when fentanyl is used to sedate patients in the ICU. Dosing is a 0.5 to 4 µg/kg IV bolus, with 1 to 2 µg/kg for repeated injections; infusion is 0.5 to 2 µg/kg/h. Time to peak effect is 5 to 6 minutes. Its short duration of effect is a result of redistribution of the drug from active sites (not its metabolism). Transmucosal fentanyl (peak effect, 30–45 minutes) is available for brief painful procedures, particularly if IV access is not readily available. Fentanyl can be administered transcutaneously by a patch in a variety of strengths (25, 50, 75, or 100 µg/h for 3 days). Fentanyl and other synthetic opioids can cause skeletal muscle rigidity, most commonly with rapid administration of large doses.

Alfentanil

Alfentanil is a potent, short-acting analog of fentanyl. It is about one-fourth as potent as fentanyl and has one-third the duration of action. It has a short half-life (1–2 hours) and high clearance. After an IV bolus dose of 10 to 20 µg/kg, the peak effect occurs in 1 to 2 minutes. Follow with smaller boluses of 5 to 10 µg/kg for short, painful procedures.

Remifentanil

Remifentanil is a potent opioid with rapid onset (<1 minute) and a very short half-life (6 minutes). Remifentanil is degraded in plasma by nonspecific cholinesterases. The context-sensitive half-time is around 4 minutes, regardless of the duration of the infusion. When given with propofol (3–4 mg/kg), excellent intubating conditions are produced within 20 to 30 seconds after a bolus of 2 to 3 µg/kg. A continuous infusion of 0.1 to 0.5 µg/kg/min provides excellent analgesia. Because of its short analgesic effects, as soon as the remifentanil infusion is discontinued, a rebound hyperalgesia syndrome can occur.

Sufentanil

Sufentanil has an intermediate half-life (2–3 hours) and a short, predictable context-sensitive half-life. Time to peak effect is 2 to 4 minutes. Dosing is a

0.2 to 0.4 µg/kg IV bolus, with repeated doses of 0.1 to 0.25 µg/kg, and an infusion of 0.1 to 0.5 µg/kg/h.

Meperidine

Meperidine is a synthetic opioid that is one-tenth as potent as morphine, with an elimination half-life of approximately 3 to 4 hours (metabolized in the liver). Meperidine has an active metabolite—normeperidine—that, if accumulated, can cause seizures. A catastrophic syndrome of excitation, delirium, hyperpyrexia, and convulsions has been described in patients on monoamine oxidase inhibitors. It is no longer used routinely for analgesia and is used rarely to treat postoperative shivering (α-2-adrenergic receptor agonist) at a dose of 0.5 to 1 mg/kg.

Methadone

Methadone is a long-acting opioid commonly used to wean patients slowly from opioids to prevent or treat iatrogenic withdrawal syndrome. It has an onset of action of 10 to 20 minutes after parenteral administration and 30 to 60 minutes after oral administration. Duration of action is 6 to 8 hours in a methadone-naive patient; but, after repeated administration, duration increases to 24 to 48 hours. It is highly protein bound, metabolized in the liver, and excreted by the kidneys. Because of wide interindividual differences, the dose needed to "convert" to methadone from other opioids is not straightforward and must be individualized. Generally, 0.05 to 0.1 mg/kg every 6 to 8 hours is adequate, but patients must be monitored closely for toxicity (CNS and respiratory depression) as well as for the need for a higher dose to prevent withdrawal. In addition, methadone prolongs the QT interval. Therefore, a 12-lead electrocardiogram should be obtained before the onset of therapy and regularly thereafter, with more frequent monitoring in patients receiving other QT-prolonging medications.

Naloxone – Opioid Antagonist

Naloxone is a pure opioid antagonist used to reverse unanticipated or undesired opioid effects. Its peak effect is seen in 1 to 2 minutes. Administration may lead to abrupt onset of pain as opioid analgesia is reversed. This may be accompanied by abrupt hemodynamic changes (hypertension, tachycardia) and seizures. Repeated administration may be needed because of its short duration of action. Dosing is a 1 to 10 µg/kg IV bolus titrated every 2 to 3 minutes as needed. Infusion at 0.25 to 1 µg/kg/h may be used to treat other opioid-related effects, including pruritus, nausea/vomiting and urinary retention.

Muscle Relaxants

There are two classes of muscle relaxants: depolarizing and nondepolarizing (Table 10.7). Succinylcholine (SCh) is the only depolarizing muscle relaxant. Nondepolarizing agents include nonsteroidal (cisatracurium) and steroidal (vecuronium, rocuronium) agents.

Table 10.7 Neuromuscular Blocking Agents

Drug	Bolus Dose	Duration of Action	Infusion Dose	Comments
Depolarizing				
Succinylcholine	1–2 mg/kg	4–6 min	NA	Suitable for RSI
Nondepolarizing				
Cisatracurium	0.15–0.2 mg/kg	30–45 min	NA	
Rocuronium	0.6–1.2 mg/kg	30–40 min	NA	Suitable for RSI at 1.2 mg/kg
Vecuronium	0.1–0.3 mg/kg	30–40 min	0.05–0.1 mg/kg/h	

NA, not applicable; RSI, Rapid sequence intubation.

Doses cited are intravenous unless otherwise specified.

Adapted from Gregory GA, Andropoulos DB. *Gregory's Pediatric Anesthesia*. 5th ed. Wiley-Blackwell, Oxford; 2012.

Muscle contraction starts by the release of acetylcholine (ACh) in the synaptic cleft of the neuromuscular junction. Calcium-dependent mechanisms are responsible for the release of ACh from presynaptic vesicles. In the synaptic cleft, ACh is degraded quickly by acetylcholinesterases; there is also reuptake of ACh by motor nerve endings. ACh works by stimulating the opening of muscle nicotinic receptors, allowing sodium and calcium to enter the cells.

Depolarizing Muscle Relaxants: Succinylcholine

SCh has many highly desirable properties, including rapid onset and short duration of action (elimination half-life, 1 minute), and is the agent of choice for emergent intubation in adults. However, the US Food and Drug Administration has issued a "Black Box" warning regarding the use of SCh in children, noting that its risk/benefit profile needs to be considered carefully, particularly regarding the risk of life-threatening hyperkalemia in children thought to be previously healthy but who have an undiagnosed myopathy. This risk may be highest among young (<8 years) males.

Pharmacokinetics

SCh induces release of ACh and muscle fasciculations. Metabolism occurs in serum, red blood cells, and liver by nonspecific esterases (pseudocholinesterases). Some patients have reduced blood pseudocholinesterase activity; such patients may remain paralyzed for hours to days following a single SCh dose.

Pharmacodynamics

When normocapnia is maintained, SCh does not increase ICP. SCh may cause bradycardia, especially after a second or subsequent dose of the drug. SCh causes potassium release that is usually minimal and has no clinical significance, unless the patient is hyperkalemic, has been immobile, or has an acute burn injury. Patients with Duchenne muscular dystrophy and other myopathies, rhabdomyolysis, and burns are at high risk of developing arrhythmias after SCh secondary to receptor upregulation in denervated muscle. SCh may cause masseter spasm and can trigger malignant hyperthermia (MH).

Dosing

The intubating dose is 1 to 2 mg/kg in children and 3 mg/kg IV in infants secondary to different volumes of distribution. The intramuscular dose of SCh for emergency tracheal intubation, if no readily available IV access is present, is 4 to 5 mg/kg.

Nondepolarizing Muscle Relaxants

Pharmacokinetics

Vecuronium is excreted unchanged in the urine and in bile (>50% is transported in bile). Patients with cholestasis have reduced clearance of vecuronium. Similarly, patients with end-stage renal failure have decreased clearance of vecuronium and a higher sensitivity to the drug. Vecuronium has a moderately active metabolite.

Rocuronium, a vecuronium derivative, has a rapid onset and duration of action similar to vecuronium. Rocuronium is excreted unchanged in the urine and feces, and its metabolism is minimal. Elimination is only slightly impaired by renal failure.

Cisatracurium is degraded spontaneously in plasma by Hoffmann elimination. It is the preferred agent when end-organ failure is present. Laudanosine— a toxic metabolite of cisatracurium—may, theoretically, increase the risk of seizures.

Pharmacodynamics

Nondepolarizing muscle relaxants (NDMRs) have little effect on CBF and ICP. Cisatracurium may release histamine and can induce bronchospasm, hypotension, and tachycardia. Rocuronium may block muscarinic receptors and induce moderate tachycardia. Acid–base disturbances (acidosis), electrolyte disturbance (hypokalemia), and hypothermia may prolong the duration of action of muscle relaxants. Various drugs commonly used in the ICU (gentamicin, calcium-channel blockers, magnesium sulfate) may enhance the block. Anticonvulsant therapy causes NDMR resistance. NDMRs can cause anaphylaxis (particularly rocuronium).

Dosing

Vecuronium dosing is 0.1 to 0.2 mg/kg, though doses of up to 0.3 mg/kg have been used to achieve faster onset of action (and produce prolonged duration of effect). It has an onset time of 1 to 3 minutes and a duration of action of 30 to 40 minutes; continuous infusion is maintained at 1 to 1.2 µg/kg/min.

Rocuronium dosing is 0.4 to 0.6 mg/kg, with an onset of 1 to 2 minutes and a duration of action of 40 to 60 minutes. If rapid-sequence induction is planned, a dose of 1.2 mg/kg provides optimal intubating conditions in less than 1 minute, but the duration of action is prolonged. Continuous infusion is maintained at 5 to 15 µg/kg/min.

Cisatracurium dosing is 0.1 to 0.2 mg/kg. Its onset is 2 to 3 minutes and its duration of action is 40 to 60 minutes. Continuous infusion is maintained at 1 to 3 µg/kg/min.

Other Medications

Multiple other medicaitons, as well as environmental measures, can be used to prevent and treat discomfort in the intensive care unit.

Topical Anesthetics - Eutectic Mixture of Local Anesthetics

A eutectic mixture of local anesthetics, or EMLA, is a mixture of lidocaine and prilocaine used for topical skin application. It is effective in reducing pain from minor painful procedures, including venous cannulation and accessing implanted central venous ports. Applying a thicker layer (2 mm) and increasing the duration of application (90–120 minutes) increases its effectiveness.

Acetaminophen

Acetaminophen is a widely used analgesic with a good safety record in pediatric patients. It has anti-inflammatory, antipyretic, and analgesic properties. Acetaminophen acts by inhibition of the cyclooxygenase enzyme. Time to peak plasma concentration is 30 to 60 minutes and 1 to 2 hours after oral and rectal administration, respectively. Bioavailability after oral administration is 85% to 95%, and usually is less than 80% after rectal administration. Approximately 90% of acetaminophen undergoes metabolism in the liver to water-soluble products, which are eliminated by the kidneys. A small part of the drug is metabolized by cytochrome P450 to a toxic metabolite (*N*-acetyl-p-benzoquinone) that may cause hepatotoxicity.

Oral dosing is 10 mg/kg in neonates and infants, and 10 to 15 mg/kg in older children. The rectal dose is 30 to 40 mg/kg secondary to decreased bioavailability. IV formulation has been approved in the United States for children 2 years or older: 10 to 15 mg/kg IV.

Ketorolac

Ketorolac is a parenteral nonsteroidal anti-inflammatory drug. The mode of action is by cyclooxygenase inhibition. It is often used as an adjuvant to opioids because of its opioid-sparing effect. Dosing is 0.25 to 0.5 mg/kg. No significant adverse effects have been reported when used postoperatively in neonates and infants. However, prolonged use may increase the risk of adverse events. Caution should be exercised as a result of the risk of bleeding from platelet dysfunction, harmful effects on bone healing, and effects on developing kidneys.

Malignant Hyperthermia

MH is a clinical syndrome characterized by uncontrolled skeletal muscle metabolism. It is triggered by volatile anesthetics and the depolarizing muscle relaxant SCh in genetically susceptible individuals. It is a disorder of the ryanodine receptor (RYR1) of the skeletal muscle and is caused by uncontrolled calcium release in skeletal muscle cells. The incidence of MH associated with general anesthesia is estimated at 1:30,000 to 1:100,000. MH can occur at any time during the anesthetic or the immediate postoperative period. Patients with various myopathies may be susceptible to MH, particularly those with central core disease and King-Denborough syndrome. The most consistent indicator of potential MH is a progressive increase in end-tidal CO_2. If untreated, MH may be lethal. Signs of MH include

- Increasing level of end-tidal CO_2
- Trunk/total body rigidity
- Masseter spasm/trismus
- Tachycardia/tachypnea
- Mixed respiratory and metabolic acidosis
- Increased temperature (late sign)
- Myoglobinuria

Dantrolene

Dantrolene is the specific treatment for MH, dosed at 2.5 mg/kg and up to a 10-mg/kg rapid IV bolus. Dantrolene inhibits the release of calcium from the sarcoplasmic reticulum by limiting the activation of the calcium-dependent ryanodine receptor. If MH is suspected, after the discontinuation of possible triggering agents, providing 100% oxygen and ventilatory support, cooling the patient, and correcting acid–base and electrolyte abnormalities are paramount. Prevention of MH in susceptible patients requiring sedation for necessary procedures consists of nontriggering sedative agents, and Sch is avoided.

In a suspected MH episode, call the MH Hotline: 1-800-644-9737.

Further Reading

Gozal D, Gozal Y. Pediatric sedation/anesthesia outside the operating room. *Curr Opin Anesthesiol*. 2008;21:494–498.

American Society of Anesthesiologists. Practice guidelines for sedation and analgesia by non-anesthesiologists. *Anesthesiology*. 2002;96(4):1004–1017.

American Academy of Pediatrics. Guidelines for monitoring and management of pediatric patients during and after sedation for diagnostic and therapeutic procedures: an update. *Pediatrics*. 2006;118(6):2587–2602.

Steur RJ, Perez RSGM, De Lange JJ. Dosage scheme for propofol in children under 3 years of age. *Pediatr Anesth*. 2004;14:462–467.

Chapter 11

Fluids and Electrolytes

Desmond Bohn

The principles that govern fluid and electrolyte physiology in children—with the exception of newborns—are, in many instances, similar to those in adults. However, because calculations for the administration of parenteral fluids have to take body size into account, the process is necessarily more complex. In addition, many of the principles used to estimate fluid losses and the requirements for replacement in children (maintenance fluids) are based on limited studies published more than 50 years ago at a time when the complexity of illness was far less than is seen today. The formulas were based on calculations for normal physiological requirements and did not take into account the fact that the hormonal and other influences that govern fluid and electrolyte balance may be seriously perturbed in critical illness. The challenge now is to rethink some of these principles in the light of new knowledge of how acute illness may influence them.

Body Water Distribution in Children

Body water content changes significantly with age in children. Total body water (TBW) is high in the fetus and preterm infant. Significant changes occur in TBW during the first year of life—from 75% of body weight at birth to 65% at 6 months and 60% at 1 year of life, where it remains through puberty in males, with a slightly lower percentage in females. Extracellular fluid (ECF) volume decreases during the first year of life—from 45% of TBW at birth to 30% at 1 year—and decreases with age thereafter, reaching adult values early in childhood. In addition, the glomerular filtration rate is lower than in the term infant, and water losses resulting from the large surface area-to-body weight ratio lead to considerable evaporative losses.

Fluid Homeostasis in Children

To achieve normal fluid homeostasis, fluid intake must balance losses. The latter consist of urine output plus insensible losses (evaporative through the skin and respiratory tract) and loss in the stool, which should be minimal in the absence of diarrhea. Insensible losses are mainly in the form of electrolyte-free water (EFW) from the respiratory tract (15 mL/100 kcal/d). This loss is minimized during humidified positive-pressure ventilation. Sweat contains mainly water

Table 11.1 Electrolyte Composition of Body Fluids (mmol/L)				
Fluid type	Na⁺, mm/L	K⁺, mm/L	Cl⁻, mm/L	HCO₃⁻, mm/L
Sweat	50	5	55	
Saliva	30	20	35	15
Gastric	60	10	90	
Bile	145	5	110	40
Duodenum	140	5	80	50
Ileum	130	10	110	30
Colon	60	30	40	20

with a small amount of sodium (Na) except in situations when sweat glands contain excessive amounts of Na (e.g., cystic fibrosis). Evaporative losses also increase with elevations in body temperature, and during thermal stress water losses may increase to as much as 25 mL/100 kcal/d.

Obligate water excretion in the urine is dependent on solute load and the ability to concentrate and dilute the urine. Infants are somewhat disadvantaged compared with the older child and adults in that they cannot maximally dilute (infant, 200 mOsm/L vs. adult, 80 mOsm/L) nor concentrate (infant, 800 mOsm/L vs. adult, 1200 mOsm/L) urine. In addition, the infant's high metabolic rate and the solute load from enteral feeding formula means they require more water excretion per unit solute amount. These factors make them prone to significant ECF contraction (dehydration) when there is excessive water loss. Typically this occurs in gastroenteritis, when reduced oral intake is combined with excessive water and electrolyte loss in the stool (Table 11.1).

Urine is the major source of electrolyte loss in the body except when there are fluid losses from the gastrointestinal tract. The commonly used values for Na and potassium (K) requirements in parenteral fluids in children have been 2 to 3 mmol/kg/d and 1 to 2 mmol/kg/d. However, in critically ill children, urinary Na and K losses may be much higher.

Intravenous Maintenance Fluids

In the normal healthy individual, water intake is regulated by thirst stimulated via osmoreceptors in the hypothalamus. Infants and small children are unable to regulate their intake because they do not have access to water for the same reasons that apply to older children or adults in coma. When oral intake is replaced by parenteral fluids in children, fluid (i.e., water) needs depend on body weight and energy expenditure. In 1957, Holliday and Segar published a formula that linked body weight to energy expenditure. In infants less than 10 kg, insensible losses and urine output averaged 100 mL/100 kcal/d. The estimates for Na (3 mmol/100 kcal/d) and K (2 mmol/100 kcal/d) in maintenance fluids were calculated from the Na and K concentrations of cow and human milk. Linking energy expenditure to weight led to the common use of the following *guidelines for daily maintenance fluid needs*:

Ten kg or less: 100 mL/kg
Ten to 20 kg: fluids for first 10 kg (1000 mL) + (kg over 10 kg) × 50 mL
More than 20 kg: fluids for first 20 kg (1500 mL) + (kg over 20 kg) × 20 mL

The article by Holliday and Segar became the standard reference for parenteral fluid administration in pediatrics. Although convenient and simple to use, the assumptions made about daily requirements for Na, K, and EFW mandate the use of hypotonic intravenous (IV) solutions, which has been almost universal practice in pediatric medicine for more than 50 years. However, stimuli for antidiuretic hormone (ADH) secretion (pain, anxiety, narcotics, positive-pressure ventilation), which inhibits the excretion of EFW, are common in critically ill patients. As a result, mild degrees of hyponatremia are common in pediatric patients receiving parenteral fluids. The nonphysiological secretion of ADH has been reported in many acute medical illnesses, including meningitis, bronchiolitis, encephalitis, traumatic brain injury, and gastroenteritis. An increasing number of publications now recommend isotonic or near-isotonic fluids for standard maintenance in pediatrics to avoid the administration of EFW, which is potentially hazardous in situations when ADH secretion is not inhibited. Hypotonic fluids should be reserved for patients with a demonstrated need for EFW (e.g., serum Na >145 mmol/L) (Table 11.2).

Table 11.2 Water and Electrolyte Content of Commonly Used Intravenous Fluids

Fluid Type	Na^+, mmol/L	Cl^-, mmol/L	Osmolality	Osmolality with 20 mmol KCl/L Added	pH	Electrolyte-Free Water/L
0.9 NaCl	154	154	308	348	5.5	0
0.45 NaCl	77	77	154	194	5.5	500
5% dextrose, 0.9 NaCl	154	154	560	600	4	0
5% dextrose, 0.45 NaCl	77	77	406	446	4	500
5% dextrose, 0.2 NaCl	34	34	321	361	4	780
4% dextrose, 0.18 NaCl	31	31	284	324	4	800
5% dextrose	0	0	252	292	4	1000
Ringers lactate	130	109	272	312	6.5	114
Ringers lactate 5%	130	109	525		6.5	114
3% NaCl	513	513	1027		5.5	0

Perioperative Fluid Management

Standard practice in intraoperative fluid management has been to replace intravascular volume loss with blood or colloid solutions and to use isotonic electrolyte solutions to provide for ongoing fluid requirements, replacement of losses from exposed serosal surfaces in open body cavities in thoracic and abdominal surgery, and losses from third-space fluid sequestration. Extra fluid is also administered frequently to treat hypotension resulting from the vasodilating effects of anesthetic agents. The preferred intraoperative electrolyte solutions used by most anesthesiologists are Ringer's lactate or isotonic saline because of concerns about the development of postoperative fluid retention and hyponatremia associated with elevated ADH levels. This inability to excrete EFW is amply illustrated in scoliosis surgery, when patients seem to be particularly at risk for the development of hyponatremia postoperatively. The degree of hyponatremia is less with use of isotonic or near-isotonic fluid, although plasma Na also decreases when Ringer's lactate is used.

Further insights to explain this observation come from a study of plasma and urine Na in adults undergoing elective surgery, all of whom received Ringer's lactate as their perioperative fluid. The authors found that the urine Na concentration was consistently more than 150 mmol/L and as high as 350 mmol/L and was associated with a significant positive water balance and a decrease in plasma Na—a process they called postoperative "desalination." This is consistent with the kidney's attempts to deal with a volume overload situation after the vasodilating effects of anesthetic agents are no longer present but ADH is still actively secreted. In this situation, it would be unwise to prescribe hypotonic fluids and impose an extra burden of more EFW to be excreted by the kidney. In prospective randomized trials comparing the use of isotonic with hypotonic saline, the incidence of hyponatremia was reduced significantly by the use of isotonic saline without development of hypernatremia.

Disorders of Sodium Homeostasis

Sodium is the principal cation of the ECF compartment (Figure 11.1). Movement of Na into the intracellular fluid (ICF) compartment is reversed by activation of the Na/K/adenosine triphosphatase pump. Na is absorbed in the proximal tubule under the influence of aldosterone. Serum Na reflects the osmolality and the ECF water volume, which is regulated tightly by ADH secretion.

Hyponatremia

Hyponatremia (serum Na <136 mmol/L) implies an expansion of the ICF compartment. It is caused by either water gain (e.g., use of hypotonic fluids)

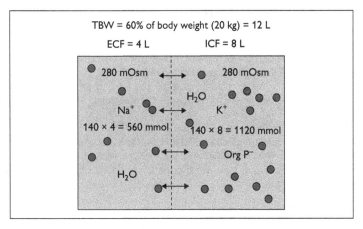

TBW = 60% of body weight (20 kg) = 12 L

ECF = 4 L   ICF = 8 L

280 mOsm   280 mOsm

H_2O

Na^+ K^+

140 × 4 = 560 mmol   140 × 8 = 1120 mmol

Org P^-

H_2O

Figure 11.1 Principal cation and anion constituents of the intracellular fluid (ICF) and extracellular fluid (ECF) compartments in a 20 kg child together with the total body water (TBW) calculation. The totals for Na^+ and K^+ content are calculated by multiplying the concentration by the volume. Water moves freely between the ICF and ECF compartment depending on the osmolar gradient.

or salt loss (e.g., gastroenteritis) (Box 11.1). Acute hyponatremia, commonly defined as a decrease in plasma Na from a normal value to less than 130 mmol/L within 48 hours, leads to rapid movement of water from the ECF to the ICF compartment and can cause cerebral edema, with catastrophic outcomes. The clinical findings are those of raised intracranial pressure (nausea, vomiting, headache), and it is frequently undiagnosed until the onset of seizures. This is usually followed by apnea resulting from brainstem herniation. Symptomatic hyponatremia is a medical emergency, and it rarely occurs unless the Na level is less than 125 mmol/L. The primary objective is to increase serum Na so that it is more than this level to prevent brainstem

---

Box 11.1 Principal Causes of Hyponatremia

Water Gain
- Excessive water ingestion
- Hypotonic fluid administration
- Syndrome of inappropriate antidiuretic hormone secreation (SIADH)
- Congestive heart failure
- Chronic renal failure

Salt Loss
- Gastroenteritis
- Cerebral salt wasting

herniation and stop seizures. This can be achieved most effectively with the use of hypertonic saline. When this threshold has been reached, serum Na can be allowed to correct by fluid restriction with or without the use of furosemide (in the event of elevated TBW) or administration of isotonic fluids (in the event of hyponatremic dehydration). IV mannitol has also been used successfully in the emergency treatment of acute symptomatic hypona-tremia. For more details, see "Treatment of Symptomatic Hyponatremia" in Chapter 12.

Chronic hyponatremia is a common finding in patients with heart failure and renal failure, and it is associated with increased TBW and salt retention. It is not associated with cerebral edema, but rapid correction of chronic hypo-natremia with isotonic or hypertonic saline has been associated with central pontine demyelination.

Hypernatremia

Hypernatremia is commonly defined as serum Na more than 145 mmol/L and is caused by either water deficit or salt gain. The former is seen in infants with severe gastroenteritis with a loss of water in excess of Na, sometimes compounded by increased solute intake from incorrect mixing of infant for-mula. Hypernatremia resulting from the absence of ADH secretion causing diabetes insipidus is seen in patients with pituitary tumors, traumatic brain injury, and central nervous system (CNS) infections. Water loss in critically ill children may also be associated with the use of loop diuretics or man-nitol. Hypernatremia secondary to salt gain is seen with the excessive use of isotonic or hypertonic saline solutions, or with the administration of IV bicarbonate (Box 11.2).

Box 11.2 Causes of Hypernatremia

Water Loss
- Gastroenteritis
- Central diabetes insipidus
- Nephrogenic diabetes insipidus
- Use of loop diuretics
- Use of osmotic diuretics
- Use of radiology contrast medium
- Excessive insensible cutaneous loss (burns, sweating)
- Diabetic ketoacidosis or hyperosmolar nonketotic diabetes

Salt Gain
- Use of high-sodium-content solutions (hypertonic saline, intravenous bicarbonate)
- Hypertonic enteral feeding formulas
- Cathartic agents

An increase in serum Na is associated with movement of water from the ICF to the ECF compartment and the development of a hyperosmolar state. In severe dehydration, brain cells adapt with an increase in electrolytes and the development of "idiogenic" osmoles (inositisol, taurine) that tend to mitigate the fluid shift, with partial restoration of intracellular osmolality and brain cell volume. Levels of Na more than 155 mmol/L are frequently associated with abnormal CNS findings, and there is an increased risk of subdural hemorrhage and infarction in infants with hypernatremic dehydration and serum Na levels more than 160 mmol/L. There is also the added danger of the development of brain edema developing during the attempt to correct these hyperosmolar states rapidly using solutions that are hypo-osmolar compared with the ICF compartment.

A similar situation exists in diabetic ketoacidosis (DKA), characterized by losses of water and electrolytes resulting from hyperglycemia-induced osmotic diuresis. The high osmolality of the ECF results in shift of water from the ICF compartment. At the time of presentation, patients are ECF contracted, and clinical estimates of the deficit are usually in the range of 7% to 10%, although shock with hemodynamic compromise is a rare event in DKA in children. The hyperglycemia in DKA results in a hyperosmolar state, but the serum Na measurement is an unreliable measure of the degree of ECF contraction because of the dilutional effect of the fluid shift from the ICF to the ECF compartment. The *effective* osmolality (2 [Na + K] + glucose, all in mmol/L [if glucose in mg/dL, then need to divide it by 18]) at the time of presentation is frequently in the range of 300 to 350 mOsm/L.

The Correction of Acute Water and Sodium Deficits in Children

Among the most common problems of acute water and electrolyte deficits in critically ill children are fluid and electrolyte deficits in acute gastroenteritis and DKA. In acute gastroenteritis, small children and infants with diarrhea are particularly vulnerable to significant losses of fluid, Na, chloride, and bicarbonate from the small intestine. They present with hypotonic, isotonic, or hypertonic dehydration, based on serum Na level. Patients with diarrheal illnesses associated with fluid loss with normal or reduced serum Na have loss of TBW and ECF with normal or increased ICF volume. Infants with hypernatremic dehydration are at greatest risk of an adverse neurological event, but seizures from severe hyponatremia have been reported in infants presenting with acute gastroenteritis resulting from oral salt-free fluids being given as a replacement. The assessment of the degree of ECF deficit is usually made on clinical grounds using the time-honored clinical signs of capillary refill time, dry mucous membranes, skin turgor, and so on. However, these are subjective and it is easy to overestimate the degree of ECF contraction in less severely ill children.

Patients with gastroenteritis whose serum is isotonic or hypotonic should be rehydrated with isotonic saline. Patients with hypernatremic dehydration resulting from gastroenteritis, and those with DKA, are at risk for the development of CNS complications because of the hyperosmolar state of the ICF compartment, where rapid rehydration results in cerebral edema. IV fluid rehydration with isotonic saline in children with gastroenteritis has been shown to protect against the development of hyponatremia without the development of hypernatremia when compared with hypotonic saline. In severe hypernatremia, serum Na should be decreased at a rate less than approximately 0.5 mmol/L/h using the following formula, which estimates the effect of 1 L of any infusate on serum Na:

$$\text{Change in serum Na} = \frac{\text{Infusate Na} - \text{Serum Na}}{\text{TBW} + 1}.$$

In severe hypernatremia (serum Na >170 mmol/L), the Na should not be corrected to less than approximately 150 mmol/L during the first 48 to 72 hours.

Similarly, the risk cerebral edema during rehydration of patients with DKA has led to the widespread adoption of the use of normal saline as a replacement fluid, focusing on a gradual reduction in elevated osmolality, which can be achieved by conservative fluid resuscitation and the avoidance of hypotonic fluids during the initial resuscitation period. A general rule is that failure of serum Na to rise during IV fluid replacement indicates too rapid a rate of infusion; the associated increase in serum Na as glucose decreases reduces effective osmolality gradually and protects against the development of cerebral edema.

Chloride

Chloride is the principal anion of the ECF compartment. It is filtered at the glomerulus, and 80% is reabsorbed in conjunction with Na in the proximal tubule. It is also reabsorbed in the ascending limb of the loop of Henle, a process blocked by furosemide. Chloride is exchanged for bicarbonate in the distal tubule. In ECF volume depletion, excess Cl along with Na is reabsorbed in the proximal tubule, resulting in lower distal delivery and less bicarbonate secretion. With chloride depletion, less Na is reabsorbed in the proximal tubule. Increased distal delivery results increased exchange with K and H^+. This contraction alkalosis is associated invariably with hypochloremia, most commonly resulting from the use of loop diuretics. Hypochloremia is also caused by gastric suctioning and respiratory acidosis. In addition, many of the conditions that cause hyponatremia also result in hypochloremia.

Hyperchloremia is seen in association with respiratory alkalosis, hypernatremic dehydration, and the administration of isotonic saline. The use of large amounts of isotonic saline used during fluid resuscitation can result in hyperchloremic metabolic acidosis. If serum chloride (or lactate) is not measured, an increased base deficit could be interpreted incorrectly as indicating inadequate volume resuscitation in shock.

Plasma chloride measurements are an integral part of the calculation of the anion gap, which is important for the diagnosis of metabolic acidosis. This is the difference between the measured cations (Na^+) and anions ($Cl^- + HCO_3^-$) and is normally in the range of 12 to 16 mmol/L. The anion gap is increased when unmeasured anions, such as lactate, are present. Normal or reduced anion gap acidosis is seen in association with hyperchloremia from saline administration, or in other situations when there is an increase in serum chloride.

Potassium

K is the major cation of the ICF compartment. The intracellular concentration is 150 mmol/L. Measurement of serum K reflects the ECF concentration, which is only 2% of total-body K. The gradient between the ICF and ECF compartments is maintained by activation of the Na^+/K^+/adenosine triphosphatase pump in the cell membrane. The movement of K from the ECF to ICF compartment is enhanced by insulin, hypothermia, alkalosis, catecholamines, and β agonists. K filtered at the glomerulus is reabsorbed in the proximal tubule and the thick ascending limb of the loop of Henle. It is secreted in the distal nephron under the influence of aldosterone, plasma K concentration, and urine flow rate.

Hypokalemia

Hypokalemia in children is commonly seen with gastroenteritis and diarrhea, in which ECF contraction leads to stimulation of aldosterone secretion. There is also total-body K depletion in DKA, although the initial measured level is high as a result of the acidosis. Adolescents with anorexia nervosa can present with profound degrees of hypokalemia, which is a known cause of sudden death in this syndrome. In the critical care setting, hypokalemia is associated most commonly with diuretic use, nasogastric suction, hypomagnesemia, and metabolic alkalosis. In acute metabolic alkalosis, each 0.1-increase in pH results in a decrease of 0.2 to 0.4 mmol/L in serum K. In chronic metabolic alkalosis, K is exchanged for a hydrogen ion in the distal nephron. Increased K output in the urine is also associated with renal tubular defects (e.g., Bartter's syndrome, renal tubular acidosis) and the use of drugs such as amphotericin, ticarcillin, carbenicillin, and steroids. K supplementation therapy in the critical care setting is usually in the form of potassium chloride because there is frequently an associated chloride deficiency. Acetate and phosphate can be used as alternative anions in the hyperchloremic state (e.g., DKA).

The clinical manifestations of hypokalemia include muscle weakness (which may prolong the effect of neuromuscular blockers), intestinal ileus, and cardiac arrhythmias. The latter are rarely a problem except in children with congenital heart disease, particularly in the postcardiopulmonary bypass setting. The potential for digoxin toxicity is enhanced with hypokalemia. In situations when hypokalemia needs to be treated in the setting of fluid restriction, high-concentration K infusions (up to 0.5 mmol/mL) can be infused through central lines with frequent measurements of serum K levels. Hypokalemia may remain resistant to treatment when significant hypomagnesemia is present.

Hyperkalemia

Hyperkalemia is caused by failure of K excretion (renal failure), excess exogenous administration, or the movement of K from the ICF to the ECF compartment. Common causes of the latter are seen in cellular breakdown or injury in tumor lysis syndrome, rhabdomyolysis, burns, and trauma; acute metabolic acidosis; use of the depolarizing neuromuscular blocker succinylcholine in this setting (or in patients with muscle dystrophy or spinal cord injury); and malignant hyperthermia (resulting from a combination of hemolysis and acidosis). Both captopril and propranolol can cause hyperkalemia by decreasing the amount of aldosterone synthesis. Propranolol also blocks β-adrenergic-mediated movement of K across the cell membrane. Severe hyperkalemia is seen frequently during cardiac arrest and cardiopulmonary resuscitation without necessarily implying causality.

Acute hyperkalemia represents a medical emergency, and serum levels in excess of 6 mmol/L can result in cardiac arrest and sudden death, particularly after cardiopulmonary bypass. Frequently, the only clinical manifestation is the finding of tall, peaked T waves and widening of the QRS complex, but the absence of these findings does not exclude the diagnosis. Patients with borderline-high levels of serum K can develop life-threatening hyperkalemia with the development of an acidosis. Because it is the extracellular K level that is harmful, emergency measures are directed at increasing the transmembrane flux from ECF to the ICF compartment, including the use of bicarbonate to correct acidemia, β agonists, and the use of glucose/insulin. The use of IV calcium chloride helps protect the heart against the development of cardiac rhythm disturbances. These are temporizing measures while steps are taken to increase K removal from the body either by using Na/K exchange resins (rectally or via nasogastric tube), acute dialysis, or diuretics that promote K excretion (e.g., furosemide).

Further Reading

Duke T, Molyneux EM. Intravenous fluids for seriously ill children: time to reconsider. *Lancet.* 2003;362(9392):1320–1323.

Holliday MA, Segar WE. The maintenance need for water in parenteral fluid therapy. *Pediatrics.* 1957;19:823–832.

Kumar S, Berl T. Sodium. *Lancet.* 1998;352(9123):220–228.

Maghnie M, Cosi G, Genovese E, et al. Central diabetes insipidus in children and young adults. *N Engl J Med*. 2000;343(14):998–1007.

Moritz ML, Ayus JC. Disorders of water metabolism in children: hyponatremia and hypernatremia. *Pediatr Rev*. 2002;23(11):371–380.

Shafiee MA, Bohn D, Hoorn EJ, Halperin ML. How to select optimal maintenance intravenous fluid therapy. *Q J Med*. 2003;96(8):601–610.

Chapter 12

Diagnosis and Management of Renal Disorders in the Pediatric Intensive Care Unit

Dana Y. Fuhrman and Michael L. Moritz

Renal disorders as primary diagnoses or secondary to other diagnoses can require management in the critical care setting. This chapter serves as a practical approach to the care of children with fluid and electrolyte emergencies and hypertensive emergencies, as well as those with acute kidney injury (AKI) with or without the need for renal replacement therapy.

Fluid and Electrolyte Emergencies

Hyponatremia

Hyponatremia, serum sodium (Na) less than 135 mEq/L, is the most common electrolyte disorder occurring in the intensive care unit (ICU) setting. Hyponatremia can occur with either a low, elevated or normal serum osmolality (Figure 12.1). Serum osmolality should be obtained to confirm there is hypo-osmolality before embarking on an extensive evaluation or treatment of hyponatremia. The evaluation of hyponatremia should include a careful history regarding changes in weight, fluid balance, and sources of free water, and an investigation of underlying conditions or medications that could lead either to impairment in free water excretion or renal or extrarenal Na losses. A urinary Na concentration greater than 30 mEq/L or a fractional excretion of Na greater than 0.5% supports a diagnosis of diuretic use, adrenal insufficiency, renal tubular dysfunction, the syndrome of inappropriate antidiuretic hormone secretion, or cerebral salt wasting. An elevated fractional excretion of urate more than 12% is highly suggestive of the syndrome of inappropriate antidiuretic hormone secretion or cerebral salt wasting even in the face of concomitant diuretic use.

Symptomatic hyponatremia is a medical emergency that can lead to death or permanent neurological impairment. The most common early symptoms of hyponatremic encephalopathy are headache, nausea, and vomiting. Later symptoms include lethargy, confusion, coma, respiratory arrest, neurogenic pulmonary edema, and seizures. Pediatric patients younger than 16 years are

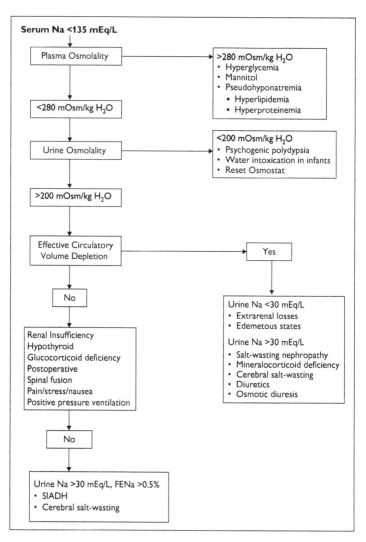

Figure 12.1 Diagnostic evaluation of hyponatremia

Na, sodium; SIADH, syndrome of inappropriate antidiuretic hormone secretion.

at particularly high risk for the development of hyponatremic encephalopathy as a result of their larger brain-to-intracranial volume ratio. Other risk factors for the development of hyponatremic encephalopathy are acute hyponatremia, underlying central nervous system disease, postmenarche in females, and hypoxia. Patients with symptomatic hyponatremia should be treated with 3% sodium chloride (NaCl; 513 mEq/L). A 5- to 6-mEq/L acute increase in serum Na is generally sufficient to reverse neurological symptoms. The correction should not exceed 20 mEq/L during the first 48 hours of therapy. During treatment for symptomatic hyponatremia, it is important to monitor serum Na values every 1 to 2 hours.

Treatment of Symptomatic Hyponatremia
- Administer a 2-mL/kg bolus of 3% NaCl over 10 minutes with a maximum volume of 100 mL.
- Repeat the bolus one to two times until symptoms improve, with a goal to increase serum Na by 5 to 6 mEq/L during the first 1 to 2 hours and to reverse neurological symptoms.
- Stop therapy with 3% NaCl when the patient is free of symptoms or has an acute increase in serum Na of 10 mEq/L during the first 5 hours of treatment.

Cerebral demyelination is a potential complication of the overcorrection of chronic hyponatremia (>48 hours). Risk factors for developing cerebral demyelination are severe hyponatremia, serum sodium less than 115 mEq/L, liver disease, hypokalemia, thiazide diuretic use, malnutrition, and overcorrection with a change in serum Na of more than 25 mEq/L during the first 48 hours of therapy.

Hypernatremia

Critical care patients have numerous risk factors for developing hypernatremia (Table 12.1) (serum Na, >145 mEq/L), such as restricted access to fluids from being non per ora, Na-containing intravenous (IV) fluids, and impaired urine concentration from loop diuretics, AKI, or chronic kidney disease. Hypernatremia is otherwise uncommon in cognitively intact individuals with unrestricted access to water because of a potent thirst mechanism triggered by hyperosmolality and hypovolemia. Hypernatremia in the outpatient setting is seen most commonly in infants, children with gastroenteritis, or cognitively impaired children who have restricted access to fluids and may be unable to communicate their increased thirst. Hypernatremia can result from a relative decrease in total body water and/or a relative increase in total body Na. A relative decrease in total body water can occur from renal losses, gastrointestinal losses, insensible fluid losses, or decreased fluid intake. Increased total body Na can occur as a result of the iatrogenic or unintended administration of an increased salt load. Hypernatremia is a maximal stimulus for vasopressin production, so a patient with hypernatremia

Table 12.1 Etiologies of Hypernatremia

Relative Decrease in Total Body Water	Relative Increase in Total Body Sodium
Renal loss	• Normal saline administration
• Diabetes insipidus (nephrogenic or central)	• Blood products
• Osmotic diuresis (e.g., hyperglycemia)	• Hypertonic saline
• Postobstructive diuresis	• Sodium bicarbonate
• Tubulopathy	• High-solute feeding
• Loop diuretics	• Sodium polystyrene
Gastrointestinal loss	• Saltwater drowning
• Diarrhea	• Salt intoxication/poisoning
• Vomiting	• Hypertonic saline irrigation
• Ostomy output	
• Malabsorption	
• Lactulose	
Insensible fluid loss	
• Fever	
• Burns	
• Respiratory illness	
• Heat injury	
Decreased fluid intake	
• Impaired thirst (hypothalamic lesion)	
• Fluid restriction	
• Ineffective breastfeeding	
• Neurological impairment	

should have maximally concentrated urine, and a water deprivation test is contraindicated. Urine osmolality of less than 800 mOsm/kg in the face of hypernatremia should be viewed as consistent with a renal concentrating defect. Any patient presenting with severe and unexplained hypernatremia, serum Na more than 160 mEq/L, should be evaluated for a renal concentrating defect and for potential iatrogenic Na overload. A gastric or stool Na concentration greater than plasma should never occur and is suspicious for salt poisoning.

Treatment of Hypernatremia
- Patients with hypernatremia are usually volume depleted, and the first step should always be to evaluate the degree of volume depletion. In general, most patients benefit from a bolus of 20 ml/kg 0.9% NaCl. Additional volume boluses and/or cardiovascular support may be needed to establish good perfusion and urine output.
- The goal in the treatment of hypernatremia is to provide the appropriate amount of free water to correct the serum Na concentration (estimate

of free water deficit: 4 mL/kg free water decreases serum Na by about 1 mEq/L).

- Urine concentration less than 800 mOsm/kg in the setting of hypernatremia is a sign of a renal concentrating defect or diuretic use.
- After initial volume expansion, the IV fluid composition should be determined based on the likely etiology and whether there are ongoing urinary free water losses:
  - 0.45% NaCl: hypernatremic dehydration with normal renal concentrating ability
  - 0.2% NaCl: hypernatremic dehydration with impaired renal concentrating ability
  - 0.1% NaCl: Congenital nephrogenic diabetes insipidus
  - D5W: hypervolemic hypernatremia
- Although critically ill patients usually require IV fluid administration, oral/enteral fluid administration is the preferred route of fluid administration in patients whose respiratory, cardiovascular, and neurological status are normal.
- Rate of correction
  - About 0.5 mEq/h or 10 mEq/24 h, not to exceed 1 mEq/h or 20 mEq/24 h
  - The rate of correction should be slower if there is concern of cerebral edema or increased intracranial pressure.
  - Stop forceful correction of hypernatremia when serum Na is less than 150 mEq/L.
- Continue with vigilant monitoring of serum Na.

Hyperkalemia

Hyperkalemia (serum potassium >5 mEq/L in infants and children, and >6 mEq/L in newborns) typically occurs in response to a potassium load in a patient with renal impairment or underlying impaired hormonal activity needed for cellular potassium uptake. Cardiac electrographic changes that are potentially life threatening generally start to occur with serum potassium levels more than 5.5 mEq/L, with an increased risk of cardiac arrhythmias occurring with potassium levels more than 6 mEq/L. A rapid increase in serum potassium or underlying cardiac disease also increases the risk of arrhythmias. The most common initial electrocardiographic changes occurring with hyperkalemia include peaked T-waves and a prolonged PR interval, which are seen best in the precordial leads. More severe hyperkalemia (>8 mEq/L) can result in the absence of the P-waves and progressive widening of the QRS complexes. Given that the first presenting symptom of hyperkalemia can be a lethal cardiac dysrhythmia, it is important to initiate therapy early if hyperkalemia is suspected, while simultaneously obtaining an electrocardiogram and seeking to identify a cause (Table 12.2).

Treatment for hyperkalemia (Table 12.3) should begin with ensuring that any ongoing exogenous administration of potassium is discontinued

Table 12.2 Etiologies of Hyperkalemia

Increased Potassium Intake	Impaired Renal Potassium Excretion	Translocation of Potassium out of the Cells

• Red blood cell transfusion
• Nutritional supplements
• Intravenous fluids
• Hyperalimentation
• Potassium for treatment of hypokalemia
	• Acute kidney injury
	• Chronic kidney disease
	• Adrenal insufficiency
	• Mineralocorticoid resistance
	• Medications
	  • Cyclosporine
	  • Tacrolimus
	  • Angiotensin-converting enzyme inhibitors
	  • Angiotensin receptor blockers
	  • Potassium-sparing diuretics
		• Acidosis (respiratory or metabolic, including diabetic ketoacidosis)
		• Rhabdomyolysis
		• Tumor lysis
		• β Blockers

immediately. Calcium should be given to reverse cardiac conduction abnormalities, especially if electrocardiographic changes are present. It is important that calcium be given through a properly functioning IV line because extravasation can cause tissue necrosis. Other available therapies for hyperkalemia work by either shifting potassium intracellularly or removing potassium from the body and include sodium bicarbonate, insulin/glucose, albuterol, furosemide, Kayexalate, and renal replacement therapy.

Hypertensive Emergencies

A hypertensive emergency is defined as a severe elevation in blood pressure, systolic and/or diastolic, that is greater than the 99th percentile plus 5 mm Hg, or a rapid increase in blood pressure associated with evidence of symptoms of acute end-organ damage. In contrast, hypertensive urgency is generally defined as an acute, significant elevation in blood pressure without symptoms or evidence of acute end-organ damage. The signs of acute end-organ dysfunction that can occur with a hypertensive emergency include

- Renal insufficiency
- Papilledema
- Heart failure
- Seizures/encephalopathy

During the evaluation of a child with a hypertensive emergency certain diagnoses should always be considered. Glomerulonephritis and hemolytic uremic syndrome can often present with significant hypertension. In addition, in a child presenting with flushing, sweating, and palpitations, a diagnosis of pheochromocytoma should be considered. Certain medications, such as

Table 12.3 Treatment of Hyperkalemia

Treatment	Dose	Onset	Duration	Notes
Stabilizes the cardiac membranes				
10% Calcium gluconate	100 mg/kg/dose IV (maximum single dose, 3000 mg)	Immediate	15–30 min	
Calcium chloride	20 mg/kg/dose IV (maximum single dose, 2000 mg)	Immediate	15–30 min	Generally given only via a central line because of the risk of severe tissue injury in the event of extravasation.
Shifts potassium into cells				
Insulin/glucose	Dextrose 0.5–1 g/kg + regular insulin 1 U for every 4–5 g dextrose given	10–20 min	2–3 h	Monitor blood glucose.
Sodium bicarbonate	1 meq/kg/dose (maximum single dose, 50 meq)	1–3 h	2 h	Monitor for a potential decrease in serum ionized calcium. Do not use if patient has refractory hypercarbia. Use only with a coinciding hyperchloremic metabolic acidosis.
Albuterol	2.5–5-mg nebulizer treatment	15–30 min	2–3 h	Can be given continuously.
Potassium removal				
Furosemide	1 mg/kg/dose IV (maximum single dose, 40 mg)	15–60 min	4–6 h	The effect depends on the renal function of the patient. May need to provide fluid bolus to avoid hypovolemia or hypotension.
Sodium polystyrene sulfonate (Kayexalate)	1 g/kg (maximum single dose, 30 g)	1–6 h	4–6 h	Oral administration has a more sustained effect, whereas rectal administration has a more rapid effect. Use with caution because of the risk of bowel necrosis.
Extracorporeal therapies (dialysis or hemofiltration)				Most definitive treatment.

IV, intravenous.

corticosteroids and calcineurin inhibitors, are known to cause hypertension. Intracranial hypertension must be considered and excluded. In addition, pain and anxiety should always be addressed in the evaluation of hypertension in the ICU. Severely elevated blood pressure should be confirmed with repeat measurements, ensuring proper size and positioning of a manual blood pressure cuff.

Considerations in the diagnostic evaluation of a hypertensive emergency should include

- Measurement of four limb blood pressures
- Laboratory studies: complete blood count with differential; serum electrolytes; blood, urea, nitrogen; creatinine; urinalysis; urine microscopy; urine culture; urine pregnancy test; urine drug screen; serum renin; serum aldosterone; thyroid function tests; urine catecholamines
- Electrocardiogram
- Echocardiogram
- Renal ultrasound with Doppler
- Technetium-99m succimer (DMSA) to evaluate for renal scarring
- Digital subtraction angiography, magnetic resonance angiography, and computed tomographic angiography, which can be used for the diagnosis of renal artery stenosis
- Head computed tomographic scan if there is a concern of intracranial trauma or mass lesion
- Magnetic resonance imaging if there is concern of stroke or posterior reversible encephalopathy syndrome

In cases of hypertensive emergency, treatment with IV antihypertensive medications should be started concurrently with the initiation of a diagnostic evaluation. If the patient is known to have usually well-controlled blood pressure and the hypertension is recent in onset, the blood pressure can be brought down more rapidly compared with a patient who is thought to have chronically untreated hypertension. The goal for blood pressure reduction should be a decrease of no more than 25% during the first 8 hours of treatment. The medications chosen for blood pressure reduction should be based on the likely underlying mechanism of the hypertension (Table 12.4).

Acute Kidney Injury

Studies indicate that the incidence of AKI in the inpatient setting is increasing. There are many etiologies of AKI in children in the ICU, with renal ischemia, sepsis, and nephrotoxic medication use being the more common causes. AKI is typically classified as resulting from decreased blood flow to the kidney (prerenal), intrinsic renal disease (renal), or obstruction of the urinary tract (postrenal). In prerenal AKI, tubular Na and urea reabsorption are increased, leading to a low fractional excretion of Na (<1%). A low fractional

Table 12.4 Treatment Options for Pediatric Hypertensive Emergencies and Urgencies

Medication	Route	Mechanism of Action	Dose	Onset	Duration	Comments
Clonidine	PO	Central α agonist	0.05–0.3 mg	15–30 min	6–10 h	Can be useful for hypertensive urgency. Monitor for sedation or rebound hypertension with abrupt discontinuation after chronic use.
Esmolol	IV	β Blocker	Loading dose, 500 μg/kg; drip, 50–250 μg/kg/min	2–10 min	20 min	Do not use if cocaine toxicity is suspected. Use with caution in children with diabetes, asthma, or congestive heart failure.
Furosemide	IV	Diuretic	Bolus, 1–2 mg/kg; drip, 0.1–0.5 mg/kg/min	15–60 min	4–6 h	Because many patients with renal disease and hypertension are volume overloaded, diuretics and/or dialysis may be needed.
Hydralazine	IV	Vasodilator	0.1–0.4 mg/kg (maximum, 20 mg)	5–15 min	3–8 h	Can cause tachycardia and flushing.
Isradipine	PO	Calcium channel blocker	0.05–0.1 mg/kg (maximum, 5 mg)	2–3 h	8–12 h	Can be useful for hypertensive urgency. Can cause tachycardia and headache.
Minoxidil	PO	Vasodilator	0.1–0.2 mg/kg (maximum, 10 mg)	30 min	Up to 2–5 days	Can be useful for hypertensive urgency. Pericardial effusion can occur with chronic use.

(continued)

Table 12.4 Continued						
Medication	**Route**	**Mechanism of Action**	**Dose**	**Onset**	**Duration**	**Comments**
Nicardipine	IV	Calcium channel blocker	0.5–5 µg/kg/min	2–5 min	2–6 h	Large volumes require central line placement. Can cause headaches and increased intracranial pressure.
Phentolamine	IV	α Blocker	0.1 mg/kg (maximum, 5 mg)	1–2 min	15–30 min	Used in catecholamine-induced hypertension.
Labetolol	IV	Alpha and Beta Blocker	Bolus: 0.2–1 mg/kg (max of 40 mg); can repeat every 15 min; Drip: 0.25–3 mg/kg/h	5 min	2–6 h	Has the potential to worsen hyperkalemia; use with caution in children with diabetes, asthma or congestive heart failure
Sodium Nitro prusside	IV	Vasodilator	0.5–1 mcg/kg/min	1–2 min	3–5 min	Thiocyanate levels should be monitored in patients on sodium nitroprusside for more than 72 hours or with renal insufficiency

IV, intravenous; PO, per ora.

excretion of urea (<35%) can aid in diagnosing prerenal AKI in patients receiving diuretics. In contrast, patients with intrinsic renal injury typically have a higher fractional excretion of Na (>2%) and urea. In addition to calculating the fractional excretion of Na, additional laboratory and radiographic tests can be done to help determine the etiology of AKI. Serum electrolytes should be sent to evaluate for the common electrolyte disturbances that can occur with AKI, such as hyperkalemia and hyperphosphatemia (Table 12.5).

For patients with AKI, it is important that nephrotoxic medications be avoided when possible and drug dosing be adjusted for glomerular filtration rate. Diuretic use can be considered for fluid management; however, it has not been shown to improve renal outcomes. The treatment of AKI in the ICU

Table 12.5 Diagnostic Evaluation of Acute Kidney Injury in the Pediatric Intensive Care Unit

Classification	Etiology	Evaluation/Comment
Prerenal	Abdominal compartment syndrome	Bladder pressure measurements
	Hepatorenal syndrome	Hypoalbuminemia, hepatic function tests
	Renal vascular thrombosis	Renal sonogram with Doppler, CT or MR angiography
	Decreased intravascular volume	Careful history, physical examination, measurement of a central venous pressure; FENa, <1%; FEU, <35%
Intrinsic	Acute tubular necrosis	Muddy brown casts, tubular cells, or casts on urine microscopy; FENa, >2%
	Glomerulonephritis	Hematuria, proteinuria, red blood cell casts, white blood cell casts on urinalysis/urine microscopy; antistreptolysin O, antinuclear antibody and antineutrophil cytoplasmic antibody, complement studies
	Tumor lysis syndrome	Serum electrolytes to evaluate for hyperphosphatemia, hypocalcemia, hyperuricemia and hyperkalemia
	Acute interstitial nephritis	Eosinophils on urine microscopy, but low sensitivity and specificity
	Hemolytic uremic syndrome	Thrombocytopenia, anemia, elevated LDH, decreased haptoglobin, hemolysis on peripheral blood smear
	Pyelonephritis	Urinalysis/urine microscopy; technetium-99m succimer (DMSA) for the detection of renal scaring
	Rhabdomyolysis	Elevated creatine phosphokinase, urine myoglobin
	Nephrotoxic medications	Common nephrotoxic medications: nonsteroidal anti-inflammatory drugs, cyclosporine, tacrolimus, aminoglycosides
Postrenal	Obstruction of a solitary kidney Bilateral ureteral obstruction Urethral obstruction	Renal ultrasound with Doppler to evaluate for urinary tract obstruction, anomalies, corticomedullary differentiation, and renal perfusion

CT, computed tomography; DMSA, dimercaptosuccinic acid); FENa, fractional excretion of sodium; FEU, fractional excretion of urate; LDH, Lactate dehydrogenase; MR, magnetic resonance.

should focus on managing fluid status as well as preventing dangerous electrolyte abnormalities and further deterioration in renal function. To achieve these goals, renal replacement therapy may be required.

Renal Replacement Therapies

Peritoneal Dialysis

Peritoneal dialysis can be used in the pediatric intensive care setting and generally causes more gradual fluid and electrolyte shifts compared with hemodialysis. This modality has the advantage of not requiring vascular access or the need for systemic anticoagulation. Peritoneal dialysis is not ideal for the treatment of severe metabolic disturbances or intoxications resulting from inefficient clearance and is contraindicated in cases of abdominal wall defects or recent abdominal surgery.

Intermittent Hemodialysis

Intermittent hemodialysis is an excellent modality for severe metabolic abnormalities, electrolyte disturbances, or toxin ingestions. However, this modality is not ideal in patients who cannot tolerate rapid changes in fluid balance. Acute hemodialysis and continuous venovenous hemofiltration requires the placement of an appropriate-size catheter (Table 12.6).

Continuous Venovenous Hemofiltration

The use of continuous venovenous hemofiltration (CVVH) is increasingly popular in the pediatric ICU. CVVH allows for a more gradual rate of solute and fluid removal, which is beneficial in patients with hemodynamic instability. Medication adjustments may be required because CVVH can alter the clearance of certain drugs especially medications that are water soluble, of lower molecular weight, or not highly protein bound. Potassium and phosphorus losses can be excessive. Appropriate electrolyte replacement can be given in the CVVH replacement fluid or in a separate IV.

Table 12.6 Vascular Access for Acute Hemodialysis

Patient Size, kg	Catheter Size
Neonate, <3	5-Fr single-lumen venous catheter
	7-Fr double-lumen dialysis catheter
3–6	7-Fr double-lumen dialysis catheter
6–30	8-, 9-Fr double-lumen dialysis catheter
>30	10-, 11-, 11.5-Fr double-lumen dialysis catheter

Further Reading

Alfonzo AV, Isles C, Geddes C, Deighan C. Potassium disorders: clinical spectrum and emergency management. *Resuscitation*. 2006;70(1):10–25.

Andreoli SP. Acute kidney injury in children. *Pediatr Nephrol*. 2009;24(2):253–263.

Flynn JT, Tullus K. Severe hypertension in children and adolescents: pathophysiology and treatment. *Pediatr Nephrol*. 2009;24(6):1101–1112.

Moritz ML. Renal replacement therapy in children. In: Kellum JA, ed. *Continuous Renal Replacement Therapy*. Oxford, UK: Oxford University Press; 2010:159–165.

Moritz ML, Ayus JC. New aspects in the pathogenesis, prevention, and treatment of hyponatremic encephalopathy in children. *Pediatr Nephrol*. 2010;25(7):1225–1238.

Moritz ML, Ayus JC. Preventing neurological complications from dysnatremias in children. *Pediatr Nephrol*. 2005;20(12):1687–1700.

Chapter 13

Hematology and Oncology

Philip C. Spinella and Jeffrey J. Bednarski II

Coagulopathy

Diagnosis

The term *coagulopathy* is most often used to describe disorders that increase the risk of bleeding (hypocoagulable state), but it can also be used to describe those disorders that increase the risk of thrombosis (hypercoagulable state). The process and regulation of coagulation occurs on cell surfaces.[1] As a result, coagulation laboratory measures that use whole blood samples should provide a more accurate representation of functional hemostasis. In vitro viscoelastic measures of coagulation, such as thromboelastogram (TEG) or ROTEM, provide global functional measures of coagulation, and are able to detect both hypo- and hypercoagulable states. Because no in vitro test of coagulation incorporates the endothelial contribution to hemostasis, no current laboratory measure of coagulation can reflect in vivo hemostasis accurately.

Prospective studies determining thresholds for increased risk of bleeding and risk of thrombosis for all methods of coagulation monitoring have not been done in children. Therefore, the diagnosis of coagulopathy, or the ability to determine whether a patient is at risk for bleeding or developing an adverse thrombotic event, is imprecise. An INR of > 1.5 is often used to define hypocoagulable coagulopathy, but this often-used definition lacks support in the literature.[2]

Thrombosis Treatment

Symptomatic thrombotic events are commonly treated with either unfractionated heparin intravenously or enoxaparin subcutaneously. Current guidelines based on limited data suggest that therapeutic unfractionated heparin in children should be titrated to achieve a target range of anti-Xa activity of 0.35 to 0.7 U/mL, or an activated partial thromboplastin time range that correlates with this anti-Xa range.[3] For neonates and children receiving either daily or twice daily therapeutic low-molecular weight heparin, current guidelines advise targeting the drug to anti-Xa activity of 0.5 to 1.0 U/mL in a sample taken 4 to 6 hours after subcutaneous injection.[3]

Blood Transfusion Indications

Specific indications for blood product use are complicated by the lack of prospective evidence indicating clinical efficacy. Red blood cell (RBC) transfusion in hemodynamically stable, critically ill children is appropriate to consider when the hemoglobin is less than 7 g/dL.[4] Cryoprecipitate or fibrinogen concentrates are advised in bleeding patients for fibrinogen values less than 100 to 150 mg/dL.[5] Platelet transfusion is recommended when platelet counts are less than 10,000/microliter in stable, nonbleeding oncology (leukemia, post-stem cell transplant, and solid tumor) patients.[6] General transfusion indications and dosing ranges are listed in Table 13.1. Table 13.2 provides definitions for blood product processing.

Current storage solutions and processing methods for blood products are based primarily on circulating survival and recovery data, and not actual function with respect to oxygen delivery or hemostasis.[7] The rate of administration of all blood products should be a balance between the urgency of correcting the deficit and the need to avoid complications of rapid administration. In hemodynamically stable patients, all blood products are generally transfused over a 2- to 4-hour period. When removed from storage and placed at the beside at room temperature, all blood product transfusions must be completed in 4 hours to reduce the risk of complications such as bacterial overgrowth. In an exsanguinating patient, blood products can be pushed manually or given with a rapid infuser. Granulocytes are always given over 2 to 4 hours and should never be given within 4 hours of amphotericin administration because of concern for acute, severe pulmonary reactions when both are used in close proximity. Caution should be exercised when using atrial catheters because potassium within stored RBC units can cause fatal dysrhythmias.

Massive Transfusion Protocols

Resuscitation from life-threatening bleeding requires rapid surgical control and application of damage control resuscitation principles.[8] Box 13.1 details these concepts. In pediatrics, massive transfusion can be defined as more than 70 mL/kg RBCs in a 24-hour period, although there is no standard well-accepted definition. Massive transfusion protocols can be applied in any immediately life-threatening bleeding scenario. Protocols that are proactive and *push* blood products to the bedside in predetermined weight-based ratios are more practical and less time-consuming than reactive protocols, which require repeated blood product orders, essentially *pulling* blood to the bedside. Typical empiric ratios for fresh frozen plasma:RBCs range from 1:1 to 1:2 U and, for random donor platelets:RBCs, from 1:1 to 1:2 U (apheresis platelet: RBCs range, 1:5–1:10 U). Frequent monitoring to prevent hypothermia, hypocalcemia, hypomagnesemia, and acidosis during massive transfusions is important. Crystalloid use promotes dilutional coagulopathy, and excessive administration should be avoided. Based on adult trauma data, tranexamic acid use in children with life-threatening traumatic bleeding can be considered.[9] The appropriate

Table 13.1 Blood Product Indication and Dosing

Product	Indication for Use	Dosing
Red blood cells	• Symptomatic anemia, physical or laboratory evidence of shock or oxygen debt • As indicated in massive transfusion protocol	• Hemodynamically stable, 10–15 mL/kg; if hemoglobin ≤5 mg/dL, then ≤5 mL/kg • Must be ABO compatible • Type O is universal donor
Platelets, random donor	• Thrombocytopenia with active bleeding or known platelet disorder • As indicated in massive transfusion protocol	• 1–2 U/10 kg or 5–10 mL/kg • 1 U ≈ 50 mL • One unit should increase the platelet count by 10,000/mm^3 • ABO compatible preferred, but not required
Platelets, single donor	• Same for random-donor platelets. • Patients at risk for platelet alloimmunization	• One single-donor unit is equal to five to six random-donor units. • 1 U = ~300 mL. • ABO compatible preferred, but not required
Fresh frozen plasma (thawed plasma)	• Active bleeding • Source of ATIII. • Therapeutic plasma exchange • Warfarin reversal in an emergent situation • As indicated in massive transfusion protocol	• 10–15 mL/kg • Must be ABO compatible with the recipient • AB plasma is universal donor
Cryoprecipitate contains fibrinogen, Factor VIII, Factor XIII, a nd von Willebrand factor	• DIC • Dysfunctional fibrinogen conditions (von Willebrand factor, Factor I, Factor VIII, and Factor XIII deficiency) • As indicated in massive transfusion protocol	• 1–2 U/10 kg • ABO compatible preferred, but not required
Fibrinogen concentrates[a]	• DIC • Dysfunctional fibrinogen conditions (von Willebrand factor, Factor I, Factor VIII, and Factor XIII deficiency) • As indicated in massive transfusion protocol	• ? 60 mg/kg? (very limited data available)
Granulocytes	• Patients with persistent neutropenia or granulocyte dysfunction with a bacterial or fungal infection who are not responding to standard therapy	• 10 mL/kg • Must be ABO compatible with the recipient • Must be irradiated and cytomegalovirus negative

ATIII, Anti-thrombin III; DIC, Disseminated intravascular coagulation.

* US Food and Drug Administration approved for congenital hypofibrinogenemia only.

Recommended guidelines to be used per physician discretion.

Table 13.2 Blood Product Processing Definitions

Term	Definition
Irradiated	• Gamma irradiation used to prevent white blood cell (WBC) replication and, as a result, graft-versus-host disease in immune-suppressed patients receiving products with viable leukocytes. • Products with potential viable leukocytes include whole blood, packed red blood cells, platelets, and granulocytes
Leukocyte reduced	• Leukopore filters are used to reduce the WBC content of blood products and to minimize the risk of transmission of cytomegalovirus. • This process removes more than 99% of WBC, which still leaves 1×10^6 WBCs.
Volume reduction	• Used in patients who, physiologically, cannot tolerate the full volume of a transfused product.

dose of tranexamic acid has not been well studied for children with traumatic injury. Some centers extrapolate from the elective surgery literature for children and use a dose range of between 25 mg/kg and 50mg/kg. A recent trial in adult trauma patients indicated reduced death from hemorrhage when a 1:1:1 U ratio of RBCs, plasma, and platelet strategy was used compared with a 2:1:1 U ratio.[10] No prospective randomized evidence exists in children to support the resuscitation approach used in massive transfusion protocols.[8]

Transfusion Reactions

Acute transfusion reactions usually occur during the first 15 minutes of the transfusion; however, reactions may occur any time during the transfusion and up to 10 hours later. Table 13.3 describes the signs and symptoms, standard actions and treatments, and potential methods to prevent transfusion reactions. If a patient exhibits any signs/symptoms of a transfusion reaction, stop the transfusion immediately, save the blood product container and tubing, and

Box 13.1 Damage Control Resuscitation Principles

- Rapid recognition of high risk for trauma-induced coagulopathy
- Permissive hypotension
- Rapid definitive/surgical control of bleeding
- Prevention/treatment of hypothermia, acidosis, and hypocalcemia
- Avoidance of hemodilution by minimizing use of crystalloids
- Early transfusion of plasma:platelets:red blood cells in a high (>1:1:2) unit ratio
- Use of thawed plasma and fresh whole blood when available
- Appropriate use of coagulation factor products (recombinant activated factor VIIa) and fibrinogen-containing products (fibrinogen concentrates, cryoprecipitate), and antifibrinolytics (tranexamic acid)
- Use of fresh red blood cells (storage age, <14 days) if available
- Thromboelastogram or other hemostasis analysis to direct blood product and hemostatic adjunct (antifibrinolytics and coagulation factor) administration

Table 13.3 Transfusion Reactions

Type/Etiology/Signs and Symptoms	Actions and Treatment	Prevention
Type: Febrile nonhemolytic transfusion reaction *Etiology*: An immune response to surface antigens on the donor white blood cells or platelets *Signs and symptoms*: Fever, chills, rigors, malaise, vomiting; headache, nausea, vomiting; hypotension or low back pain typically not present	• Stop the transfusion. • Change all IV tubing containing blood. • Treat with acetaminophen. • Resume the transfusion at a slower rate if indicated.	Acetaminophen 30–60 minutes before transfusion, leukocyte-reduced or washed blood products (for recurrent febrile nonhemolytic transfusion reaction)
Type: Acute hemolytic transfusion reaction *Etiology*: ABO incompatibility *Signs and symptoms:* Fever; chills; feeling of uneasiness; pain in low back, flank, chest, infusion vein; hypotension; bleeding; disseminated intravascular coagulation renal failure *Laboratory findings*: free hemoglobinemia, hemoglobinuria	• Stop the transfusion. • Change all IV tubing containing blood. • Monitor hemodynamics closely. • Treat symptomatically. • Obtain blood samples such as direct antiglobulin test/Coombs test, lactate dehydrogenase, haptoglobin, bilirubin, repeat patient ABO, and urine samples.	Strict adherence to patient identification procedures from proper labeling of type and cross samples at the bedside to confirming product and patient identification at the bedside with 2 nurses
Type: Allergic transfusion reaction *Etiology:* Usually in patients who have had previous transfusion, and the recipient's anti-IgA antibodies react with some IgA subtypes in donor blood product *Signs and symptoms*: Urticaria, pruritis, flushing, facial edema, angioedema, wheezing, stridor, dyspnea, cough. hypotension, loss of consciousness, nausea, vomiting, abdominal cramps	• If no accompanying fever, slow the rate of the transfusion. • If fever appears, stop the transfusion. • Stay with the patient, call for medical assistance, change the IV tubing (containing blood product) down to the needleless connector or hub of catheter and keep vein open with normal saline. • Diphenhydramine (IV/per ora) • Nebulized albuterol for bronchospasms if ordered	Antihistamines 1 hour prior to transfusion. For moderate to severe reactions, corticosteroids may be indicated.

(Continued)

Table 13.3 Continued

Type/Etiology/Signs and Symptoms	Actions and Treatment	Prevention
Type: Anaphylaxis *Etiology*: IgE-mediated hypersensitivity allergic reaction *Signs and symptoms*: Immediate respiratory distress, upper airway obstruction, lower airway bronchospasm (wheezing, retractions, shortness of breath), hypotension, loss of consciousness	• Stop the transfusion. • Change all IV tubing containing blood product. • Obtain frequent vital signs. • Treatment may require oxygen, epinephrine, diphenhydramine, methylprednisolone, albuterol, and ranitidine.	Autologous blood donation for elective surgery; IgA-deficient or washed blood components
Type: Transfusion-related acute lung injury, increased permeability *Signs and symptoms*: Dyspnea, hypoxemia, cyanosis, hypotension, fever, decreased intravascular volume	• Stop the transfusion. • Change all IV tubing containing blood product. • Symptomatic therapy often requires mechanical ventilation and circulatory support.	Use of pooled plasma products, plasma with low HLA antibodies, red blood cells of decreased storage age
Type: Transfusion-associated cardiac overload, increased hydrostatic pressure *Signs and symptoms*: Dyspnea, hypoxemia, cyanosis, hypotension, Increased intravascular volume	• Stop the transfusion. • Symptomatic therapy often requires mechanical ventilation. • Diuresis and fluid restriction	Slow transfusion rate, use of diuretics for patients at high risk of poor cardiac function

Ig, immunoglobin; IV, intravenous.

return any remaining blood and the administration set to the transfusion service. If respiratory symptoms occur, consider obtaining a chest X-ray, blood gas analysis, and brain natriuretic peptide level to assist with evaluation of transfusion-related acute lung injury (TRALI) or transfusion-associated circulatory overload (TACO).

TRALI is defined as an acute syndrome including dyspnea, hypoxemia, and interstitial pulmonary infiltrates presenting within 6 hours of transfusion in the absence of other detectable causes. Although TRALI is treatable with supportive care, delayed recognition of the clinical manifestations can lead to death. TRALI has been attributed primarily to donor leukocyte antibodies that are thought to interact with recipient neutrophils, resulting in activation and aggregation in pulmonary capillaries, release of local biological response modifiers causing capillary leak, and lung injury. An alternate mechanism termed the *two-hit* or *neutrophils-priming hypothesis* postulates that a pathway to neutrophil activation and aggregation can occur without leukocyte anti-bodies. A first event such as sepsis or trauma can induce pulmonary endothe-lial activation, release of cytokines, and priming of neutrophils. A subsequent second event such as exposure to lipids, cytokines, or antibodies in a blood component would then cause activation of adherent neutrophils and a release of bioreactive molecules leading to lung injury. These proposed mechanisms are not mutually exclusive in that donor leukocyte antibodies can be pathogenic in both models and have implications for new strategies to prevent TRALI.[11]

TACO occurs with transfusion in the setting of hypervolemia and car-diac dysfunction. Pulmonary edema occurs as a result of increased pulmo-nary hydrostatic pressure, which is distinct from TRALI, in which there is increased pulmonary capillary permeability. There is no sentinel feature that distinguishes TRALI from TACO. Developing a thorough clinical profile—including presenting signs and symptoms, fluid status, cardiac status (includ-ing measurement of brain natriuretic peptide), and leukocyte antibody testing—is the best strategy currently available to distinguish between the two disorders.[12]

Abnormal Cell Counts

Critically ill patients can have numerous underlying disorders that contribute to abnormal circulating blood cell counts. The significance and clinical relevance of the changes in blood cell counts depends on etiology and the clinical status of the patient. In the simplest terms, altered cell counts are a consequence of changes in the production or destruction of the specific cell lines. Decreases in bone marrow production often affect all cell lines whereas destructive pathol-ogies most often affect specific cell populations. Understanding the underlying pathology is essential to selecting the most appropriate treatment interven-tion (Table 13.4).

Etiologies in the Intensive Care Unit Setting

Table 13.5 describes some factors that commonly cause abnormal cell counts in an intensive care unit (ICU) setting.

Bone Marrow Suppression Secondary to Acute Illness or Infectious Processes

Many infectious processes, including sepsis, can suppress bone marrow production while simultaneously increasing cell turnover rates. The result is combined leukopenia, anemia, and thrombocytopenia. The increased cell loss is typically secondary to inflammatory processes that reduce cell half-lives rather than immune- or vascular-mediated destruction of cells. Supportive care with transfusions as needed, until resolution of the

Table 13.4 Age-Based Norms for Cell Counts

Age	Mean Leukocyte Count, ×10³/mm³ (Range)	Mean Hemoglobin, g/dL (−2 SDs)	Mean Hematocrit, % (−2 SDs)	Mean Platelet Count × 10⁹/L ± SD
3–6 mo	11.9 (6.0–17.5)	11.5 (9.5)	35 (29)	365 ± 49
6 mo–2 y	10.9 (6.0–17.5)	12.0 (10.5)	36 (33)	314 ± 78
2–6 y	9.1 (5.0–17.5)	12.5 (11.5)	37 (34)	304 ± 66
6–12 y	8.1 (4.5–13.5)	13.5 (11.5)	40 (35)	295 ± 58
12–18, y, female	7.8 (4.5–13.0)		41 (36)	234 ± 48
male		14.0 (12.0) 14.5 (13.0)		

SD, standard deviation.

Data from Orkin SH, Nathan DG, Ginsburg D, Look TA, Fisher DE, Lux SE IV, eds. *Nathan and Oski's Hematology of Infancy and Childhood*. 7th ed. Saunders Elsevier: Philadelphia; 2009.

underlying etiology, is generally sufficient. There are no data to support the routine use of erythropoietin in critically ill children except in the setting of chronic renal failure.

Anemia of Inflammation

In response to both acute and chronic illness, inflammatory cytokines, particularly interleukin 6, stimulate increased liver production of hepcidin, an iron-regulating hormone.[13,14] Hepcidin binds to and inhibits the iron export channel on macrophages, hepatocytes, and enterocytes. Consequently, iron scavenged by phagocytes and absorbed by enterocytes cannot be released. The result is low serum iron levels, similar to iron deficiency anemia, and decreased RBC production. Erythrocytes are generally normochromic and normocytic, but can be mildly hypochromic and microcytic. Laboratory evaluation often demonstrates increased total iron binding capacity, but normal ferritin. Treatments are directed at resolution of the underlying pathology, which ultimately reduces hepcidin production and allows release of stored iron, increased RBC production (increased reticulocyte count), and resolution of the anemia.

Heparin-Induced Thrombocytopenia

Heparin-induced thrombocytopenia (HIT) is an immune-mediated response to heparin that triggers production of antibodies against platelet factor 4. HIT occurs in approximately 1% to 2% of pediatric patients, with a higher incidence in ICU patients.[15] Notably, low-molecular weight heparin (enoxaparin) is associated with a much lower incidence of HIT than unfractionated heparin.[16] Onset is 5 to 10 days after heparin administration and is marked by thrombosis and thrombocytopenia (>50% decrease).[15] Importantly, the absence of thrombocytopenia does not exclude a diagnosis of HIT. Current testing uses

Table 13.5 Common Causes of Abnormal Cell Counts in the Intensive Care Unit Setting

Cell Line	Increased	Decreased	
		Decreased Production	Increased Destruction
Neutrophils	• Infection • Steroids	• Infection • Medications • Cyclic neutropenia • Leukemia • Hemophagocytic lymphohistiocytosis	• Autoimmune neutropenia • Alloimmune neutropenia
Hemoglobin	• Hemoconcentration from intravascular volume contraction • Chronic hypoxemia	• Infection • Medications • Kidney failure • Anemia of inflammation • Iron deficiency	• DIC • Immune-mediated hemolysis • Mechanical hemolysis (ECMO or dialysis) • Red blood cell defect (G6PD, spherocytosis) • Blood loss • Splenic sequestration
Platelets	• Acute-phase response to infection	• Infection • Medications	• Increased consumption (fever, mechanical destruction [e.g., by ECMO circuit]) • DIC • Budd-Chiari • Heparin-induced thrombocytopenia • ITP

DIC, disseminated intravascular coagulation; ECMO, extracorporeal membrane oxygenation.

detection of antiplatelet factor 4 antibodies. Treatment includes discontinuation of heparin and initiation of alternative anticoagulants, such as argatroban or lepirudin.[16] However, there are no clinical trials evaluating optimal therapy for HIT in pediatric patients.

Sickle Cell Disease

A single mutation in the β-hemoglobin chain is responsible for the abnormal hemoglobin in sickle cell disease (SCD). In the deoxy conformation, sickle hemoglobin polymerizes rapidly, leading to the characteristic RBC deformation, increased RBC rigidity and oxidative damage to the RBC membrane. Increased RBC lysis releases free hemoglobin, which binds plasma nitric oxide, thereby preventing smooth muscle relaxation, resulting in vasoconstriction. The combination of vasoconstriction and increased RBC rigidity leads to decreased blood flow, hypoxia, and endothelial wall injury. The result is vascular injury plus acute and chronic inflammation that, ultimately, cause organ damage. The clinical manifestations of SCD are determined by the genetic basis of a patient's disease (Table 13.6) in association with other (mostly nondescribed) genetic and environmental modifiers.

Veno-occlusive Event

Pain crises (also called *veno-occlusive events*) are secondary to intravascular sickling with tissue infarction and are the most common complication of SCD. Although rarely a reason for admission to the ICU, pain is a frequent comorbidity. Management includes aggressive pain control with narcotics and nonsteroidal anti-inflammatory drugs plus continuous intravenous fluids to maintain hydration. Blood transfusions are rarely indicated in the management of veno-occlusive events, but can be beneficial in severe, unremitting pain episodes. Inadequate management of pain can exacerbate other disease complications, particularly acute chest syndrome. For example, increased chest pain

Table 13.6 Genetics of Sickle Cell Disease

Type	Genetic Basis	Clinical Severity
HbSS	Two copies of the β chain with the S mutation	Anemia is more pronounced with lower baseline Hb concentration. Clinical course is generally more severe.
HbSC	One copy of S and one copy of C mutation in the β-chain	Anemia is less with higher baseline Hb concentrations than HbSS. Clinical course is generally less severe.
HbC	Two copies of the β-chain with C mutation	No clinical problems
HbS β⁰-thalassemia	One copy of S mutation and other β-chain locus has a mutation that eliminates expression	Clinically similar to HbSS
HbS β⁺-thalassemia	One copy of S mutation and other β-chain locus has a mutation that causes decreased expression	Clinically similar to HbSC
Persistent fetal Hb	Mutations in the γ-chain gene that result in increased expression of fetal Hb	Generally associated with less severe phenotype in all of the sickle hemoglobinopathies

Hb, hemoglobin; HbC, disseminated intravascular coagulation HbS, hemoglobin-S; HbSC, hemoglobin-SC HbSS, hemoglobin-SS.

results in splinting and decreased lung volumes, leading to hypoxemia, further vasoconstriction, and RBC sickling.

Acute Chest Syndrome

The diagnostic criteria for acute chest syndrome include evidence of a new pulmonary infiltrate in combination with one or more of the following: chest pain, fever, tachypnea, cough, new-onset hypoxemia, and/or increased work of breathing.[17] Importantly, not all of these symptoms need to be present to diagnose acute chest syndrome. Any patient with SCD and new respiratory symptoms *must* be evaluated for acute chest syndrome. Treatment (Table 13.7) centers on improving oxygenation and decreasing Hemoglobin S (HbS) polymerization and associated vasoconstriction.[17,18]

Table 13.7 Treatment of Acute Chest Syndrome

Intervention	Purpose	Additional Information
Supplemental oxygen	Reverse hypoxemia	Noninvasive support or intubation may be necessary in severe cases.
Intravenous fluids	Improve hydration and decrease viscosity	Maintain infusion rates. Monitor for pulmonary edema and maintain even fluid balance.
Red blood cell transfusion	Improve oxygenation	Simple transfusion is used early and for patients with hemoglobin < 9 g/dL
Exchange transfusion	Improve oxygenation and reduce percent Hemoglobin-S to less than 30%	Indicated if worsening hypoxia or rapid deterioration
Antibiotics	Treat underlying infections that may be triggered	Third-generation cephalosporins plus azithromycin to treat mycoplasma or chlamydia
Bronchodilator	Improve bronchospasm and bronchoconstriction	Trial for all patients with ACS is reasonable, but should be stopped if no improvement. For patients with asthma, should be continued in combination with steroids.
Oral steroids	Treat asthma	Used only in patients with concomitant asthma. Minimal benefit in ACS without asthma.

ACS, acute chest syndrome.

Data from Vichinsky EP, Styles LA, Colangelo LH, Wright EC, Castro O, Nickerson B. Acute chest syndrome in sickle cell disease: clinical presentation and course: cooperative study of sickle cell disease. *Blood.* 1997;89(5):1787–1792; Vichinsky EP, Neumayr LD, Earles AN, et al. Causes and outcomes of the acute chest syndrome in sickle cell disease: National Acute Chest Syndrome Study Group. *N Engl J Med.* 2000;342(25):1855–1865; Sobota A, Graham DA, Heeney MM, Neufeld EJ. Corticosteroids for acute chest syndrome in children with sickle cell disease: variation in use and association with length of stay and readmission. *Am J Hematol.* 2010;85(1):24–28.

Splenic Sequestration

An acute decrease in hemoglobin with a rapidly enlarging spleen is consistent with splenic sequestration in patients with SCD. This process can progress very rapidly and may lead to death shortly after onset of symptoms as a result of trapping a significant portion of the RBC mass. Splenic sequestration is one of the leading causes of death in patients with SCD.[19] This acute crisis typically occurs in patients younger than 5 years, before autosplenectomy, but can occur in older patients with hemoglobin-SC (HbSC) or HbS-β-thalassemia, as splenic infarction may not have occurred. Associated symptoms include dyspnea, lethargy, left-side abdominal pain, and vomiting. Laboratory studies demonstrate a 2 g/dL or more decrease in hemoglobin concentration and moderate to severe thrombocytopenia.[19] Early recognition, close monitoring, and urgent intervention at signs of progression are essential to prevent complications. Treatment consists of emergent blood transfusions to restore circulating intravascular volume. Small-volume transfusions (5–10 mL/kg) of RBCs used as relief of sequestration result in a rapid return of sequestered hemoglobin to the circulation. Overly aggressive transfusion can result in hyperviscosity and associated complications, including stroke. A single episode of splenic sequestration is an indication for splenectomy, which should be performed after resolution of the acute event.[20]

Stroke

Acute neurological events in patients with SCD require emergent intervention to prevent progression and to minimize long-term devastation. Hemiparesis, focal seizures, gait dysfunction, and speech defects are the most common presenting signs. A detailed neurological examination is beneficial for differentiation from other etiologies and for documentation of neurological deficits. The best initial radiographic examination is noncontrast computed tomography to evaluate for hemorrhage. Magnetic resonance imaging is better for identifying infarction, but changes may not be present at the initial presentation. Treatment should be based on clinical determination of stroke and should not be delayed to obtain the magnetic resonance image. The standard treatment for stroke in SCD is immediate exchange transfusion with the goal of reducing the HbS concentration to less than 30%, without increasing viscosity or overall blood volume.[21]

Critical Complications of Oncological Disorders

Hyperleukocytosis

Leukemia can be associated with a very high white blood cell count (>100,000/mm³). Hyperleukocytosis is associated with massive tumor lysis (discussed in the next section) and hyperviscosity, which can lead to renal failure, central nervous system hemorrhage, and pulmonary leukostasis with decreased blood oxygenation. Hydration with intravenous fluids at 3000 mL/m^2/d and leukopheresis are essential to minimize complications of leukocytosis and acutely decrease the white blood cell count.

Tumor Lysis Syndrome

Tumor lysis syndrome is a constellation of metabolic abnormalities that occur with a massive breakdown of tumor cells, either spontaneously or in response to treatment (Table 13.8). It is the most common emergent oncological complication and occurs most frequently in diseases with high tumor burden, such as leukemia (hyperleukocytosis) and Burkitt's lymphoma. The triad of hyperkalemia, hyperuricemia, and hyperphosphatemia occurs in tumor lysis syndrome. Importantly, these metabolic derangements are exacerbated by acute renal injury from hyperuricemia. Treatment is targeted at optimizing renal clearance and preventing complications from the electrolyte disturbances.[22,23]

Table 13.8 Tumor Lysis Abnormalities and Treatment	
Abnormality	**Treatment**
Prevention	• D5 ¼ NS + 40 mEq/L NaHCO$_3$ (without potassium) at 3000 mL/m^2/d • Keep urine pH between 7.0 and 8.0 • Maintain urine output at 2–4 mL/kg/h
Hyperuricemia	• Allopurinol 100 mg/m^2/dose three times daily *or* rasburicase 0.2 mg/kg/dose intravenously • Allopurinol blocks uric acid production; it does not decrease current serum uric acid level, but it does prevent the generation of more toxin. Rasburicase catabolizes uric acid, resulting in an immediate reduction in serum levels. Check G6PD prior to starting rasburicase.
Hyperkalemia	• Sodium polystyrene (Kayexalate) 1 g/kg orally every 6 hours • Albuterol nebulization • Furosemide • Insulin (0.1 U/kg) with concurrent 25% dextrose (2 mL/kg) • Calcium gluconate (100–200 mg/kg)
Hyperphosphatemia	• Aluminum hydroxide 15–30 mL per ora every 6 hours • Renagel (sevelamer)
Hypocalcemia	• Calcium gluconate (50–100 mg/kg/dose)
Renal failure	• Renal dialysis may be necessary for control of tumor lysis syndrome. Indications are the same as for other causes of renal failure, but initiation should be early to avoid further complications.

Data from Coiffier B, Altman A, Pui CH, Younes A, Cairo MS. Guidelines for the management of pediatric and adult tumor lysis syndrome: an evidence-based review. *J Clin Oncol.* 2008;26(16):2767–2778; Mullen E, Whangbo J, Vrooman LM. Oncologic emergencies. In: Orkin SH, Nathan DG, Ginsburg D, Look TA, Fisher DE, Lux SE IV, eds. *Nathan and Oski's Hematology of Infancy and Childhood.* 7th ed.

Saunders Elsevier, Philadelphia; 2009:1121–1143.

Neutropenic Fever and Sepsis

Neutropenia and immune suppression from chemotherapy increase the risk of bacterial infection. The highest risk is during the period of neutropenia that follows each cycle of chemotherapy. Importantly, many episodes of fever and neutropenia in oncology/bone marrow transplant patients are culture negative, despite clear clinical signs of sepsis. These patients should continue to be treated as if they are bacteremic with sepsis. Broad-spectrum antibiotics are started immediately and should be tailored to possible sources of infection. For example, if skin abscesses are present, vancomycin should be started to treat Gram-positive organisms, in addition to broad-spectrum Gram-negative coverage (e.g., cefepime). Antifungal therapy should be considered if fevers and symptoms persist for 3 to 4 days despite appropriate antibiotic coverage. Patients should be supported aggressively with fluid resuscitation, inotropes, and filgrastrim (granulocyte-colony stimulating factor to support neutrophil production) as needed. In severe cases, granulocyte infusions should be considered if neutrophil recovery is not expected for more than 7 days and the patient has an infection that has been resistant to or has progressed despite appropriate antimicrobial therapy.[24,25] Patients with septic shock and a history of adrenalectomy or substantial steroid therapy should be started on stress doses of hydrocortisone early during the resuscitation. Overall, oncology patients with septic shock treated in the ICU have the same survival rate as nononcology patients with similar clinical pictures.[26]

Veno-occlusive Disease

Veno-occlusive disease has also been termed *sinusoidal obstructive syndrome* and is defined by tender hepatomegaly, fluid retention with weight gain, and elevated serum bilirubin levels.[27] Other findings include platelet consumption (similar to DIC), ascites, and jaundice. Doppler ultrasound of the portal vein can show reversal of flow, but this is a late finding and is not essential to the development of the clinical picture or to the diagnosis.[27] Underlying pathology is unclear, but vascular endothelial injury in the liver is believed to be the inciting factor, followed by microthrombosis, venular narrowing, and sclerosis. The clinical course can progress to multiorgan failure, including the kidneys, lungs, and heart. Strict fluid management with a goal of maintaining euvolemia is essential to minimizing organ injury.[27,28] Defibrotide, a fibrinolytic, is beneficial in improving outcomes in patients with veno-occlusive disease and should be started at the earliest signs of disease.[28] Risks include gastrointestinal and cranial hemorrhage, but incidence is low. The addition of ursodiol has also been associated with clinical benefit.[29]

Graft-Versus-Host Disease

Recipients of allogeneic (related or unrelated) bone marrow transplants are at risk of graft-versus-host disease (GVHD), in which donor immune cells attack the recipient's organs (Table 13.9). The pathophysiology of GVHD involves

Table 13.9 Graft-Versus-Host Disease Presentation

Organ	Symptoms	Adjuvant Treatment (Added to Systemic Immune Suppression)
Skin	Acute: dry, pruritic, erythematous maculopapular rash; typically starts on the palms and soles, and progresses to trunk and face Chronic: thickening, discoloration	• Moisturizing cream • Topical steroids • Topical calcineurin inhibitors
Eyes	Decreased tear production resulting in dry, painful eyes; conjunctival injection	• Ophthalmic steroids • Ophthalmic calcineurin inhibitors
GI	Common presenting symptoms: vomiting (upper GI disease) and diarrhea (lower GI disease) along with abdominal; diarrhea can cause fluid losses of liters per day, with significant electrolyte abnormalities	• Nothing by mouth • Oral beclomethasone • Octreotide
Liver	First signs: elevated bilirubin, GGT, and alkaline phosphatase; can progress to fulminant liver failure	• Ursodiol
Lungs	Presentation: shortness of breath with excursion, wheezing, cough. Can have obstructive (decreased forced expiratory volume in 1 s) or restrictive (decreased forced vital capacity (FVC), total lung volume) pattern; progresses to fibrosis, such as bronchiolitis obliterans	• Inhaled steroids • Montelukast • Azithromycin • Albuterol

GI, gastrointestinal.

Data from Baird K, Cooke K, Schultz KR. Chronic graft-versus-host disease (GVHD) in children. *Pediatr Clin North Am*. 2010;57(1):297–322; Carpenter PA, Macmillan ML. Management of acute graft-versus-host disease in children. *Pediatr Clin North Am*. 2010;57(1):273–295.

immune activation and tissue inflammation. Treatment centers on aggressive immune suppression to dampen the graft response and an attempt to reeducate the donor cells to accept the host as "self." Front-line therapy includes high-dose steroids (2 mg/kg/d) and calcineurin inhibitors (cyclosporine, tacrolimus).[30,31] Additional agents may be added to target inflammatory cytokines or deplete lymphocytes. GVHD is a significant cause of morbidity and mortality following engraftment of donor cells.[30,31] Early recognition and initiation of treatment are critical to resolving disease and minimizing long-term complications and death. Importantly, many manifestations of GVHD overlap with other pathologies, including infections. Infections must be excluded before escalation of immune suppression to avoid acceleration of the infectious process.

Hemophagocytic Lymphohistiocytosis

Hemophagocytic lymphohistiocytosis (HLH) is a disorder of dysregulated innate immunity with uncontrolled proliferation and activation of cells

Box 13.2 Diagnostic Criteria for Hemophagocytic Lymphohistiocytosis

Diagnosis of hemophagocytic lymphohistiocytosis is established by either

1. Molecular or genetic diagnosis consistent with hemophagocytic lymphohistiocytosis (determined by flow cytometry or genetic testing) or
2. Fulfilling five of the following eight criteria

- Fever
- Splenomegaly
- Cytopenias (affecting ≥2 cell lines)
  - Hemoglobin <9 g/dL
  - Platelets <100 × 10^9/L
  - Neutrophils <1000/mm^3
- Hypertriglyceridemia and /or hypofibrinogenemia (change of ≥3 standard deviations for age)
  - Fasting triglycerides ≥265 mg/dL
  - Fibrinogen ≤1.5 g/L
- Hemophagocytosis in bone marrow, spleen, or lymph nodes
- Low or absent natural killer cell function
- Elevated ferritin >500 µg/L
- Elevated soluble interleukin 2 receptor (CD25) ≥2400 U/mL

Data from Henter JI, Horne A, Arico M, et al. HLH-2004: diagnostic and therapeutic guidelines for hemophagocytic lymphohistiocytosis. *Pediatr Blood Cancer.* 2007;48(2):124–131.

in the monocyte–macrophage lineage.[32] HLH is a challenging diagnosis because of diverse clinical presentations that can overlap with many other disease processes In critically ill patients. Timely diagnosis and treatment is essential, because a delay in therapy affects outcomes adversely. Diagnosis is based on the criteria presented in Box 13.2.[33] Although many disease processes can have individual abnormalities in any of the listed parameters, only patients with HLH have the complete constellation of findings. Importantly, a ferritin level of more than 10,000 µg/L is nearly pathognomonic for HLH.[34] Treatment consists of high-dose steroids and early initiation of etoposide.[33]

References

1. Hoffman M. A cell-based model of coagulation and the role of factor VIIa. *Blood Rev.* 2003;17(suppl 1):S1–S5.

2. Dzik WH. The James Blundell Award lecture 2006: transfusion and the treatment of haemorrhage: past, present and future. *Transfus Med.* 2007;17(5):367–374.

3. Monagle P, Chan AK, Goldenberg NA, et al. Antithrombotic therapy in neonates and children: Antithrombotic Therapy and Prevention of Thrombosis, 9th ed: American

College of Chest Physicians Evidence-Based Clinical Practice Guidelines. *Chest.* 2012;141(2)(suppl):e737S–e801S.

4. Lacroix J, Hebert PC, Hutchison JS, et al. Transfusion strategies for patients in pediatric intensive care units. *N Engl J Med.* 2007;356(16):1609–1619.

5. Rossaint R, Bouillon B, Cerny V, et al. Management of bleeding following major trauma: an updated European guideline. *Crit Care.* 2010;14(2):R52.

6. Agency for Healthcare Research and Quality. Guideline for platelet transfusion thresholds for pediatric hematology/oncology patients. http://www.guideline.gov/content.aspx?id=34608. Published 2011. Accessed September 5, 2012.

7. Spinella PC, Doctor A, Blumberg N, Holcomb JB. Does the storage duration of blood products affect outcomes in critically ill patients? *Transfusion.* 2011;51(8):1644–1650.

8. Spinella PC, Holcomb JB. Resuscitation and transfusion principles for traumatic hemorrhagic shock. *Blood Rev.* 2009;23(6):231–240.

9. CRASH-2 Trial Collaborators, Shakur H, Roberts I, et al. Effects of tranexamic acid on death, vascular occlusive events, and blood transfusion in trauma patients with significant haemorrhage (CRASH-2): a randomised, placebo-controlled trial. *Lancet.* 2010; 376(9734):23–32.

10. Holcomb JB, Tilley BC, Baraniuk S, et al. Transfusion of plasma, platelets, and red blood cells in a 1:1:1 vs a 1:1:2 ratio and mortality in patients with severe trauma: the PROPPR randomized clinical trial. *JAMA.* 2015;313:471–482.

11. Triulzi DJ. Transfusion-related acute lung injury: an update. *Hematology Am Soc Hematol Educ Program* 2006:497–501. https://dx.doi.org/10.1182/asheducation-2006.1.497

12. Skeate RC, Eastlund T. Distinguishing between transfusion related acute lung injury and transfusion associated circulatory overload. *Curr Opin Hematol.* 2007;14(6):682–687.

13. Ganz T, Nemeth E. Hepcidin and disorders of iron metabolism. *Annu Rev Med.* 2011;62:347–360.

14. Weinstein DA, Roy CN, Fleming MD, Loda MF, Wolfsdorf JI, Andrews NC. Inappropriate expression of hepcidin is associated with iron refractory anemia: implications for the anemia of chronic disease. *Blood.* 2002;100(10):3776–3781.

15. Risch L, Huber AR, Schmugge M. Diagnosis and treatment of heparin-induced thrombocytopenia in neonates and children. *Thromb Res.* 2006;118(1):123–135.

16. Martel N, Lee J, Wells PS. Risk for heparin-induced thrombocytopenia with unfractionated and low-molecular-weight heparin thromboprophylaxis: a meta-analysis. *Blood.* 2005;106(8):2710–2715.

17. Vichinsky EP, Styles LA, Colangelo LH, Wright EC, Castro O, Nickerson B. Acute chest syndrome in sickle cell disease: clinical presentation and course: Cooperative Study of Sickle Cell Disease. *Blood.* 1997;89(5):1787–1792.

18. Vichinsky EP, Neumayr LD, Earles AN, et al. Causes and outcomes of the acute chest syndrome in sickle cell disease. *N Engl J Med.* 2000;342(25):1855–1865.

19. Seeler RA, Shwiaki MZ. Acute splenic sequestration crises (ASSC) in young children with sickle cell anemia: clinical observations in 20 episodes in 14 children. *Clin Pediatr (Phila).* 1972;11(12):701–704.

20. Kinney TR, Ware RE, Schultz WH, Filston HC. Long-term management of splenic sequestration in children with sickle cell disease. *J Pediatr*. 1990;117(2):194–199.

21. Hulbert ML, Scothorn DJ, Panepinto JA, et al. Exchange blood transfusion compared with simple transfusion for first overt stroke is associated with a lower risk of subsequent stroke: a retrospective cohort study of 137 children with sickle cell anemia. *J Pediatr*. 2006;149(5):710–712.

22. Coiffier B, Altman A, Pui CH, Younes A, Cairo MS. Guidelines for the management of pediatric and adult tumor lysis syndrome: an evidence-based review. *J Clin Oncol*. 2008;26(16):2767–2778.

23. Mullen E, Whangbo J, Vrooman LM. Oncologic emergencies. In: Orkin SH, Nathan DG, Ginsburg D, Look TA, Fisher DE, Lux SEIV, eds. *Nathan and Oski's Hematology of Infancy and Childhood*. 7th ed. Saunders Elsevier: Philadelphia; 2009:1121–1143.

24. Atay D, Ozturk G, Akcay A, Yanasik M, Anak S, Devecioglu O. Effect and safety of granulocyte transfusions in pediatric patients with febrile neutropenia or defective granulocyte functions. *J Pediatr Hematol Oncol*. 2011;33(6):e220–e225.

25. Bishton M, Chopra R. The role of granulocyte transfusions in neutropenic patients. *Br J Haematol*. 2004;127(5):501–508.

26. Pound CM, Johnston DL, Armstrong R, Gaboury I, Menon K. The morbidity and mortality of pediatric oncology patients presenting to the intensive care unit with septic shock. *Pediatr Blood Cancer*. 2008;51(5):584–588.

27. Bearman SI. The syndrome of hepatic veno-occlusive disease after marrow transplantation. *Blood*. 1995;85(11):3005–3020.

28. Corbacioglu S, Kernan N, Lehmann L, et al. Defibrotide for the treatment of hepatic veno-occlusive disease in children after hematopoietic stem cell transplantation. *Exp Rev Hematol*. 2012;5(3):291–302.

29. Tay J, Tinmouth A, Fergusson D, Huebsch L, Allan DS. Systematic review of controlled clinical trials on the use of ursodeoxycholic acid for the prevention of hepatic veno-occlusive disease in hematopoietic stem cell transplantation. *Biol Blood Marrow Transplant*. 2007;13(2):206–217.

30. Baird K, Cooke K, Schultz KR. Chronic graft-versus-host disease (GVHD) in children. *Pediatr Clin North Am*. 2010;57(1):297–322.

31. Carpenter PA, Macmillan ML. Management of acute graft-versus-host disease in children. *Pediatr Clin North Am*. 2010;57(1):273–295.

32. Verbsky JW, Grossman WJ. Hemophagocytic lymphohistiocytosis: diagnosis, pathophysiology, treatment, and future perspectives. *Ann Med*. 2006;38(1):20–31.

33. Henter JI, Horne A, Arico M, et al. HLH-2004: diagnostic and therapeutic guidelines for hemophagocytic lymphohistiocytosis. *Pediatr Blood Cancer*. 2007;48(2):124–131.

34. Allen CE, Yu X, Kozinetz CA, McClain KL. Highly elevated ferritin levels and the diagnosis of hemophagocytic lymphohistiocytosis. *Pediatr Blood Cancer*. 2008;50(6):1227–1235.

35. Orkin SH, Nathan DG, Ginsburg D, Look TA, Fisher DE, Lux SE IV, eds. *Nathan and Oski's Hematology of Infancy and Childhood*. 7th ed. Saunders Elsevier: Philadelphia; 2009.

36. Sobota A, Graham DA, Heeney MM, Neufeld EJ. Corticosteroids for acute chest syndrome in children with sickle cell disease: variation in use and association with length of stay and readmission. *Am J Hematol*. 2010;85(1):24–28.

Chapter 14

Nutrition and Gastrointestinal Emergencies

Renán A. Orellana and Jorge A. Coss-Bu

Nutrition Practice in Pediatric Intensive Care

Infants and children need a continuous supply of nutrients to meet energy requirements for activity, immunological defense and tissue repair, and growth. Their needs vary across stages of development. Inadequately nourished patients are more likely to experience complications, prolonged mechanical ventilation, longer time in the intensive care unit, and an increased risk of death. Near 50% of pediatric intensive care unit (PICU) patients may have chronic conditions associated with undernutrition and frequent hospital admissions.

Nutrition Assessment in the Pediatric Intensive Care Unit

Determination of nutritional risk helps identify baseline nutritional deficits that may be exacerbated by critical illness. The American Society for Parenteral and Enteral Nutrition recommends that critically ill children undergo nutrition screening to identify malnutrition and to develop an individualized nutrition plan. Cohorts of children likely to be at nutritional risk may include those in Table 14.1.

Critically ill patients are in a dynamic metabolic state that fluctuates with the evolution of their disease. Thus, requirements must be reassessed frequently. A nutrition support plan should aim to provide adequate calories, protein, and micronutrients to support a positive protein–energy balance during the specific stage of the critical illness, including enough nutrients to maintain a positive nitrogen balance, to correct deficits, to replace ongoing losses, and to sustain age-appropriate growth if possible.

Table 14.1 Patients at High Risk for Nutritional Deficiencies	
Cohort	Examples
Chronic illness	Congenital heart disease, severe encephalopathy, chronic respiratory insufficiency with ventilator dependence, chronic organ system failure, transplant or chemotherapy recipients
Chronic feeding intolerance	Short-gut and other malabsorption syndromes, history of omphalocele/gastroschisis, severe gastroesophageal reflux disorder
Anorexia/cachexia	Cancer, immunological disorders
Excess requirements	Nutrient losses or abnormal use: proteinuria, burns, metabolic disorders
Risk for refeeding syndrome	Starvation secondary to neglect, anorexia
Obesity	Body mass index ≥95th percentile for age

Assessment of Nutritional Status

History and physical examination identify patients with wasting syndromes, obesity, and growth stunted by chronic malnutrition. Body mass index, head circumference (up to 3 years of age), weight-for-height by reference charts, and historically charted weight velocity provide important information. Examination reveals the presence of edema, anasarca, signs of dehydration, muscle bulk, excess or limited subcutaneous fat, and skin changes associated with micronutrient deficiencies. A weight obtained in the PICU may be altered by fluid overload and acute compartmental shifting, not reflecting dry body weight.

Assessment of Nutritional Status by Laboratory Markers

Initial values change in response to nutrition therapy and the evolution of the disease process. Understanding glucose and protein metabolism, the endocrine milieu, and biochemical regulation of enzymes and metabolites during critical illness is required to interpret the clinical relevance of these values.

Assessment of Carbohydrate Metabolism

Hyperglycemia may result from overfeeding if the patient is in a hypometabolic state and calories are provided in excess. Although insulin resistance may cause hyperglycemia, pediatric patients with critical illness often have normal or low insulin levels. Thus, a *reduction in glucose delivery, rather than initiation of insulin therapy* may be appropriate. Ketone bodies in urine or plasma may establish whether low glucose levels are associated with starvation or whether high glucose levels reflect a relative hypoinsulinemic state and merit an insulin infusion.

Assessment of Protein Metabolism

Circulating visceral proteins such as albumin, prealbumin, and retinol-binding protein are often used to evaluate nutritional status. However, anabolism and catabolism during critical illness may be driven by the systemic inflammatory response and not necessarily by the availability of substrates. During inflammatory conditions, the liver makes acute phase reactants preferentially, such as C-reactive protein, rather than normal visceral proteins. In these cases, visceral proteins do not reflect losses or gains in total body protein accurately, and protein wasting may occur despite adequate visceral protein concentrations.

Blood urea nitrogen (BUN) decreases during starvation and states of low muscle mass. Major nitrogen losses may occur in the urine, thoracic or peritoneal output, or during dialysis. BUN is elevated during dehydration, renal insufficiency, or in the presence of excessive dietary protein or gastrointestinal (GI) blood. Rapidly changing physiology in critical illness limits the value of 24-hour urinary nitrogen excretion to assess nitrogen balance and protein metabolism.

Assessment of Lipid Metabolism

Triglycerides (TGs) are measured to monitor for excessive elevation when intravenous (IV) lipids are used. The plasma enzyme that controls TG concentrations (lipoprotein lipase) is downregulated during acute inflammation and upregulated in the presence of circulating TG. Thus, in the presence of a mildly elevated plasma TG level, the appropriate intervention is to provide lipids.

Nutritional Requirements in the Pediatric Intensive Care Unit

Estimation of Energy Requirements

Nutrition support should supply recommended caloric proportions for normal conditions (50%–60% of calories from carbohydrates, 25%–35% from protein, and 10%–25% from fat). Calories should match resting energy expenditure (REE), which is best measured by indirect calorimetry (IC). IC is recommended in patients ventilated for more than 7 days to avoid the risk of overfeeding or underfeeding. If IC is not available, energy provision may be based on published formulas or nomograms for dietary intake, total energy expenditure, or basal metabolic rate for healthy children. Note that these estimates commonly *overestimate* REE. Calories provided should meet 50% of REE by 48 hours and 100% by days 3 through 5. Energy requirements may increase by 12% to 30% over REE for conditions associated with hypermetabolism, such as fever, respiratory distress, surgery, and sepsis. Unlike adults, critically ill children are often hypometabolic. Paralyzed, sedated patients may have remarkably low caloric requirements.

Estimation of Protein Requirements

Table 14.2 provides protein intake recommendations for critically ill children. Protein intake should meet 50% of protein requirements by 48 hours and 100% by day 3, with adjustments made to supplement deficits from chronic

Table 14.2 Pediatric Protein Requirements Recommended by the American Society for Parenteral and Enteral Nutrition (ASPEN) for Critically Ill Children and the World Health Organization (WHO) for Healthy Children.

Child's status	Age Group				
	<1 y	1–2 y	2–3 y	3–12 y	13–18 y
Critically ill (ASPEN), g/kg/d	2.0–3.0	2.0–3.0	1.5–2.0	1.5–2.0	1.5
Healthy (WHO), g/kg/d	1.5	1.2	1.05	0.95	0.85

illness and nitrogen losses. "Nonprotein calories" are calories provided by carbohydrates and fat. The recommended ratio is 130 to 150 kcal (nonprotein)/ g nitrogen (1 g protein = 6.25 g nitrogen). Calories from protein should be included in the total estimated energy requirements to avoid overfeeding.

Estimation of Fat Requirements

Lipids have high caloric density (9 kcal/g) and can help achieve caloric goals not met by carbohydrates (4 kcal/g) in the setting of fluid restriction or hyperglycemia. They prevent essential fatty acid deficiency. Fat calories should not exceed 60% of the total intake to reduce the risk of ketosis.

Estimation of Micronutrient Requirements

Micronutrient requirements for critically ill children are not known. Levels should be checked in chronic malabsorption or if a deficit is suspected. Provide supplementation in conditions associated with increased use or loss. Because humans do not store zinc, constant adequate intake is required; severe compromise of the skin and GI tract integrity may require additional zinc supplementation. Multivitamins should be added to enteral nutrition (EN) and parenteral nutrition (PN).

Functional Considerations for Individualized Nutrition Support in Critically Children

In critically ill children with adequate GI function, EN is preferable to PN because of its lower cost and lower risk of nosocomial infection. However, a variety of factors may prompt a decision to use PN or a combination of the two.

A combination of EN and PN may help supply nutrients as soon as the patient has been stabilized. When feeding critically ill children consider

1. *Limitations to oral intake*: risk of aspiration, dysphagia, gastroesophageal reflux disease (GERD), respiratory instability, noninvasive mechanical

ventilation, sedation, anorexia, or chronic EN using orogastric (OG), naso-gastric (NG), or transcutaneous feeding tubes.

2. *Limitations to use of the GI tract*: paralytic ileus, primary GI disease, intestinal obstruction, severe food allergies, gastric/duodenal ulcer disease and GI bleeding, symptomatic pancreatitis and malabsorption syndromes. Total parenteral nutrition (TPN) or supplemental PN should be used.

3. *Frequent interruptions of EN resulting from medical procedures*: TPN should be used.

4. *Inadequate GI perfusion*: TPN should be used.

5. *Obesity*: Critically ill, obese pediatric patients are at risk of overfeeding. Predicted energy need estimations vary considerably, and use of ideal body weight underestimates resting metabolic rate. Measurement by IC, or estimation of energy needs based on actual weight, without adjustment for the degree of metabolic stress, is recommended. Caloric restriction proposed for critically ill obese adults does not apply to pediatric patients. Protein and fat should not be restricted.

6. *Feeding intolerance and intestinal failure*: Intestinal failure reflects a clinical state of malabsorption necessitating dependence on TPN or supplemental PN. Diminished GI motility, impairment of digestive enzymes or enteral surface capacity, congenital defects (e.g., omphalocele, gastroschisis), infections (e.g., *Clostridium difficile*), inflammatory bowel disease, or surgical resection (e.g., for volvulus) can lead to impaired absorption of nutrients and dumping syndrome (high-output enteral losses). In short-bowel syndrome, enteral feeding remains beneficial for long-term bowel adaptation, and patients should receive small volumes provided continuously with slow advancement, while monitoring ostomy, fistula, and fecal output. Although these patients usually have normal REE, those receiving EN must consume excess calories, usually provided by lipids, and protein to compensate for malabsorption.

Enteral Nutrition

Enteral feeding is the most important stimulus for villous growth, bile flow, intestinal motility, and bowel adaptation. Patients recovering from shock or on extracorporeal membrane oxygenation may be fed with caution when cardiac output and end-organ perfusion appear adequate. Infants may present more risk of feeding intolerance and gut ischemia when perfusion is compromised.

OG, NG, or nasoduodenal feeding tubes provide access to the GI tract. Feeding tubes with a distal weight allow peristalsis to advance the distal tip into the intestine. Contraindications to feeding tube placement may include upper respiratory tract or esophagus surgery, GI perforation, suspected basilar skull fracture (cribiform plate), maxillofacial trauma, and thermal or chemical injury to the face, upper respiratory tract, or esophagus. After insertion, position of the feeding tube should be confirmed by radiographic studies.

Intermittent (bolus) feeding replicates the normal pattern of nutrient consumption required for circadian and hormonal homeostasis, but data supporting intermittent gastric meals over continuous EN are not available. Intermittent feedings require a feeding tube in the stomach and tolerance to high-volume bolus meals. Continuous tube feeding requires less volume tolerance and may allow a critically ill patient to reach delivery of full nutrient requirements more quickly, with improved caloric intake. Continuous feeding may be gastric or postpyloric. Postpyloric feeding should be considered when gastric feeding has not been tolerated or causes distension, discomfort, large residuals, or aspiration. However, small bowel feeding may not prevent abdominal distension, diarrhea, or aspiration.

Trophic feedings are continuous, small-volume infusions intended to prevent or treat small bowel mucosal atrophy that may occur when bowel mucosa does not receive nutrients. Trophic feeds should not be inferred to satisfy significant nutrient requirements.

To provide full nutrition via the enteral route

1. Determine energy and protein requirements.
2. Determine maximum fluid volume.
3. Select the appropriate enteral formula, based on age, carbohydrate and protein concentrations, and osmolarity. Age-inappropriate formulas may lead to diarrhea, feeding intolerance, hyperglycemia, increased protein load to the kidney, and higher risk of necrotizing enterocolitis in infants. Children with normal bowel function and fluid requirements can tolerate a lactose-free enteral formula based on intact protein and long-chain triglycerides (LCTs). Most pediatric enteral formulas contain a caloric density of 1 kcal/mL. More energy-dense (1.5–2 kcal/mL) formulas help meet caloric needs during fluid restriction or the need for increased calories and protein.

   • *Formulations for malabsorption*: Peptide-based (hydrolyzed protein) formulas contain simple carbohydrates and a mixture of medium-chain triglycerides (MCTs) and LCTs, and are designed for patients with inadequate digestion or abnormal bowel function. Free amino acid-based formulas contain simple carbohydrates and a mix of MCTs and LCT oils, and are appropriate for malabsorption syndromes and milk allergies. Formulas for fat malabsorption contain 55% or more MCT oil supplemented with essential fatty acids, intact protein, and simple carbohydrates. They are valuable for patients with liver failure, cystic fibrosis, or chylothorax.

   • *Formulations for organ insufficiency*: Pulmonary formulas are designed to meet higher caloric requirements and to prevent protein wasting in children with chronic lung disease. They are protein rich and energy dense, but their high caloric density is supplied primarily by lipids to minimize carbon dioxide production from carbohydrates. Renal formulas are designed for patients with renal failure who have ongoing nitrogen losses and require fluid and electrolyte restriction. They have a higher caloric and protein density provided primarily by carbohydrates, oligopeptides, and free amino acids. They have low renal solute loads, with low phosphorus, potassium, and sodium. Metabolic formulas are disease-specific for inborn errors of metabolism and are used with the guidance of a metabolic specialist. Gluten-free formulas should be considered in patients with inflammatory bowel disease.

4. Supplement enteral formulas to reach caloric requirements if necessary. Simple carbohydrate or glucose polymers (4 kcal/g) or vegetable oil (9 kcal/g fat) can be added to increase the caloric density of the formula. MCT oils are absorbed directly into the portal system, may preserve reticuloendothelial bacterial clearance, and do not require bile salts and lipase for digestion and absorption. Indications for their use include malabsorption syndromes and chylothorax. They lack essential fatty acids, which should be provided as well. Protein or amino acid mixtures can be used to reach protein requirements.

Breast milk (20 kcal/30 ml) can be given to the acutely ill infant when available, and can be enriched to meet the estimated nutritional requirements.

Withholding or Limiting Enteral Nutrition

Undigested formula aspirated from the feeding tube may suggest feeding intolerance. However, feeding residuals should not be interpreted as intolerance in the absence of other clinical signs. Withholding EN may be indicated if the amount of residuals is equal to or more than twice the hourly rate on continuous feedings or 50% or more of previous bolus feeding. Bowel rest is indicated for severe abdominal distension or discoloration, signs of gastric or bowel perforation or peritonitis, bilious gastric residuals or emesis, apnea/bradycardia, cardiopulmonary instability, and significant elevation of pancreatic enzymes. For decreased intestinal motility and mild feeding tolerance, a bowel regimen with stool softeners, laxatives, and prokinetics may improve peristalsis and promote stool evacuations until narcotic dosing can be decreased and patient ambulation is possible. In the absence of need for bowel rest, residuals can be measured and reinstilled before resuming feedings.

With significant intestinal losses resulting from malabsorption or intestinal failure, nutrient absorption may be better with continuous tube feeding than with bolus meals. Hydrolyzed protein may be more digestible and is absorbed easily proximal to the mid jejunum. Although enteral lipids slow GI motility, steatorrhea increases losses of calcium, zinc, and magnesium. Children with cystic fibrosis and pancreatic failure suffer from fat malabsorption and loss of fat-soluble vitamins. They require pancreatic enzyme supplementation before and after bolus feeding. For continuous enteral tube feeding, pancreatic enzymes should be provided every 4 hours.

Parenteral Nutrition

Failure of, or contraindication to, EN should prompt initiation of PN. Supplemental PN should be considered if EN does not cover the estimated energy and protein requirements because of slow advancement or limited tolerance. If low-volume EN is started and is inadequate to meet nutritional needs, supplemental PN should continue and be decreased as EN is advanced until the full volume of enteral feeds is reached.

PN is dependent on availability of venous access. Peripheral IVs are adequate for PN with low dextrose concentrations ($\leq$12.5%), but the high osmolarity of high dextrose concentrations require infusion into a central vein. Essential fatty acid deficiency may occur within 7 days of lipid-free PN. Although PN is not associated with increased mortality, it is associated with an increased infection rate and increased risk of volume overload, metabolic acidosis, and electrolyte abnormalities. Relative contraindications for PN are unstable glucose needs (as occurs in hyperinsulinism or metabolic disorders), suspicion of metabolic disorders that could be worsened by parenteral amino acids, and allergy to components in the IV lipid formulation.

To provide nutrient requirements via PN

1. Determine energy and protein requirements.
2. Determine maximum fluid volume.
3. Determine caloric requirements and energy intake partition. Caloric requirements are met by dextrose (4 kcal/g; 50%–60% of caloric needs) and lipid emulsions (9 kcal/g; 15%–20% of caloric requirements). Circulating TGs should be monitored. Levels of more than 350 mg/L call for discontinuation of IV lipids.
4. Determine protein requirements (Table 14.2).
5. Determine need for specific micronutrients.
6. Monitor tolerance to and adequacy of PN. On initiation of PN, base-line electrolyte levels, blood glucose concentrations, liver function tests, and TG levels should be obtained and then monitored approximately one to three times weekly. If the patient is undergoing dialysis, nitrogen losses in the dialysate should be included in the estimation of the protein needs.

Gastrointestinal Emergencies

Critical illness may be caused by, or associated with, gastrointestinal or other abdominal crises, including both surgical and nonsurgical conditions. Because many patients are unable to provide an adequate history, a high index of suspicion along with careful physical examination, laboratory testing, and radiographic evaluation are essential.

Acute Abdomen

Presentation

The initial evaluation of abdominal pain and/or distension in critically ill children must differentiate between surgical and nonsurgical conditions. Nonverbal patients with static encephalopathy are at risk of abdominal catastrophe without early ominous signs, and heavily sedated patients may be unable to describe symptoms.

Elevated fever and white cell count, with neutrophil and immature form predominance suggest infection, such as peritonitis, appendicitis, or a perforated viscus. A high plasma lactate level and persistent acidosis despite improved perfusion after resuscitation may indicate bowel necrosis. Markedly elevated pancreatic enzymes (more than three times normal) suggest pancreatitis, but may reflect a pancreatic response to other acute conditions.

Evaluation and Management

Plain abdominal radiography may suggest volvulus (intestinal gas centered in the abdominal cavity), or show evidence of a perforated viscus (free air in the abdomen) or pneumatosis intestinalis and air in the portal system, which are associated with necrotizing enterocolitis and with bowel necrosis resulting from mesenteric ischemia. Bedside abdominal ultrasonography can detect free peritoneal fluid; hematomas in solid abdominal viscera; appendicitis; pancreatitis; cystic collections; abscesses; hepatic, biliary, and gallbladder disease; hydronephrosis; cholelithiasis; renal stones; and ovarian and uterine diseases. Doppler imaging can also visualize blood flow to solid organs. An abdominal computed tomographic (CT) scan provides a more detailed evaluation of abdominal structures, but patients require transfer to a CT suite and use of IV contrast, which may be detrimental in the presence of acute kidney injury, or oral contrast, which may not be tolerated.

Immediate stabilization and treatment of shock is essential. Patients should be made NPO (nothing by mouth), with an OG/NG tube placed for decompression, and surgical consultation and radiological evaluations should be obtained. Acute anemia or coagulopathy may require treatment as part of the initial stabilization. Broad antibiotic coverage for Gram-positive and -negative aerobic and anaerobic bacteria should be initiated empirically. If surgery is required, continued resuscitation in the operating room may be necessary.

Abdominal Compartment Syndrome

Presentation

Tense abdominal distension may accompany surgical and nonsurgical conditions (including peritonitis, pancreatitis, liver or kidney failure with ascites, and trauma). Intra-abdominal pressure exceeding 20 mm Hg may compromise perfusion of intra-abdominal organs and lead to renal failure, impaired lung function, and decreased venous return to the heart.

Management

In addition to making the patient NPO and placing an NG tube, close monitoring of bladder pressures, renal function, and urine output is essential. Central venous pressure should be monitored in the superior vena cava. Systemic blood pressure support with vasoactive agents may be necessary to maintain adequate organ perfusion pressures. Persistent, high blood lactate levels in the setting of adequate mixed venous oxygen saturation and distal perfusion suggests bowel ischemia. Surgical consultation should be obtained. Abdominal decompression by paracentesis is appropriate if there is free fluid, and decompression may be necessary.

Upper Gastrointestinal Hemorrhage

Presentation

Hematemesis or bright red blood in the gastric tube indicates upper GI bleeding (proximal to the ligament of Treitz). Hemodynamic instability may develop. The most common causes in infants and children include esophageal and gastric varices, gastric or duodenal ulcers, and esophagitis or gastritis (including *Helicobacter pylori* infection).

Evaluation and Management

Hemodynamic stabilization is essential, but volume resuscitation should not be excessive. Targeting a central venous pressure less than or equal to 10 mm Hg minimizes the risk of recurrent bleeding, especially from varices. Hemoglobin concentration should be monitored every 2 to 4 hours initially, depending on the severity of bleeding. Packed red blood cells should be transfused to maintain intravascular volume and hemoglobin greater than 7 g/dL. Transfusion of plasma and/or platelets may be required in the presence of coagulopathy, platelet dysfunction, thrombocytopenia, or heparinization (in which case protamine may also be needed). Patients should be NPO, should have an OG/NG tube placed to minimize aspiration risk and provide gastric access, and should receive proton pump inhibitors or H2 blockers for acid suppression. Administration of octreotide (1–5 μgm/kg/h) or vasopressin (0.002–0.01 U/kg/min) to decrease splanchnic blood flow is a routine element of treatment. Vitamin K (1–10 mg IV) can be used to ensure adequate substrate for coagulation factor synthesis and recombinant factor VIIa (90–270 μg/kg) for uncontrolled life-threatening bleeding, although supporting data are limited. Radionuclide scans with radioactively tagged red blood cells can be used to locate the site of GI bleeding.

Persistent life-threatening bleeding may require emergency therapeutic endoscopy in the operating room for cauterization of a bleeding vessel, with surgical availability in case of the need for an urgent laparotomy. The use of β blockers is not recommended in acute GI hemorrhage.

The presence of hematochezia or melena indicates lower GI bleeding. Although rarely massive, life-threatening lower GI bleeding may require an emergent laparotomy and colectomy.

Gastroesophageal Reflux Disease

Presentation

Severe GERD and bronchial aspiration can lead to acute life-threatening events: apnea and bradycardia in infants, severe pneumonia, and hypoxemic respiratory failure.

Evaluation

A multichannel study such as the oxycardiorespirogram can be performed with simultaneous measurement of the esophageal pH, heart rate, and resting rate to correlate derangements in vital signs with decreases in esophageal pH that occur during gastroesophageal reflux. Direct laryngoscopy may show signs of vocal cord swelling, supraglottic granulation, and mucosal erosive changes in upper airways from acid injury. A fluoroscopic upper GI study with swallowed contrast may show laryngeal penetrance and severe GERD. Aspiration may be demonstrated when suctioning the endotracheal tube (and finding formula or food particles) or during bronchoscopy/bronchial aspiration (lipid-laden macrophages).

Management

Patients require heart rate, resting rate, blood pressure, and saturated oxygen monitoring and may need intubation and mechanical ventilation. Management includes thickened feedings, raising the head of the bed to 30° to 45°, and the use of acid-suppressing medications. Metoclopramide, a prokinetic agent, may also have value but is associated frequently with neurological side effects. If these steps fail, gastric fundoplication may be indicated

Pancreatitis

Presentation

Most patients have severe abdominal pain (usually epigastric) and elevation of pancreatic enzymes, and may have periumbilical or flank ecchymosis. Severe pancreatitis can lead to a systemic inflammatory response, shock, severe capillary leak, hypocalcemia, and acute respiratory distress syndrome.

Evaluation and Management

Severe disease requires placement of an OG/NG tube for decompression, aggressive pain management, and radiological evaluations. Bedside abdominal ultrasound can evaluate cystic collections; abscesses; and hepatic, biliary, and gallbladder disease. An abdominal CT scan provides a more detailed evaluation of biliary structures. Early nutrition appears to improve outcome; in adults, it is associated with decreased infection and multiorgan failure, decreased mortality, and shorter hospital stay. EN is superior to PN, but some patients will require TPN, or continuous tube feeding in the third portion of the duodenum with or without PN until abdominal pain subsides. Surgical consultation is appropriate, particularly for patients with hemorrhagic necrosis, but surgical intervention is not usually required.

Acute Liver Failure

Presentation

Acute liver failure is often rapidly progressive and associated with multiorgan system dysfunction. The most threatening of these is acute hepatic encephalopathy. Patients may transition rapidly from normal brain function through fatigue and listlessness and/or irritability, to coma (associated with severe cerebral edema), herniation, and brain death. Severe coagulopathy, respiratory insufficiency, hypoglycemia, and renal failure are also common. Because progression is so often very rapid, early consultation by a pediatric gastroenterologist and referral to a transplant center is strongly recommended.

Chronic liver failure, often with cirrhosis, may prompt admission to the PICU for an episode of variceal bleeding, progressive renal dysfunction, infection (including peritonitis), or respiratory compromise.

Evaluation and Management

Patients often develop rapidly progressive jaundice and deteriorating mental status. Ascites is uncommon unless acute liver failure is occurring with a background of chronic disease. In patients with new-onset liver failure, studies to identify the cause may include those listed in Table 14.3. Laboratory evaluation and ongoing monitoring also should include complete blood count with platelets, prothrombin time/partial thromboplastin time, serum electrolytes, calcium, magnesium, phosphate, glucose, BUN and creatinine, total protein, albumin, transaminases, bilirubin, ammonia, amylase, and lipase. Acid–base evaluation is also important. Abdominal ultrasound for evidence of vascular or biliary abnormalities, liver size, and possible mass lesions is indicated. Head computed tomography may help assess the severity of cerebral edema.

In most cases, treatment is nonspecific; early evaluation for liver transplantation is appropriate. Close respiratory and hemodynamic monitoring guides ventilatory and cardiovascular support. Norepinephrine may be particularly valuable for hypotension related primarily to vasodilatation.

IV fluid administration with close attention to serum glucose levels is essential; 5 to 8 mg/kg/min or more of dextrose may be needed. Interruptions of dextrose delivery must be avoided. Hypokalemia and hypophosphatemia are common and can be corrected with potassium phosphate. Avoiding cerebral edema while maintaining adequate renal perfusion can be challenging. Isotonic fluids are appropriate to maintain intravascular volume and urine output. Furosemide (1–3 mg/kg/d, increased as needed) may be necessary. Episodes of hypovolemia and/or hypotension secondary to hemorrhage or excessive fluid restriction may precipitate the hepatorenal syndrome. Prevention of GI hemorrhage with proton pump inhibitors (e.g., pantoprozole 0.5–1.0 mg/kg/g for patients weighing less than 20 kg) or H2 blocking agents (e.g., ranitidine 1–3 mg/kg every 6 hours) is appropriate.

If coagulopathy is severe and associated with bleeding, common recommendations include administration of fresh frozen plasma (15–20 mL/kg), although it is not clear there is significant value except in instances of significant

Table 14.3 Evaluation of Acute Liver Failure		
Age	**Routine evaluation**	**Consider**
≤3 mo	• Ferritin • Herpes simplex virus PCR • Enterovirus PCR • CMV PCR • Acylcarnitine profile	• Lactate • Pyruvate • Blood culture • Urine culture	• Galactose 1-phosphate uridyltransferase (red blood cell assay) • Transthoracic echocardiogram (hypoplastic left heart)
>3 mo	• Hepatitis A, B, C serology • HSV PCR • Acetaminophen level • Acylcarnitine profile • Lactate • Pyruvate	• Antinuclear antibody, Smooth muscle antibody, Anti-liver/kidney microsome antibodies • Immunoglobulin G • Blood culture • Urine culture • Urine drug screen	• Enterovirus PCR • Epstein-Barr virus PCR • CMV PCR • Fibrinogen • Ferritin (very high in HLH, nonspecific) • Triglyceride (high in HLH) • Hepatitis E antibody • Halogenated hydrocarbons • Other drugs
For children >3–5 years, add	• Ceruloplasmin		

CMV, cytomegalovirus; HLH, Hemophagocytic Lymphohistiocytosis

PCR, polymerase chain reaction.

bleeding or in preparation for invasive procedures. Recombinant factor VIIa usually corrects coagulopathy for 6 to 12 hours, but is extremely expensive; its use is usually limited to preparation for invasive procedures or in a patient with life-threatening hemorrhage. Fresh frozen plasma administration represents a large volume load; hemofiltration or plasma exchange may help avoid hypervolemia.

Hepatic encephalopathy has no specific treatment. Measures to minimize serum ammonia include avoiding GI bleeding and administering lactulose (1–2 mL/kg every 4–6 hours), neomycin (50–100 mg/kg/d), or rifaximin (10–30 mg/kg/d, orally, to a maximum of 1200 mg/d, divided every 8 hours). Minimizing both stimulation and pharmacological sedation, especially benzodiazepines, as well as fever, is appropriate. Endotracheal intubation (typically with narcotics and neuromuscular blockade) and mechanical ventilation are commonly necessary as hepatic encephalopathy progresses to grade III (Table 14.4), as well as for primary respiratory dysfunction commonly

Table 14.4 Grades of Hepatic Encephalopathy	
Grade	Description
I	Patient demonstrates confusion and mood changes
II	Patient is drowsy or shows inappropriate behavior
III	Patient is sleepy or stuporous but obeys simple commands
IVa	Patient is comatose but arousable with painful stimuli
IVb	Patient is in a coma and not arousable

complicating acute liver failure. Aside from adequate oxygenation, the appropriate goal of ventilation is uncertain. A partial pressure of carbon dioxide of 35 mm is sometimes recommended, but may not be sufficient ventilation to avoid intracranial hypertension in a child who has been breathing spontaneously to a much lower partial pressure of carbon dioxide. Monitoring intracranial pressure may be desirable, but is associated with significant risk because of the coagulopathy. There may be value to moderate hypothermia.

Patients with severe multisystem dysfunction may benefit from plasma exchange or continuous hemofiltration, with or without dialysis. Goals include maintenance of appropriate intravascular volume, correction of electrolyte concentrations and acid–base balance, improved coagulation, and administration of nutrition without worsening hyperammonemia.

Further Reading

Alberda C, Gramlich L, Jones N, et al. The relationship between nutritional intake and clinical outcomes in critically ill patients: results of an international multicenter observational study. *Intensive Care Med.* 2009;35(10):1728–1737.

Bechard LJ, Parrott JS, Mehta NM. Systematic review of energy and protein intake on protein balance in critically ill children. *J Pediatr.* 2012.

Carcillo JA, Michael DJ, Holubkov R, et al. The randomized comparative pediatric critical illness stress-induced immune suppression (CRISIS) prevention trial. *Pediatr Crit Care Med.* 2012;13(2):165–173.

Coss-Bu JA, Klish WJ, Walding D, et al. Energy metabolism, nitrogen balance, and substrate utilization in critically ill children. *Am J Clin Nutr.* 2001;74(5):664–669.

Heidegger CP, Darmon P, Pichard C. Enteral vs. parenteral nutrition for the critically ill patient: a combined support should be preferred. *Curr Opin Crit Care.* 2008;14(4):408–414.

Heyland DK, Cahill NE, Dhaliwal R, et al. Impact of enteral feeding protocols on enteral nutrition delivery: results of a multicenter observational study. *JPEN J Parenter Enteral Nutr.* 2010;34(6):675–684.

Hulst JM, van Goudoever JB, Zimmermann LJ, et al. The effect of cumulative energy and protein deficiency on anthropometric parameters in a pediatric ICU population. *Clin Nutr.* 2004;23(6):1381–1389.

Meert KL, Daphtary KM, Metheny NA. Gastric vs small-bowel feeding in critically ill children receiving mechanical ventilation: a randomized controlled trial. *Chest.* 2004;126(3):872–878.

Mehta NM, Compher C. A.S.P.E.N. clinical guidelines: nutrition support of the critically ill child. *JPEN J Parenter Enteral Nutr.* 2009;33(3):260–276.

Mziray-Andrew CH, Sentongo TA. Nutritional deficiencies in intestinal failure. *Pediatr Clin North Am.* 2009;56(5):1185–1200.

Narkewicz MR, Olio DD, Karpen SJ, et al. Pattern of diagnostic evaluation for the causes of pediatric acute liver failure: an opportunity for quality improvement. *J Pediatr.* 2009;155:801–806

Srinath AI, Lowe ME. Pediatric pancreatitis. *Pediatr Rev.* 2013;34:79–90.

Sundaram SS, Alonso EM, Narkewicz, MR, et al. Characterization and outcomes of young infants with acute liver failure. *J Pediatr.* 2011;159:813–818.

van Waardenburg DA, de Betue CT, Goudoever JB, Zimmermann LJ, Joosten KF. Critically ill infants benefit from early administration of protein and energy-enriched formula: a randomized controlled trial. *Clin Nutr.* 2009;28(3):249–255.

Verbruggen SC, Coss-Bu J, Wu M, et al. Current recommended parenteral protein intakes do not support protein synthesis in critically ill septic, insulin-resistant adolescents with tight glucose control. *Crit Care Med.* 2011;39(11):2518–2525.

Verbruggen SC, Schierbeek H, Coss-Bu J, et al. Albumin synthesis rates in post-surgical infants and septic adolescents: influence of amino acids, energy, and insulin. *Clin Nutr.* 2011;30(4):469–477.

World Health Organization. *Protein and Amino Acid Requirements in Human Nutrition.* Report no. 935. Geneva: WHO Press; 2007.

Chapter 15

Infections in the Intensive Care Unit

Samina Afreen, Hector R. Wong, and Marian G. Michaels

General Principles

The major types of infection to consider in the intensive care unit (ICU) are (1) community infections requiring initial ICU management and (2) nosocomial infections complicating hospitalization. In addition, special consideration should be given to infections in the immunocompromised host.

Community-acquired organisms requiring ICU admission can often be predicted by the patient's age or disease manifestations. Nosocomial infections in the ICU are often a result of the disruption of the normal barriers of the body, such as that found with the presence of invasive catheters or surgical procedures. Finally, immunocompromised hosts can present to the ICU with a wide variety of microbial organisms that would be nonpathogenic in a healthy host.

Antimicrobial Use

In the era of increasingly resistant bacteria, it is critical to obtain cultures before administering antimicrobials to inform subsequent therapy, with the aim of narrowing antibiotics as soon as possible. Not only does this impact the child positively by limiting exposure to unnecessary antimicrobials, but also it decreases resistance in the hospital environment and reduces overall healthcare dollars.

Antibiotics are evaluated by their pharmacokinetics and pharmacodynamics as well as their mode of bacterial killing. Microbiology laboratories usually give a standard interpretation of an organism being sensitive or resistant to a particular drug based on the following properties:

- *Pharmacokinetics*: Measures how the body handles the drug regarding absorption, distribution, metabolism, and excretion
- *Pharmacodynamics*: Evaluates how the drug affects the body at the level needed to attack the organism (e.g., safety profile and mechanism of action)
- *Minimal inhibitory concentration*: the minimal amount of drug needed to inhibit bacterial growth, taking into account the general amount of drug level achieved safely in the body

The safety profile, ability to kill bacteria in the site found, and interactions with other medications all need to be considered when deciding on empiric antibiotics.

Infections Leading to Intensive Care Unit Hospitalization

Sepsis and Bacteremia

Bacteremia leading to sepsis can be a major cause of morbidity and mortality. The timeliness of administration of appropriate therapy impacts morbidity and mortality. Septic shock is covered in detail in Chapter 8, so this chapter deals with bacteremia in general. Wide use of immunizations in the United States has decreased episodes of bacteremia (and meningitis) significantly but has not eliminated them completely. Bacteremia requiring ICU admission is usually associated with systemic inflammatory response syndrome and cardiovascular or respiratory dysfunction. Common risk factors and laboratory evaluation follow.

Predisposing Factors
- Prematurity, particularly those with very low birth weight
- Age younger than 1 year
- Unimmunized status
- Underlying illnesses
  - Immunodeficiency
  - Splenic dysfunction
  - Congenital heart disease
  - Primary organ dysfunction (e.g., renal, hepatic, or pulmonary disease)
- Intravascular device

Investigations
- Before antibiotic therapy, if possible, obtain
  - Two blood cultures, at least one drawn percutaneously
  - Cultures of other sites as indicated clinically (e.g., urine with urine analysis, cerebrospinal fluid [CSF], wounds, respiratory secretions, or other bodily fluids)
- Complete blood count (CBC) with differential and platelets
- Complete metabolic panel (electrolytes, blood urea nitrogen [BUN], creatinine, liver function tests)
- Arterial blood gas (in the setting of severe respiratory distress and/or hemodynamic instability)
- Fibrinogen, coagulation factors (prothrombin time, partial thromboplastin time)
- C-reactive protein or procalcitonin levels (controversial, but often obtained to assist with following course)
- Consider lactate level

Treatment: Antibiotic Therapy

Intravenous antibiotics should be started as soon as possible for severe sepsis, ideally after obtaining appropriate cultures. However, technical difficulties in obtaining appropriate cultures should not delay antibiotic administration. The empiric antimicrobial therapy should be based on the likely pathogen and should be able to penetrate the presumed source of infection. Antibiotics should be modified on the basis of culture results, with therapy targeting the microbe with as narrow a spectrum as possible. In general, for bacteremia, bactericidal antibiotics are preferred over bacteriostatic ones (Table 15.1). In addition to appropriate antibiotic treatment, adequate management often requires source control as listed below.

Source Control
- Drainage of abscess or local focus of infection
- Debridement of necrotic tissue
- Removal of a device identified as infected

Oropharyngeal and Neck Infections

Oropharyngeal and neck infections are associated frequently with airway obstruction and may be associated with sepsis/septic shock and/or involvement of mediastinal structures (Table 15.2).

Community-Acquired Pneumonia

Worldwide, pneumonia is a major cause of mortality and morbidity in children younger than 5 years. Diagnostic evaluation is limited because of the inability to sample lung specimens noninvasively. In the United States, viruses are the major cause of community-acquired pneumonia in children younger than 5 years, although bacteria such as *Streptococcus pneumoniae* and *Staphylococcus aureus* need to be considered in those with more severe community-acquired pneumonia requiring ICU care. Bacteria are more likely if there is a lobar

Table 15.1 Community-Associated Bacteremia		
Age Group, mo	**Microorganisms**	**Empiric antibiotics**
<2	Group B streptococcus *Listeria monocytogenes* Enteric Gram-negative rods	Ampicillin and aminoglycoside or third-generation cephalosporin
>2	*Streptococcus pneumoniae* *Neisseria meningitidis* *Staphylococcus aureus* *Streptococcus pyogenes*[a]	Third- or fourth-generation cephalosporin Add vancomycin if MRSA or meningitis suspected

MRSA, methicillin-resistant *S. aureus*.

[a] Less frequent causes of bacteremia.

Table 15.2 Oropharyngeal and Neck Infections in the Pediatric Intensive Care Unit

Disease	Usual Age	Clinical Features	Usual Organisms	Treatment
Ludwig's angina: sublingual cellulitis	Adolescents–young adults	Acute onset; fever, chills, odynophagia, drooling, bull neck, brawny boardlike edema of the submandibular region; tongue elevation	Polymicrobial, oral anaerobes predominate: *Staphylococcus aureus, Streptococcus viridans*	Airway management, IV antibiotics against mouth flora (e.g., clindamycin or ampicillin–sulbactam), prompt surgical drainage
Epiglottitis	2–12 y	Acute onset; fever, pharyngitis, drooling, odynophagia, stridor; preference for sitting in tripod position	*Haemophilus influenzae* in unimmunized children, *Streptococcus Pneumoniae*, other streptococcal species, non–Type B encapsulated *H. influenzae* species, *S. aureus*	Person experienced in intubation should secure the airway (usually under inhalational anesthesia); IV antimicrobial therapy: ampicillin–sulbactam, cefuroxime; in areas with high rates of MRSA, third-generation cephalosporin and vancomycin or clindamycin
Bacterial tracheitis	6 mo–8 y	Acute onset fever following upper respiratory viral infection, cough, tachypnea, stridor, hoarseness, preference to lie flat	*S. aureus* predominates, *Streptococcus Pneumoniae*, *Streptococcus pyogenes*, *Moxarella catarrhalis, H. influenzae*	Airway management, frequent suctioning; IV antibiotics directed against *S. aureus* and other common bacteria; empiric therapy should usually include treatment of MRSA, with adjustment made after culture results available; third-generation cephalosporin and vancomycin or clindamycin; consider ampicillin–sulbactam, cefuroxime; inhaled bronchodilators, racemic epinephrine, and steroids are not indicated

Condition	Age group	Clinical features	Microbiology	Treatment
Suppurative jugular thrombophlebitis (Lemierre's syndrome)	Adolescents–young adults	Pharyngitis; high fever; unilateral neck pain and swelling; torticollis; signs of thrombotic spread to lungs, liver, spleen, kidney, or meninges	Fusobacterium necophorum (90%), less commonly other mouth anaerobes, S. aureus, S. pyogenes	Ampicillin–sulbactam if no central nervous system involvement; clindamycin with third-generation cephalosporin ± metronidazole; heparin anticoagulation
Retropharyngeal abscess/phlegmon	<5 y	Preceding URI, nontoxic; fever, decreased oral intake, pharyngitis, drooling, torticollis; asymmetric bulge in posterior pharyngeal wall may be seen	Polymicrobial infection is common, S. pyogenes and anaerobes predominate, S. aureus infrequent	Airway management, IV antimicrobials (ampicillin–sulbactam or clindamycin); surgical drainage if not responsive or progressed to abscess stage
Peritonsillar abscess	Older children, adolescents	Fever, chills, drooling, odynophagia, cervical lymphadenopathy, unilateral swelling of affected tonsillar area, shift of uvula, edema of palatine tonsils, torticollis	S. pyogenes predominates, S. aureus, H. influenzae, mouth anaerobes	IV antibiotics (ampicillin–sulbactam, clindamycin, or clindamycin and third-generation cephalosporin); surgical drainage if not responsive

IV, intravenous; MRSA, methicillin-resistant S. aureus.

presentation or complications such empyema, necrotizing pneumonia, or lung abscess. Mycoplasma should be considered in older children but rarely requires ICU care. Causes of pneumonia in the immunocompromised host are broader, including bacteria, atypical bacteria, viruses, and fungi. Tuberculosis should be considered in travelers and children exposed to high-risk adults (Table 15.3). Complications frequently associated with a need for intensive care and laboratory assessment follow.

Complications
- Pleural effusion
- Necrotizing pneumonia
- Empyema
- Lung abscess
- Pneumothorax
- Sepsis/septic shock
- Respiratory failure/acute respiratory distress syndrome (ARDS)

Table 15.3 Causes of Pneumonia in the Intensive Care Unit		
Age Group	**Common Pathogens**	**Empiric Antimicrobials**
0–3 mo[a]	Group B streptococcus Listeria monocytogenes Bordetella pertussis Viruses (in particular, respiratory syncytial virus, influenza) Chlamydia trachomatis Mycoplasma hominis Ureaplasma urealyticum Treponema pallidum	Ampicillin and aminoglycoside or third-generation cephalosporin No antimicrobials for most viruses in this age group Macrolides for atypical pneumonias Penicillin for T. pallidum
>4 mo–5 y	Viruses: adenovirus, influenza, parainfluenza Streptococcus pneumoniae Staphylococcus aureus	Oseltamivir for influenza Ampicillin for susceptible S. pneumoniae; third-generation cephalosporin for presumed resistant S. pneumoniae or Haemophilus influenza Vancomycin or clindamycin for suspected S. aureus
> 5 years	S. pneumoniae Mycoplasma pneumoniae Chlamydophila pneumoniae Viruses	Ampicillin for susceptible S. pneumoniae; third-generation cephalosporin for presumed resistant S. pneumoniae Macrolide addition for presumed atypical pneumonia Vancomycin or clindamycin for suspected S. aureus

[a] Excluding premature infants in the neonatal intensive care unit.

Investigations
- Chest radiograph
  - Bilateral, perihilar, or interstitial patterns suggest viral etiology
  - Lobar or segmental pattern, or pleural effusion suggest bacterial etiology
- Blood culture
- Bacterial culture of tracheal secretions from initial intubation (Gram stain and culture)
- Viral assays on nasopharyngeal wash or flocculated nasopharyngeal swab or tracheal aspirate
- Nucleic acid testing for *Mycoplasma pneumoniae* and *Bordetella pertussis*
- Pulse oximetry and arterial blood gas monitoring
- CBC with differential and platelet
- C-reactive protein, procalcitonin

Criteria for Intensive Care Unit Admission[1]
- Invasive ventilatory support (e.g., intubation)
- Noninvasive positive-pressure ventilation (e.g., continuous positive airway pressure)
- Pulse oximetry less than 92% on a fraction of inspired oxygen ≥0.50
- Impending respiratory failure
  - Increased work of breathing
  - Recurrent apnea
- Cardiovascular insufficiency
  - Sustained tachycardia
  - Blood pressure support refractory to fluid resuscitation
- Altered mental status resulting from hypercarbia or hypoxemia

Toxic Shock Syndrome

Children with suspected toxic shock syndrome (TSS) should be admitted to the pediatric intensive care unit (PICU) early during their course for anticipatory management of multisystem organ failure and hemodynamic instability. The two major causes are *S. aureus* and *Streptococcus pyogenes*. Although distinct mechanistically, both are caused by toxigenic strains of bacteria with overlapping clinical presentations. Staphylococcal TSS is usually associated with an inconsequential site of initial infection or retained foreign body whereas streptococcal TSS most often involves an ongoing wound infection or a complication of varicella; *S. aureus* can also complicate varicella. Criteria for the diagnosis of staphylococcal and streptococcal TSS and approach to management follow.

Case Definitions

Staphylococcal Toxic Shock Syndrome[2,3]
- *Fever*: temperature of 38.9°C or more
- *Cutaneous*: diffuse macular erythroderma
- *Desquamation*: 1 to 2 weeks after onset

- *Hypotension*
  - Systolic blood pressure of 5% or less for age in children younger than 16 years
  - Orthostatic drop in diastolic blood pressure of 15 mm Hg or more from lying to sitting
  - Orthostatic syncope or dizziness
- Multisystem organ involvement with three or more of the following:
  - *Gastrointestinal*: vomiting or diarrhea at onset of illness
  - *Muscular*: severe myalgia or creatinine phosphokinase level more than two times the upper limit of normal
  - *Mucous membrane*: vaginal, oropharyngeal, or conjunctival hyperemia
  - *Renal*: BUN or creatinine level more than two times the upper limit of normal or urinary sediment with five or more white blood cells (WBCs) per high-power field in the absence of a urinary tract infection
  - *Hepatic*: Bilirubin, or liver enzymes more than two times the upper limit of normal
  - *Hematological*: platelet count of $100,000/mm^3$ or less
  - *Central nervous system*: disorientation or altered level of consciousness without focal neurological signs when fever and hypotension are absent
- Negative laboratory criteria
  - Bacterial cultures of blood, CSF, or throat (except *S. aureus*)
  - Serology for Rocky Mountain spotted fever, leptospirosis, measles

Probable case: negative laboratory criteria and four of the five clinical criteria
Confirmed case: Negative laboratory criteria and all five clinical criteria, unless patient dies before desquamation could have occurred

Streptococcal Toxic Shock Syndrome[3]
- Isolation of *S. pyogenes* from
  - Normally sterile site (e.g., blood, CSF, biopsy; *required to meet definitive diagnostic criteria*)
  - Nonsterile site (e.g., throat, vagina, skin lesion)
- Hypotension
  - *Organ systems*: involvement of two or more
  - *Renal*: creatinine level two times or more than the upper limit of normal for age
  - *Hematological*: platelet count of $100,000/mm^3$ or less, or disseminated intravascular coagulation
  - *Hepatic*: Bilirubin, or liver enzymes two times or more than the upper limit of normal for age
  - *Pulmonary*: ARDS
  - *Cutaneous*: generalized erythematous, macular rash
  - *Soft tissue necrosis*: necrotizing fasciitis, myositis, gangrene

Toxic Shock Syndrome Management
- Fluid management and hemodynamic stabilization (Chapter 8)
- Location and drainage of infected sites
  - Removal of foreign materials
- Identification and susceptibility testing of bacteria
- *Empiric antibiotics*: Because it is difficult to distinguish staphylococcal from streptococcal TSS definitively, initial antibiotics should include an antistaphylococcal β-lactam agent (e.g., oxacillin, nafcillin, cefazolin) and a protein synthesis-inhibiting drug (e.g., clindamycin)
  - Vancomycin can be used in areas with high rates of methicillin-resistant *S. aureus* (MRSA)
  - Modification based on identification and susceptibility
  - Continuation of protein synthesis inhibitor for at least several days to stop enzyme or toxin production
- Duration of therapy is 10 to 14 days, depending on the underlying focus of infection.
- Consider intravenous immunoglobulin as adjunctive therapy.

Necrotizing Fasciitis and Soft Tissue Infections

Necrotizing soft tissue infections (NSTIs) are rapidly progressive bacterial infections affecting the dermis, subcutaneous tissue fascia, fat, or muscle fascia. Although infrequent, they have high case fatality rates, particularly if there is a delay in diagnosis with subsequent delay in debridement. All soft tissue infections should be evaluated to rule out a necrotizing component. Early consideration should be given when pain appears disproportionate to clinical findings or when crepitus is present.

Microbiology

NSTIs can be from polymicrobial infection with anaerobes (*Bacteroides* spp., *Peptostreptococcus* spp., or *Clostridium* spp.) and streptococci or Gram-negative rods, or from *S. pyogenes* or *S. aureus* as monomicrobial. *Vibrio* spp. have been reported with seawater or marine mammal exposure.

Predisposing factors include prior surgery, penetrating wounds, varicella (particularly for *S. pyogenes*), diabetes, burns, or underlying immune deficiencies. On rare occasions, necrotizing fasciitis can complicate minor insults to the skin. Evaluation and basic approach to management are included below.

Investigations for Suspected NSTI[4]
- Hematological
  - CBC differential and platelet count, prothrombin time, and partial thromboplastin time
    - Leukocytosis common
    - Thrombocytopenia common
    - Coagulopathy possible
- C-reactive protein, often elevated significantly

- Radiographs
  - Plain films may show gas or soft tissue edema
  - Magnetic resonance images preferred to delineate extent of disease but should not delay surgery
- Surgical evaluation/operative findings
  - Cloudy fluid in the wound
  - Gray fascia without bleeding
  - Lack of resistance to digital exploration of normally adherent fascia
- Pathological examination
  - Neutrophilic infiltration in deeper parts of the dermis, subcutaneous tissue, and fascia
  - *Early*: superficial epidermal hyaline necrosis with dermal and pannicular edema and hemorrhage
  - *Later*: necrosis of all layers of tissue as well as eccrine sweat glands and ducts
- Gram stain and bacterial cultures for aerobes and anaerobes

Treatment
- Aggressive surgical debridement
  - Scheduled frequent debridement should be performed until no further necrosis is noted.
  - Amputation is sometimes required.
- Antimicrobial therapy
  - Broad-spectrum antibiotics should be given emergently to cover Gram-positive and anaerobic bacteria empirically while cultures are pending. *Pseudomonas* coverage should be added if neutropenia is present.
  - *Monotherapy drugs*: carbapenems, piperacillin–tazobactum, or ampicillin–sulbactam
  - Clindamycin added for suspected *S. pyogenes* or *S. aureus* for antitoxin effect
  - Vancomycin or linezolid added for suspected MRSA
- Supportive care
  - Cardiovascular support for sepsis and multiorgan failure (see Chapters 8)
  - Pain control
- Adjuvant therapy
  - Hyperbaric oxygen, should not delay surgical intervention
  - Intravenous immunoglobulin (controversial and lacking randomized controlled studies)

Central Nervous System Infections in the Intensive Care Unit

Meningitis, encephalitis, or a combination of the two account for the main infections of the central nervous system that require ICU care.

Meningitis

Viruses and bacteria are the major causes of meningitis in the previously healthy child. Treatment varies depending on the etiology (Table 15.4). The incidence of bacterial meningitis in the United States has decreased substantially by vaccinations against *Haemophilus influenzae* type b and S. *pneumoniae*. When present, bacterial meningitis has an acute onset that requires prompt antimicrobial treatment. Viral meningitis is usually self-limited and infrequently requires ICU care. Tuberculous meningitis has a subacute clinical course but often requires ICU management and should be considered with appropriate epidemiological exposures and when the CSF has a high protein level, significant hypoglycorrhachia, but negative bacterial culture. Lyme meningitis rarely requires ICU care. Unusual causes of meningitis in previously healthy children such as sporotrichosis, or cryptococcal or amoebic meningitis can be considered in specific epidemiological circumstances.

Clinical Features

Fever, vomiting, mental status changes, lethargy, irritability, decreased activity and appetite, and seizures are clinical features of meningitis. In addition, neonates can have nonspecific signs and present with hypothermia, bulging fontanel, or apnea. Older children are more likely to have headache, neck stiffness, and photophobia. Petechiae or purpuric rash suggests meningococcus. Dexamethasone should be considered for unimmunized children with suspected *H. influenzae* type b meningitis. Laboratory evaluation should include the following:

Investigations
- Lumbar puncture
  - Cell count
  - Glucose
  - Protein
  - Gram stain/bacterial culture
  - Consider polymerase chain reaction (PCR) for enterovirus, herpes simplex virus (HSV)
  - Acid-fast bacilli stain/culture when considering tuberculosis

Table 15.4 Common Causes of Meningitis in the Intensive Care Unit

Age Group, mo	Microorganisms	Empiric Antibiotics
<2	Enterovirus Group B streptococcus *Listeria monocytogenes* Enteric Gram-negative rods Herpes simplex virus[a]	Ampicillin and aminoglycoside or cefotaxime Acyclovir[a]
>2	*Streptococcus pneumoniae* *Neisseria meningitidis*	Third- or fourth-generation cephalosporin and vancomycin

[a] Consider in babies ≤4 weeks, particularly in those presenting with seizures or vesicles.

- Bacterial blood culture
- CBC, differential and platelets
- Electrolytes, BUN, creatinine, glucose
  - Serum glucose just prior to lumbar puncture to compare CSF glucose
- Monitoring of urine output and electrolytes for syndrome of inappropriate antidiuretic hormone secretion

Neurologic complications and other organ system dysfunction often accompany or follow meningitis.

Complications of Meningitis
- Sensorineural hearing loss
- Syndrome of inappropriate antidiuretic hormone secretion
- Neurological deficits
  - Seizures
  - Impaired motor or cognitive functioning
  - Hydrocephalus
  - Cranial nerve palsy
- Renal or cardiac dysfunction, ARDS, Disseminated intravascular coagulation (DIC), adrenal hemorrhage, arthritis

Encephalitis

Infectious encephalitis is usually of viral etiology. Although supportive care is required for all, HSV encephalitis also requires immediate administration of high-dose intravenous acyclovir. It should be considered in all cases of encephalitis, but particularly in those children presenting with focal seizures or temporal lobe changes on magnetic resonance imaging or electroencephalogram. Diagnosis is confirmed by HSV PCR testing of the CSF. Treatment of neonates should be for a minimum of 21 days, whereas 14 to 21 days is recommended for older children and adults. Repeat CSF examination toward the end of therapy, with continuation if HSV PCR remains positive, is recommended.

Other causes of encephalitis in children include arboviruses, enterovirus, other herpes viruses, and respiratory viruses. Rabies remains a rare cause of encephalitis in the United States as a result of the attention paid to vaccination of domestic animals and postexposure prophylaxis. When symptoms occur, survival is rare. Protocols for treatment of proven rabies can be found at the Medical College of Wisconsin website (www.mcw.edu/rabies).

Nosocomial Infections in the Intensive Care Unit and Preventive Strategies

Healthcare-associated infections (HAIs) are an important patient safety threat facing children in the ICU.

Central Line-Associated Bloodstream Infections

Central line-associated bloodstream infections (CLABSIs) are among the most common HAIs affecting children in PICUs, and 65% to 70% of CLABSI may be preventable. Common risk factors and preventive measures are listed below.

Risk Factors
- Lack of appropriate catheter care practices
- Central venous access duration of more than 7 days
- Underlying oncological diseases, abdominal surgery, or intestinal insufficiency
- Patient characteristics (e.g., genetic syndromes, congenital malformations)
- Multiple ICU interventions (e.g., blood transfusion)
- Extracorporeal therapy (e.g., renal replacement therapy, extracorporeal membrane oxygenation)
- Additional risks in cardiac ICU
  - Noncardiac comorbidities
  - Unscheduled medical admission

Microbiology
- Approximately 90% of CLABSIs are caused by a single organism
- Coagulase-negative *Staphylococcus* predominates
- Gram-positive cocci > Gram-negative rods > fungal > Gram-positive bacilli

Basic Interventions to Reduce CLABSI Rates
- Hand hygiene
- Skin antisepsis with chlorhexidine
- Maximal sterile barriers during catheter insertion
- Attention to catheter maintenance and dressing changes
- Minimizing entry into catheters (e.g., by clustering times of blood sampling for laboratory studies)
- Reassessment of central access need
- Prompt removal of unnecessary catheters

Adjunctive (But More Costly) Interventions to Prevent CLABSI
- Antibiotic-coated catheters
- Antiseptic-impregnated sponges
- Antibiotic or ethanol lock or flush solutions

Ventilator-Associated Pneumonia

Pneumonia is second most common HAI in the PICU. Understanding the risk factors allows for strategies to prevent ventilator-associated pneumonia (VAP). Note that the definitions are somewhat controversial, and the Centers for Disease Control and Prevention (CDC) have combined radiological, clinical, and microbiological criteria to improve sensitivity and specificity.

Classification
- *Early VAP*: less than4 days ventilation
- *Late VAP*: more than 4 days ventilation

Pathogenesis

Tracheal colonization with pathogenic bacteria from the upper airway or the endotracheal tube leads to tracheobronchitis and then to VAP.

Microbiology

S. aureus and *Pseudomonas aeruginosa* are the most commonly isolated pathogens.

Risk Factors
• Underlying factors
  • Genetic syndrome
  • Female
  • Neuromuscular weakness
  • Immunodeficiency
  • Narcotic use
• Nosocomial factors
  • Enteral, nasoenteral feeds
  • Immunosuppression
  • Nebulizers or manipulation of ventilatory circuits
  • Surgery
  • H2 blocking agents (and possibly Proton Pump Is)
  • Reintubation
• Transport out of PICU while intubated

Diagnosis

Direct examination and culture of lung tissue is the gold standard but is rarely available. Instead, diagnosis is based on indirect criteria using a constellation of patient characteristics

Diagnostic Criteria Based on CDC Algorithms
• Mechanical ventilation for more than 2 days and CDC clinically defined pneumonia
  • Two or more serial chest radiographs with new or progressive and persistent radiographic infiltrates, consolidation, cavitation, or pneumatoceles for infants younger than 12 months (one or more radiographs is sufficient for children without underlying disease)
• *Plus* three of the following
  • Children between 1 year and 12 years
    • *Temperature*: hypothermia, less than 36.5°C; fever, more than 38.4°C
    • *Peripheral WBC count*: less than 4000/mm^3 or more than 15,000/mm^3
    • New onset of purulent sputum, or increased respiratory secretions or suctioning requirements
    • New onset or worsening cough, dyspnea, apnea, or tachypnea
    • Rales or bronchial breath sounds
    • Worsening gas exchange

Table 15.5 Major Immunodeficiencies Requiring Intensive Care Unit Care

Type of Immunodeficiency	Clinical and Laboratory Findings	Comments/Treatment Issues
Combined immunodeficiency disorders		
Severe combined immunodeficiencies	Present during the first 6 mo of life with severe fungal, bacterial, viral, or opportunistic infections (e.g., PCP); can have persistent thrush, chronic diarrhea, pneumonia, failure to thrive	Consider in infants with severe lymphopenia Require aggressive investigation of fevers and treatment of infections Require HSCT Irradiated and CMV-negative blood products Avoid live vaccines
Hematopoietic stem cell transplant recipients	Broad immunosuppression of all cell lines until engraftment; GVHD impairs immune reconstitution and interrupts mucosal integrity	Preengraftment (0–30 d): bacteria predominate Empiric coverage for *Streptococcus viridans* and Gram-negative rods, including pseudomonas Postengraftment (30–100 d): opportunistic infections predominate Late: GVHD a major determinant of infection, invasive fungal risk
HIV/AIDS	Without antiretroviral therapy, recurrent bacterial infections, PCP, recalcitrant thrush, failure to thrive, chronic diarrhea, dermatitis; can have high levels of IgG, but dysfunctional	Significantly decreased in United States because of routine prenatal screening of pregnant women and treatment to prevent mother-to-child transmission Consider in children with PCP, or those with serious bacterial processes, particularly if mother not screened during pregnancy PCP prophylaxis until 1 y of age regardless of CD4 count
Ig deficiency disorders		
X-linked gamma globulinemia	Recurrent encapsulated bacterial infections, sinopulmonary infections, mycoplasma arthritis, chronic enteroviral encephalitis; can have associated dermatomyositis	Can present to ICU with severe infection from encapsulated organisms (*Haemophilus influenzae b, Streptococcus pneumoniae*) Require Ig replacement

(Continued)

Table 15.5 Continued

Type of Immunodeficiency	Clinical and Laboratory Findings	Comments/Treatment Issues
Common-variable immunodeficiency	Recurrent bacterial infections, chronic pulmonary disease, chronic giardiasis, intestinal malabsorption, autoimmune diseases	Variable presentations; can present to ICU with bacterial processes
X-linked immunodeficiency with hyper-IgM syndrome	Recurrent bacterial infections, opportunistic infections, pneumonia, PCP, CMV, *Aspergillus*, *Cryptosporidium*	Aggressive treatment of infection
Primary T-cell deficiency		
DiGeorge syndrome (chromosome 22q11 deletion)	Congenital cardiac defects, particularly those involving the great vessels; dysmorphic facies; hypocalcemic tetany; variable T-cell deficiency based on thymic function	Cardiac repair HSCT or thymic transplant Irradiated and CMV-negative blood products Avoidance of live vaccines
Ataxia–telangiectasia	Cerebellar ataxia, oculocutaneous telangiectasia, recurrent sinopulmonary infection leading to bronchiectasis, lymphomas	Avoidance of radiation exposure, live vaccines, and blood transfusions Supportive care
Solid-organ transplantation	T-cell immunity affected more than humoral immunity	Early infections (0–30 d): bacteria predominate; associated with surgical procedures and indwelling devices Middle period (30–180 d): opportunistic infections, reactivation of latent herpes viruses or donor-associated viruses, CMV and Epstein–Barr virus/PTLD Late period: influenced by chronic rejection and organ transplanted; PTLD risk persists
Phagocyte defects		
Chronic granulomatous disease	Serious infection with organisms that do not produce hydrogen peroxide (e.g., *Streptococcus. aureus*, *Serratia* spp., *Burkholderia cepacia*), invasive *Aspergillus*	Interferon γ, trimethoprim sulfamethoxasole, fungal prophylaxis Aggressive treatment of bacterial and fungal infections Consider white blood cell transfusions for invasive *Aspergillus*

Table 15.5 Continued

Type of Immunodeficiency	Clinical and Laboratory Findings	Comments/Treatment Issues
Chediak-Higashi syndrome	Partial albinism, variable neurological defects; recurrent severe infection with *S. aureus* that eventually culminates in lymphoproliferation with hemophagocytosis, which is often fatal	HSCT, antibiotics to control infections Surgery to drain abscesses
Leukocyte adhesion defect	Delayed separation of umbilical cord, invasive bacterial infections first 6 mo of life, poor wound healing, severe periodontal disease	Aggressive antibiotic therapy HSCT Irradiated and CMV-negative blood products
Cyclic neutropenia	Fever, stomatitis, periodontitis, skin infections during periods of low neutrophil count; most are benign and recover without therapy; however, necrotizing fasciitis from *Clostridium septicum* and other anaerobes can lead to ICU admission and is a surgical emergency	Present to ICU with necrotizing fasciitis Intravenous antibiotic therapy Granulocyte-colonizing stimulating factor Prompt evaluation of rapidly spreading cellulitis
Complement deficiency		
Defects of terminal complement components (C5–C9)	Susceptibility to recurrent *Neisseria* infections	Immunize against *Neisseria meningitidis* and treat with intravenous antibiotics
Deficiency of C2, C3, C4	Increased risk of developing rheumatic disorders; can present with severe infection with encapsulated bacteria	Immunize against encapsulated bacteria and treat infections aggressively
Deficiency of factor H	Familial relapsing hemolytic uremic syndrome	Hemolytic uremic syndrome management Consider eculizumab

CMV, cytomegalovirus; GVHD, graft-versus-host disease; HSCT, hematopoietic stem cell transplantation; ICU, intensive care unit; Ig, immunoglobin; PCP, *Pneumocystis jiroveci* pneumonia; PTLD, posttransplant lymphoproliferative disorder.

- Children 1 year or younger
  - Temperature instability
  - *Peripheral WBC count*: less than 4000/mm^3 or more than 15,000/mm^3 and left shift (≥10% band forms)
  - New onset of purulent sputum, or increased respiratory secretions or suctioning requirements
  - Apnea, tachypnea, nasal flaring with retraction of chest wall, or grunting
  - Wheezing, rales, or rhonchi
  - Cough
  - Bradycardia (<100 beats/min) or tachycardia (>170 beats/min)

Prevention Measures
- Ventilator bundle
  - Elevating the head end of the bed to 30° to 45°
  - Sedation vacation (daily scheduled interruptions in sedation)
- Deep Venous Thrombosis (DVT) prophylaxis
- Daily assessment of readiness to extubate
- Age-appropriate comprehensive mouth care

Antimicrobial Therapy
Empiric therapy should cover *S. aureus* and *P. aeruginosa*, such as carbapenems, cefepime, or piperacillin–tazobactam. Vancomycin or linezolid can be added in facilities with high rates of MRSA or for critically ill children in whom MRSA is prevalent. Daptomycin should not be used for lung disease with MRSA because of surfactant inhibition. Antibiotic coverage should be adjusted after identifying pathogens. Treatment duration is 5 to 7 days in patients with uncomplicated disease. Longer treatment courses may be warranted for critically ill children infected with multidrug-resistant organisms.

Infections in Immunocompromised Host

Children with known primary or acquired immune deficiencies are at risk for serious infections that influence treatment and management in the ICU setting. In addition, children presenting with specific infections may require evaluation of their immune competence. Table 15.5 highlights some of the major immune deficiencies and types of infections that lead to ICU care.

References

1. Bradley JS, Byington CL, Shah SS, et al. The management of community-acquired pneumonia in infants and children older than 3 months of age: clinical practice guidelines by the Pediatric Infectious Diseases Society and the Infectious Diseases Society of America. *Clin Infect Dis*. 2011;53(7):e25.

2. Chuang Y-Y, Huang Y-C, Lin T-Y. Toxic shock syndrome in children: epidemiology, pathogenesis, and management. *Pediatr Drugs*. 2005;7(1):11–25.

3. American Academy of Pediatrics. *Staphylococcus aureus* toxic shock syndrome, streptococcal toxic shock syndrome. In: Pickering LK, Baker CJ, Kimberlin DW, Long SS, eds. *Red Book: 2012 Report of the Committee on Infectious Diseases* Elk Grove Village, IL: Academy of Pediatrics; 2012:654–670.

4. Anaya DA, Patchen Dellinger E. Necrotizing soft-tissue infection: diagnosis and management. *Clin Infect Dis*. 2007;44:705–710.

5. Venkatachalam V, Hendley JO, Wilson DF. The diagnostic dilemma of ventilator-associated pneumonia in critically ill children. *Pediatr Crit Care Med*. 2011;12:286–296.

Chapter 16

Endocrine Disorders in Pediatric Critical Care

Carmen L. Soto-Rivera and Michael S. D. Agus

Hypernatremia

Diabetes Insipidus

Diabetes insipidus (DI) is caused by an inability of the kidneys to concentrate urine either because of a deficiency of antidiuretic hormone (ADH) secretion from the hypothalamus and posterior pituitary gland (central) or renal unresponsiveness to ADH (nephrogenic). Nephrogenic DI in children is most commonly X-linked recessive, presenting in males during early infancy.

Pathophysiology

Central DI (lack of ADH) can result from hypothalamic or pituitary lesions resulting from congenital (e.g., septo-optic dysplasia, holoprosencephaly, midline craniofacial defects) or acquired causes (e.g., trauma, neoplasms including as a complication of their removal, infiltrative processes, drugs). In the absence of ADH, urine is inappropriately dilute, and a hyperosmolar state develops. If this happens abruptly, it may lead to dehydration of neural tissues, which can cause serious neurological sequelae or result in death. The pons is particularly sensitive to this effect, which results in central pontine myelinolysis.

Clinical Manifestations

In DI, failure of water reabsorption results in increased urine excretion (polyuria), frequently presenting as enuresis or nocturia. Provided the thirst mechanism is intact and fluids are accessible (and the child is developmentally capable of reaching them), the child can compensate for the water loss by drinking more (usually up to 3–4 L/m^2/day). If fluids are not available or if fluid intake is interrupted because of an illness, hypertonic dehydration ensues rapidly. Failure to compensate for fluid losses can also present as chronic dehydration and failure to thrive. However, if the cries of the infant are interpreted as hunger rather than thirst, the infant with DI may be obese.

Physical examination may be normal, or signs of dehydration may be present. Because of the hyperosmolarity, the degree of dehydration may be underestimated on physical examination. Symptoms of increased intracranial pressure, visual fields defects, and papilledema may be present from a craniopharyngioma or optic nerve glioma. Hypothalamic or pituitary lesions can lead to other endocrine abnormalities such as secondary hypothyroidism and growth failure.

Laboratory Workup and Usual Findings

DI is diagnosed by demonstrating that the kidneys fail to concentrate urine when fluid intake is restricted. High urinary output (>4 mL/kg/h or >3 L/m^2/day), despite significant dehydration, may provide the first and most convincing evidence for DI. This condition can be difficult to prove in children. Criteria for the diagnosis of DI include

- Elevated serum osmolality (>300 mOsm/L)
- Elevated serum sodium concentration ([Na]; >145 mmol/L)
- Inappropriately dilute urine (osmolality <600 mOsm/L)
- Polyuria persisting for more than 30 minutes
- Other causes of polyuria are ruled out (e.g., diuretics, osmotic contrast agents, hyperglycemia)

The definitive diagnosis may be made by a formal water deprivation test, but an intensive care unit (ICU) patient is unlikely to tolerate this in the acute setting. More commonly, important ICU considerations are current volume status (central venous pressure, clinical measures of right atrial filling, and peripheral perfusion), as well as a detailed clinical history of intake and output, particularly in the operating room.

Management

Acute management is directed toward correction of the dehydration and the hyperosmolar state. In the hypotensive child or in the child with a serum Na$^+$ greater than 160 mmol/L, initial volume expansion is necessary, using 20 mL/kg normal saline during the first hour or more rapidly, if needed. After restoration of end-organ perfusion, further fluid replacement should be accomplished slowly because overly rapid volume correction can cause cerebral edema, seizures, and death resulting from osmotic shifts.

Free-Water Replacement
- Free water deficit can be estimated with the formula [(Actual Na – Target Na)/Target Na] × 0.6 × weight in kg. The total should be delivered over at least 48 hours in addition to maintenance fluids.
- Free water deficit should be replaced with the lowest osmolality possible. If replacing enterally, water may be administered. Intravenously, 5% Dextrose with ¼ normal saline should be used for the replacement.
- Serum [Na] should be targeted to decrease at a maximum of 0.5 mEq/L/h.

Treatment with Vasopressin or 1-Deamino-8-D-Arginine Vasopressin (DDAVP)

In the ICU, if DI is strongly suspected, starting a vasopressin infusion may be appropriate:

- Vasopressin (aqueous pitressin) infusion should start at 2.5 mU/kg/h and the rate increased slowly (every 5–10 minutes; maximum, 10 mU/kg/h) to decrease urine output to < 2 mL/kg/h. It is difficult to titrate vasopressin

to a particular urine output; rather, its effect should be approached as either "on" or "off."
- When patients have responded to vasopressin, they can no longer excrete excess water and should be considered to be effectively in syndrome of inappropriate ADH secretion (SIADH) physiology. Therefore, maintenance fluids should be restricted to 1000 mL/m^2/d (equivalent to two-thirds maintenance). Fluid required to replete the initial estimated free water deficit over 48 hours may be added to this total.
  - Do not replace urine output with additional fluids.
  - Monitor serum [Na] and serum osmolality every 1 to 2 hours.
  - Monitor urine osmolality to confirm renal tubular response to vasopressin.
  - When restricting fluids, ensure that all intravenous (IV) and enteral fluids are accounted for, including medications.

When the child is able to tolerate oral fluids, 1-Deamino-8-D-Arginine Vasopressin (DDAVP) may be started either enterally (longer onset, more reliable absorption), intranasally (rapid onset, less reliable absorption), or subcutaneously.

Failure to respond to either form of ADH suggests the possibility of renal tubular unresponsiveness to ADH (nephrogenic DI).

Hyponatremia

Syndrome of Inappropriate Antidiuretic Hormone Secretion

The overall incidence of SIADH in childhood is unknown, but it is common in certain disease states. More than 50% of children with bacterial meningitis, up to 20% of patients on positive-pressure ventilation, and up to 70% of children with Rocky Mountain spotted fever develop some degree of SIADH. ADH secretion can be elevated, however, by numerous physiological stresses, including pain, nausea, and infection (most notably pneumonia).

Pathophysiology

Disorders of the central nervous system (CNS) may cause excessive ADH secretion by producing either a local disturbance of the hypothalamic osmoreceptors or some undetermined nervous stimuli. Many intrathoracic conditions are associated with SIADH, probably as a result of the vestigial ability of the lung to produce ADH. Excessive secretion of ADH prevents free water clearance by the collecting tubules of the kidneys. The retained water expands the intravascular compartment, dilutes all plasma constituents, and lowers the plasma osmolality.

Clinical Manifestations

Most patients with SIADH are asymptomatic until the plasma [Na] decreases to <125 mmol/L. When this threshold is reached, symptoms can progress from anorexia, headache, nausea, vomiting, irritability, disorientation, and weakness to seizures and coma, leading, ultimately, to death.

Laboratory investigations for diagnostic purposes are outlined in Table 16.1. Diagnostic criteria for SIADH include (1) hyponatremia in the context of low serum osmolarity; (2) inappropriately elevated urine osmolality; (3) excessive urine [Na] (usually >18 mmol/L) in the presence of hyponatremia; (4) normal renal, adrenal, and thyroid function; and (5) euvolemic to hypervolemic state. As a consequence of the patient's volume status, aldosterone is suppressed and urine potassium is low, as measured by the transtubular potassium gradient.

Hyperlipidemia may lower laboratory measurement of [Na] falsely. Hyperglycemia and hypoproteinemia, however, lead to true hyponatremia. Renal salt wasting, secondary to adrenal insufficiency, is accompanied by hyperkalemia and dehydration. Cerebral salt wasting is extremely rare and is characterized by hypovolemia and a high urine output, as long as renal perfusion remains intact.

Management
Severely Symptomatic Children
Patients in whom hyponatremia is severe enough to cause neurological symptoms, such as lethargy, seizures, or coma, need urgent treatment. Seizures should be treated with the usual antiepileptics as first-line therapy. Hypertonic (3%) saline is the only agent that increases serum [Na] directly and acutely. Infusing small amounts of 3% saline in the range of 3 mL/kg every 10 to 20 minutes until symptoms remit is a reasonable approach; 12 mL/kg 3% saline raises serum [Na] by approximately 10 mmol/L. A single dose of furosemide (1 mg/kg) also can be administered IV. Fluid balance, plasma and urinary [Na], potassium, and osmolality should be monitored closely during treatment.

Asymptomatic or Mildly Symptomatic Children
In asymptomatic or mildly symptomatic patients, rigorous fluid restriction is the most effective treatment. Fluid input should be sharply limited, often below insensible losses, until serum Na and osmolality begin to increase, unless the patient's vascular status is compromised. When the initial serum Na level is less than 125 mmol/L, all fluids must be withheld. As improvement occurs, with increasing serum Na and decreasing urine osmolality, the rate of fluid administration can be increased gradually up to a maximum of $1 \text{ L/m}^2/\text{d}$, as long as SIADH remains. Close monitoring of neurological status, fluid balance, plasma electrolytes, and osmolality is of utmost importance. Patients with chronic or recurrent episodes of SIADH may require treatment with demeclocycline or a specific vasopressin receptor antagonist (conivaptan IV, tolvaptan by mouth). The underlying cause should be identified and treated as possible.

Disruption of Water and Sodium Metabolism in the Child with Traumatic Brain Injury
A "triphasic response" can result from traumatic brain injury and from neurosurgery when there is an insult to the pituitary. During the acute or first phase,

Table 16.1 Causes of Hyponatremia and Associated Findings

		Cause of Hyponatremia			
	Dehydration/↓Effective Volume	SIADH	Cerebral Salt Wasting	Water Intoxication	Adrenal Insufficiency
Frequency	Common	Uncommon	Very rare	Rare	Rare
Intravascular volume (CVP)	Low	Normal/high	Low	High	Low/normal
Serum osmolarity	Normal/high	Low	—	Low/normal	High/normal
Urine osmolarity/concentration	High/concentrated	Maximally concentrated	—	Low/diluted	—
Urine sodium, mEq/L	Low, <20	High, >100	>200	Normal	High
Urine output	Low	Decreased, normal	Very high	Increased	Normal/low if dehydrated
AVP level	High (because of high osmolarity)	High	High	Low	High
Aldosterone	Increased if low blood pressure	Low	Normal/high	Low	Low
Other	High BUN, tachycardia	Low BUN, high A/B-NP (volume overload)	Low A/B-NP, HR unreliable	Low BUN	BUN normal

A/B-NP, atrial/brain natriuretic peptide; AVP, arginine vasopressin; BUN, blood, urea, nitrogen; CVP, central venous pressure; SIADH, syndrome of inappropriate antidiuretic hormone secretion.

diabetes insipidus ensues, believed to be from blunted ADH release secondary to edema. It is commonly transient, lasting from 0.5 to 2 days. The second phase involves remission of DI and superimposed SIADH, as ADH stores are released from necrotic tissues, and can last up to 10 days. The third phase is characterized by cell loss, resulting in stable DI. When present, it is likely permanent. Careful monitoring, with an expectation of rapid changes in serum Na levels and urine concentration, is essential to make prompt changes in fluid replacement according to each phase and prevent morbidity.

Acute Adrenal Insufficiency

Acute adrenal insufficiency is a life-threatening event that usually manifests during an intercurrent infection or after trauma when the adrenal cortex fails to produce enough glucocorticoid and mineralocorticoid in response to metabolic stress.

Pathophysiology

The adrenal glands are responsible for producing corticosteroids, mineralocorticoids, and androgens. Corticotropin-releasing hormone is released from the hypothalamus to stimulate adrenocorticotropic hormone (ACTH) release from the pituitary, which in turn controls cortisol release from the adrenal glands. Cortisol stimulates gluconeogenesis and is essential for vascular responsiveness to cathecholamines and for the suppression of inflammatory and immune responses.

Mineralocorticoids, especially aldosterone, play an important role in salt and water homeostasis by promoting salt resorption and potassium excretion in the distal renal tubules and collecting ducts. Their production is regulated primarily by the renin–angiotensin system.

Individuals at risk for adrenal insufficiency are those with a disruption in any of these pathways from either an adrenal (primary) or hypothalamic–pituitary (secondary) disorder.

Primary Adrenal Insufficiency

Primary adrenal insufficiency may result from adrenal dysgenesis, impaired steroidogenesis (congenital adrenal hyperplasia), or adrenal destruction (autoimmune process, X-linked adrenoleukodystrophy, adrenal hemorrhage). Waterhouse-Friderichsen syndrome, acute adrenal infarction, should be considered in a patient with fulminant sepsis and hypotension unresponsive to vasopressors or inotropes, especially if a result of meningococcemia.

Rapid decompensation in the face of metabolic stress is often the first clue of adrenal insufficiency. In primary adrenal insufficiency, both corticosteroid and mineralocorticoid production are disrupted. Affected children are more likely to have a gradual onset of symptoms of glucocorticoid deficiency, such as fasting hypoglycemia, increased insulin sensitivity, decreased gastric acidity, nausea, vomiting, and fatigue. Mineralocorticoid deficiency can manifest similarly, with fatigue and gastrointestinal symptoms, as well as muscle weakness, weight loss, anorexia, salt craving, hypotension, hyperkalemia, hyponatremia, and acidosis.

Findings on physical examination are more likely to be characteristic of the precipitating illness or trauma rather than specifically suggestive of adrenal insufficiency. Hyperpigmentation is characteristic of primary adrenal insufficiency as a result of high melanocyte stimulating hormone levels as it is cosecreted with ACTH.

Secondary Adrenal Insufficiency

Hypothalamic–pituitary causes of ACTH deficiency and, thus, secondary adrenal insufficiency include CNS tumors, neurosurgical procedures, head trauma, and radiation therapy involving the pituitary. Exogenous administration of glucocorticoids, particularly in patients treated with high doses of corticosteroids for chronic disease (e.g., nephrotic syndrome, acute lymphoblastic leukemia, asthma), is a common cause of suppression of the adrenal–pituitary axis—an effect that often lasts well beyond cessation of therapy.

Patients with secondary adrenal insufficiency present with symptoms of glucocorticoid deficiency as mentioned, resulting from the lack of stimulation from corticotropin-releasing hormone and/or ACTH. However, because mineralocorticoid production is regulated primarily by the renin–angiotensin system, adrenal insufficiency resulting from hypothalamic–pituitary causes is not associated with a lack of aldosterone; therefore, hyponatremia and hyperkalemia are not part of the constellation.

Laboratory Workup and Usual Findings

In primary adrenal insufficiency, findings include hyponatremia, hyperkalemia, and acidosis from mineralocorticoid deficiency and significantly elevated ACTH levels resulting from a lack of negative feedback from cortisol. Mild hypercalcemia may be present.

Cortisol deficiency both from primary and secondary causes can manifest as hypoglycemia during stress or fasting. Definitive diagnosis depends on the demonstration of an inappropriately low level of cortisol in the serum. Because cortisol is secreted in a pulsatile manner with a specific diurnal rhythm that has its highest peak in the morning, an 8 AM *plasma cortisol* is the preferred initial test to evaluate for adrenal insufficiency. However, it is not often practical because of loss of diurnal rhythm during critical illness. A random cortisol level is only helpful in ruling out adrenal insufficiency if it is markedly elevated (>18 μg/dL) during stress. A low random cortisol level taken later during the day is difficult to interpret.

A high-dose *ACTH stimulation test* is done by measuring total cortisol and ACTH at baseline (hour 0), then administering 250 μg synthetic ACTH (i.e., cosyntropin) IV or intramuscularly and measuring total cortisol 60 minutes later. In infants, 62.5 to 125 μg of cosyntropin may be used. A cortisol level of more than 18 μg/dL post-stimulation rules out primary adrenal insufficiency. In the setting of critical illness, an increase in cortisol by 9 μg/dL or more is also considered a sufficient response.

In early secondary adrenal insufficiency, if adrenal atrophy has not occurred, a "high-dose" ACTH stimulation test can be normal. Many experts recommend a "low-dose" stimulation test using 1 μg cosyntropin and measuring total cortisol 30 minutes after administration. A normal response is considered to be more than 18 μg/dL. Both tests can be combined such that the "high-dose" ACTH is administered after measuring the 30-minute cortisol post-"low dose."

Management

Treatment of adrenal crisis requires rapid volume expansion and the administration of glucocorticoids. Improvement in peripheral circulation and blood pressure should occur quickly with therapy. Because adrenal crisis is commonly brought on by another stress such as infection, the symptoms of malaise, anorexia, and lethargy may take longer to resolve.

Acute Phase

Treatment of the acute phase of adrenal crisis includes steroids (hydrocortisone) and volume expansion.

- Hydrocortisone
  - Immediate treatment: 50 to 100 mg/m^2/dose hydrocortisone IV
  - Subsequent treatment: hydrocortisone 50 mg/m^2/24 h given IV continuously or divided every 6 hours
- Volume expansion as needed, keeping in mind that Na needs may be particularly elevated with mineralocorticoid deficiency and that dextrose should be included because of the propensity for hypoglycemia.

Mineralocorticoid therapy is rarely important during the acute phase, provided fluid therapy is adequate, because high-dose hydrocortisone provides sufficient mineralocorticoid activity. Hypertonic saline should be considered only if there is neurological deterioration.

Specific therapy directed toward correction of hyperkalemia is required if there are electrocardiogram (ECG) changes (peaked T wave, prolonged QRS duration) or arrhythmias.

Long-Term Treatment

High-dose glucocorticoid therapy should be continued for 48 hours or at least 24 hours after the patient is clinically stable. After that, physiological replacement for a patient confirmed to have adrenal insufficiency can be achieved with 6 to 10 mg/m^2/d hydrocortisone. Patients with primary adrenal insufficiency need replacement with fludrocortisone—a mineralocorticoid for long-term management. Initial dose of 0.1 mg orally is usually sufficient, except in younger patients who sometimes require higher doses.

Calcium Disorders

About 98% of the body's calcium is contained within bones, with only 2% circulating either as free ionized calcium (50%) or protein-bound calcium (50%), mainly to albumin. Tight regulation of the ionized calcium within a narrow range is maintained through parathyroid hormone (PTH) secretion, 1,25-(OH)2-vitamin D production, and renal handling of calcium.

Hypocalcemia

Pathophysiology

Under normal circumstances, hypocalcemia turns off the calcium-sensing receptor in the parathyroid glands, which stimulates PTH secretion. PTH promotes calcium reabsorption at the distal renal tubule while increasing phosphate excretion into the urine at the proximal tubule. In bone, PTH increases the release of calcium by promoting the differentiation of osteoclasts. PTH also stimulates the conversion of 25-vitamin D to 1,25-vitamin D by upregulating 1-alpha-hydroxylase activity in the kidney. 1,25-Vitamin D acts to increase calcium and phosphorus absorption in the intestine and promotes osteoclastic bone resorption.

Etiology

Hypocalcemia develops as a consequence of either decreased absorption of calcium from bone, kidney, or the gastrointestinal tract, or excessive loss of calcium into the urine, bone, or stool. Total serum calcium decreases 0.8 mg/dL for every 1 g/dL decrease in albumin below 4 g/dL; thus, this is important to confirm true hypocalcemia.

There are several causes of hypocalcemia listed in Box 16.1.

Clinical Manifestations

Hypocalcemia can lead to a prolonged QT interval, with risk of life-threatening arrhythmias, and neuromuscular excitability, presenting as paresthesias and muscle cramps. Severe hypocalcemia may lead to tetany, seizures, and laryngospasm. Careful physical examination may show a positive Chvostek sign (tapping the facial nerve causes twitching of the circumoral and orbicularis oculi) and/or Trousseau sign (inflated sphygmomanometer above systolic blood pressure for more than 3 minutes causes carpopedal spasm). Lenticular cataracts are associated with long-standing hypocalcemia of any cause.

Laboratory Evaluation and Usual Findings

When hypocalcemia is confirmed, a systematic approach is recommended to elucidate the cause. Labs should be obtained while the calcium level is abnormal. Use of age-appropriate normal ranges is essential (Table 16.2).

Management

Acute management for life-threatening hypocalcemia involves IV calcium gluconate (200–500 mg/kg/d as a continuous infusion or in four divided doses; maximum, 2000–3000 mg/dose).

In nutritional vitamin D deficiency rickets, high-dose oral vitamin D (ergocalciferol, cholecalciferol) in addition to oral calcium supplements is recommended.

In hypoparathyroidism, long-term management consists of treatment with the active analog of vitamin D, calcitriol ($1,25\text{-}(OH)_2D_3$) at 0.01 to 0.05 µg/kg/d. Supplemental oral calcium is almost always necessary.

Box 16.1 Endocrine Causes of Hypocalcemia

Neonatal Hypocalcemia

Early onset (<5 days old)
  Insufficient parathyroid hormone (PTH) release or sensitivity
    Prematurity
    Infant of diabetic mothers
    Preeclampsia
    Perinatal stress
    Maternal hypoparathyroidism
Late onset (5–10 days old)
  PTH resistance
  Transient hypoparathyroidism
  Increased phosphate load
  Vitamin D deficiency
  Hypomagnesemia

Disorders Associated with Low or Inappropriately Normal PTH

Alterations in calcium sensing
Hypoparathyroidism
  Parathyroid agenesis/dysfunction
    Familial forms of isolated PTH deficiency
    DiGeorge syndrome
    Kenney-Caffey syndrome
  Acquired hypoparathyroidism
    Autoimmune
    Radiation exposure/postsurgical
    Idiopathic
  Abnormal PTH secretion
    Hypomagnesemia
    Critical illness
  Peripheral resistance to PTH
    Pseudohypoparathyroidism

Disorders Associated with High PTH

Vitamin D deficiency
  Nutritional deficiency
  Liver disease
  Iatrogenic
Vitamin D resistance
  Hydroxylase deficiencies
  Vitamin D receptor dysfunction

Table 16.2 Causes of Hypocalcemia and Associated Findings

| | Diagnosis | | | |
	Vitamin D Deficiency	Vitamin D-Dependent Rickets	Hypoparathyroid States	PHP
Calcium	Low/normal	Low	Low	Low/normal
Phosphorus	Low/normal	Low	High	High
25-Vitamin D	Low	—	Normal	Normal
1,25-Vitamin D	Low/normal	1-Alpha-hydroxylase deficiency: low 1,25-Vitamin D resistance: high	Low/normal	Normal
PTH	High	High	Low	High
Urine spot Ca/Cr	Low	Low	High	High

Ca, calcium; Cr, creatinine; PHP, pseudohypoparathyroidism; PTH, parathyroid hormone.

Hypercalcemia

Pathophysiology

Under normal circumstances, hypercalcemia stimulates calcium-sensing receptors, suppressing PTH, which in turns decreases calcium reabsorption at the kidney.

Etiology

Hypercalcemic conditions in children are relatively rare. In neonates, iatrogenic causes are most common, usually related to inadequate phosphate intake or excessive calcium or vitamin D supplementation, diuretics, and/or extracorporeal membrane oxygenation. Causes of hypercalcemia can be subdivided in those with suppressed PTH or elevated/inappropriately normal PTH. The following is a discussion of the endocrine causes of hypercalcemia.

Clinical Manifestations

Hypercalcemia is often an incidental finding. It can manifest as hypotonia, myopathy, weakness, listlessness, anorexia, weight loss, failure to thrive, constipation, and vomiting, and, in the neonate, respiratory distress and apnea. The child may develop hypertension, shortened QTc interval on ECG, polyuria (resulting from renal unresponsiveness to ADH), and, rarely, encephalopathy with seizures. Less commonly, diffuse bone pain or renal colic may be present. Certain characteristic features, including hypertelorism, broad forehead, epicanthal folds, prominent upper lip, an underdeveloped nasal bridge, and a small mandible, have been associated with idiopathic hypercalcemia in infancy, but have been noted in infants with hyperparathyroidism as well.

Management

Acute management of hypercalcemia depends on the level of calcium and the presence of signs and symptoms. In the asymptomatic patient with serum calcium less than 12 mg/dL, careful follow-up is recommended.

For severe or symptomatic hypercalcemia, the initial approach should be to increase the urinary excretion of calcium by correcting dehydration, if present, and maximizing glomerular filtration rate with IV fluids. Normal saline is commonly used as a first-line agent. Furosemide and other loop diuretics are rarely necessary, but can be used carefully. Excessive diuresis and further dehydration may worsen hypercalcemia.

Calcitonin (2–4 U/kg every 12 hours intramuscularly or subcutaneously) is effective as an emergency treatment, but tachyphylaxis is common and occurs quite rapidly.

The nitrogen-containing bisphosphonates, in consultation with a specialist, can be an alternative. Therapy should be initiated early during the course because onset of action can be delayed for up to 3 days. Patients must be monitored carefully, because they can develop severe hypocalcemia, hypophosphatemia, and hypomagnesemia, in addition to an acute-phase reaction on first administration in up to 20% of patients. Potential long-term adverse effects in children are still under study.

Parathyroid surgery is recommended for all children with primary hyperparathyroidism, especially in the case of an adenoma, in which removal of the single affected gland is curative.

Thyroid Storm

Life-threatening thyrotoxicosis, or thyroid storm, is an extremely rare disorder in children and adolescents. It occurs in only 1% of patients with hyperthyroidism. Precipitating factors include intercurrent infection, trauma, thyroid, or nonthyroidal surgery in a patient with unrecognized or inadequately treated thyrotoxicosis, diabetic ketoacidosis, concomitant use of sympathomimetics (e.g., pseudoephedrine), abrupt cessation of antithyroid drugs, and, rarely, radioactive iodine therapy. Thyroid storm is characterized by multisystem involvement and a high mortality rate if not recognized immediately and treated aggressively.

Pathophysiology

The exact mechanisms of progression from uncomplicated hyperthyroidism to storm are not known. One hypothesis is an increase in the amount of free thyroid hormones. Thyroid hormone released suddenly into the circulation causes uncoupling of oxidative phosphorylation and/or increased lipolysis, resulting in excessive thermogenesis. Another theory that may explain the pathogenesis of thyroid storm is a possible increase in β-adrenergic receptor density and an enhanced adrenergic response. Tachycardia is caused by both the hyperthermia and the direct action of thyroid hormones on the cardiac conduction system. Insensible fluid loss increases as a result of increased metabolism and sweating.

Clinical Manifestations

Most commonly, thyroid storm occurs in patients with known hyperthyroidism. Characteristic clinical findings include goiter (>95%), exophthalmos, tachycardia, bounding pulses, and systolic hypertension. Diastolic hypotension, tremulousness, and restlessness may be present. The primary features distinguishing thyroid storm from uncomplicated hyperthyroidism are the presence of high fever, often as high as 41°C (105.8°F) and CNS changes ranging from mania or delirium to frankly psychotic behavior. The marked increase in cardiac workload may result in high-output cardiac failure and may lead to hypotension and pulmonary edema.

Laboratory Workup and Usual Findings

Thyroid studies reveal elevated free thyroxine (free T_4) as well as total triiodothyronine (T_3). Alternatively, total T4 can be used if analyzed in the context of a T_3 resin uptake. Most commonly there is a primary cause that results in thyroid stimulating hormone suppression (<0.1 mU/L). Values overlap with those found in uncomplicated hyperthyroidism; therefore, diagnosis relies on clinical criteria. A chest radiograph and ECG are helpful in evaluating and following cardiac status. In many cases, therapy must be initiated on the basis of clinical evidence if results are not available on an emergency basis.

Management

Initial treatment is directed toward lowering the metabolic rate and reducing the cardiac workload. Subsequent treatment is directed toward controlling thyroid hormone production. Aggressive cooling should be implemented to decrease metabolic rate. Aspirin should not be used because of its potential to uncouple oxidative phosphorylation and exacerbate the hypermetabolic state. Volume resuscitation and adequate hydration are essential.

Treatment of Exaggerated Adrenergic Effects
- Propranolol starting at 10 µg/kg IV over 10 to 15 minutes. Maintenance dosing of propranolol is 2 mg/kg/d divided every 6 hours in neonates and 10 to 40 mg every 6 hours in older children.
- Esmolol infusion is initiated with a loading dose of 500 µg/kg/min over 1 minute with a subsequent continuous infusion of 50 to 250 µg/kg/min.
- ECG monitoring for heart rate and arrhythmias is recommended.

Limiting the Amount of Thyroid Hormone Available
- *Methimazole*: 0.5 to 0.7 mg/kg/d divided into three oral doses
  - Inhibits iodine oxidation in the thyroid gland.
  - Blocks iodine's ability to combine with tyrosine to form T_4 and T_3.
  - Reduction in thyroid levels may take several days to weeks.
  - Propylthiouracil was a first-line agent but, because of its association with pediatric liver failure, is now contraindicated in children.
- *Iodide therapy*: Lugol's iodide (sold under the brand name Saturated Solution of Potassium Iodide [SSKI]) 3 to 5 drops once every 8 hours orally or Na iodide 125 to 250 mg/d intravenously over 24 hours

- Should be given at least 1 hour after the first dose of methimazole to avoid further increasing synthesis of thyroid hormone.
- Rapidly terminates thyroid hormone release within 24 hours; however, this effect is overcome after 3 to 5 days of iodide therapy.
- Decreases the vascularity of the thyroidal arterial supply; is useful as preoperative agent.
- Glucocorticoids
  - Dexamethasone 0.2 mg/kg or hydrocortisone 5 mg/kg can be given parenterally during the acute phase.
    - Appear to inhibit thyroid hormone release from the thyroid and decrease the peripheral conversion of T_4 to T_3.

Treatment of Precipitating Factors

- Broad-spectrum antibiotics should be considered while awaiting the results of cultures; there is a documented association between thyrotoxicosis and pneumococcal bacteremia.

Improvement should be seen within a few hours after the initiation of treatment with β blockers, especially in terms of cardiovascular status. Full recovery and adequate control of the underlying thyroid disease take several days to achieve. For the patient presenting with thyroid storm, serious consideration should be given to permanent treatment of the hyperthyroidism, either by surgery or radioiodide ablation.

Diabetic Ketoacidosis

Pathophysiology

Diabetic ketoacidosis (DKA) is a result of severe insulin deficiency. It occurs most commonly in children with undiagnosed type 1 diabetes or when patients on treatment omit insulin doses either accidentally or deliberately. It can also develop in patients with type 1 diabetes during acute illness when there are increased metabolic demands despite the patient taking the usual amount of insulin. Less commonly, children with monogenic diabetes or type 2 diabetes can also develop DKA.

DKA develops when there is insufficient circulating insulin in the setting of increased counterregulatory hormones such as cortisol, catecholamines, glucagon, and growth hormone in response to metabolic stress, resulting in a catabolic state. During this process there is increased gluconeogenesis and glycogenolysis in the liver coupled with impaired glucose uptake in peripheral tissues, which eventually leads to worsening hyperglycemia and hyperosmolarity. Severe insulin deficiency promotes lipolysis and ketogenesis from fatty acids in an attempt to combat starvation and generate fuel for the brain to use, which causes ketonemia and metabolic acidosis. When the plasma glucose level exceeds the renal threshold of about 180 mg/dL, glucosuria ensues, followed by osmotic diuresis and further dehydration if untreated. Vomiting, caused by severe ketosis and acidosis, can worsen dehydration and leads to loss of other electrolytes as well. If the child is septic or severely hypoperfused, lactic acidosis can also develop.

Clinical Manifestations

Children with DKA present with variable degrees of dehydration. Severe depletion of water and electrolytes happens from both intra- and extracellular fluid compartments. Blood pressure is mostly maintained or may even be elevated. Increased urine output resulting from glucosuria and osmotic diuresis is common, but oliguria and acute renal failure can occur when there is extreme water depletion and a significant decrease in renal blood flow. Tachypnea and Kussmaul respirations (deep, rapid breathing) are common findings. Patients usually have nausea, vomiting, and abdominal pain, and assessing whether there is a superimposed acute abdominal condition is important. Drowsiness is common, but significant mental status changes such as confusion, lethargy, obtundation, and loss of consciousness, as well as cranial nerve palsy, bradycardia, and decorticate or decerebrate posturing are ominous signs of cerebral edema.

Laboratory Workup and Usual Findings

DKA is defined as having (1) hyperglycemia with a blood glucose level of 200 mg/dL or more (11 mmol/L), (2) metabolic acidosis with a venous pH <7.3 or bicarbonate levels less than 15 mmol/L, and (3) ketonemia (blood β-hydroxybutyrate ≥3 mmol/L) and ketonuria (moderate or large).

The severity of DKA can be defined by the degree of acidosis: mild (venous pH <7.3 or bicarbonate <15 mmol/L), moderate (venous pH <7.2 or bicarbonate <10 mmol/L), or severe (venous pH <7.1 or bicarbonate <5 mmol/L).

A blood sample should be obtained to measure serum or plasma glucose, electrolytes, blood urea nitrogen, creatinine, serum osmolality, venous pH, venous carbon dioxide, hemoglobin, hematocrit, and complete blood count. Albumin, calcium, phosphorus, and magnesium levels are also recommended. β-Hydroxybutyrate can be measured in blood if available, or urinalysis can be sent for ketones. A hemoglobin A1C can help establish duration of hyperglycemia (>6.5% diagnostic for diabetes mellitus). If there is fever and/or signs of infection, blood, urine, or throat cultures should be obtained, although isolated white blood cell count elevation in DKA is extremely common even without a diagnosed infection.

DKA is characterized by total-body potassium depletion, mostly from intracellular losses. Hypertonicity and glycogenolysis cause potassium shifts, insulin deficiency and acidosis cause potassium efflux from cells, vomiting causes gastrointestinal losses, and osmotic diuresis exacerbates urinary losses of the ion. When insulin is given, potassium is driven back into the cells, decreasing serum levels.

Intracellular phosphate is also depleted as a result of osmotic diuresis and can be exacerbated when insulin is initiated as phosphate is driven into the cells; therefore, insulin boluses at the initiation of therapy ought to be avoided.

Management

A careful clinical evaluation should assess neurological status (level of consciousness with Glasgow Coma Scale), respiratory compromise, severity of dehydration, and urine output and identify possible infection. It is important to determine the current weight for treatment calculations. A blood sample should be obtained to measure electrolytes, blood glucose, renal function, and venous gases. Either blood β-hydroxybutyrate measurement if available or urinalysis should be obtained to determine ketonemia. A complete blood count should be evaluated, keeping in mind that DKA itself, in the absence of infection, can result in leukocytosis. An ECG is useful in assessing changes of hypo- or hyperkalemia before blood concentrations are available.

Emergency management should follow Pediatric Advanced Life Support guidelines. It is important to manage DKA in a unit with experienced nursing staff and clinicians. In severely obtunded patients, particular consideration should be given to securing the airway and emptying the stomach to prevent aspiration. Oxygen should be given as needed. The patient should be under cardiac monitoring, and at least one peripheral IV catheter inserted. Central venous catheters are usually avoided because of an increased risk of thrombosis in the child with DKA. If there is a high suspicion of concurrent infection, antibiotics should be initiated after cultures are taken.

Studies have shown that clinical estimates of fluid deficit in children with DKA are often inaccurate. For this reason, current guidelines recommend using 5% to 7% dehydration in moderate DKA and 7% to 10% in severe DKA. Crystalloids are recommended. Our protocol starts with a 10-mL/kg normal saline fluid bolus that occasionally may be repeated or increased at the discretion of the clinician. Some centers use lactated Ringer's solution for volume expansion. The initial 4 to 6 hours of fluid replacement should be with an isotonic solution that can then be switched to a tonicity of 0.45% NaCl or more with added potassium (chloride, phosphate, or acetate) depending on the patient's hydration status, serum Na, osmolality, and mental status (keeping in mind that the risk of cerebral edema may increase with administration of fluids containing less than isotonic saline). Rehydration is usually planned for 48 hours, with frequent reassessment of the patient's volume status. However, patients are generally switched to oral hydration after 12 hours of therapy. Ongoing clinical trials are expected to determine whether the rate or composition of IV fluids during rehydration affect outcomes, comparing 1-time versus 1.5-times versus 2-times maintenance rates and different Na concentrations.

Insulin should be initiated after initial volume expansion (1–2 hours after rehydration is started) at 0.05 to 0.1 U/kg/h of IV regular insulin. A recent randomized controlled trial showed no superiority of using standard-dose (0.1 U/kg/h) versus low-dose (0.05 U/kg/h) insulin, but further studies are needed. During initial volume expansion, plasma glucose is expected to decrease rapidly as renal perfusion is augmented. When insulin is started, this decline in plasma glucose continues and dextrose should be provided in IV fluids when glucose decreases to 250 to 300 mg/dL. Initially, 5% dextrose can be added to fluids and titrated up to maintain blood glucose above 200 mg/dL and to prevent hypoglycemia while acidosis corrects. The maximum concentration of dextrose given peripherally should be 12.5%. In places where continuous IV infusion is not possible, or in patients with uncomplicated DKA, hourly intramuscular or 2 to 3 hourly subcutaneous short-acting or rapid-acting insulin can be considered (such as insulin lispro or aspart).

Potassium replacement should be started along with initial volume expansion before starting insulin, except in the rare patient with hyperkalemia or acute renal failure. A concentration of 40 mmol/L can be the starting point, titrated depending on the patient's status, added to rehydration fluids but not to the initial rapid bolus (normal saline bolus). Phosphate replacement should also be considered, which can be done by providing some of the potassium replacement as potassium phosphate. Careful monitoring of calcium during phosphate replacement is important to prevent hypocalcemia.

The main goals of therapy are to correct the acidosis and reverse the ketosis, while correcting dehydration. Treatment restores near-normal blood glucose levels, but preventing hypoglycemia while enough insulin is provided to correct the acidosis is key. Another main aspect of treatment is careful monitoring to identify and treat precipitating events that can lead rapidly to complications. The most common complications of DKA and its treatment are inadequate rehydration, hypoglycemia, hypokalemia, hyperchloremic acidosis, and cerebral edema.

Diffuse cerebral edema occurs more frequently than previously thought and can be present in brain imaging in otherwise asymptomatic patients. Clinically evident cerebral edema is the most common fatal complication of DKA in children and carries a mortality rate of 21% to 24%. The pathophysiology of cerebral edema and precipitating factors are still under study. Fluid shifts resulting from abrupt changes in osmolarity have been proposed, with recent evidence suggesting there might also be a component of hypoperfusion–reperfusion CNS injury and permeability changes in the blood–brain barrier. Changes in neurological status should prompt immediate evaluation and treatment with a hyperosmolar agent (mannitol 0.5–1 g/kg IV over 10–15 minutes or hypertonic 3% saline 2.5–5 mL/kg IV over 10–15 minutes). Head imaging may be considered *after* treatment has been initiated.

When the acidosis is corrected, as indicated by a reduction in the anion gap to normal (12–14 mmol/L) or β-hydroxybutyrate concentration less than 1 mmol/L, and there is clinical improvement in the patient's symptoms, transition to subcutaneous insulin and oral fluids should occur in consultation with a pediatric endocrinologist.

Further Reading

August GP. Treatment of adrenocortical insufficiency. *Pediatr Rev*. 1997;18(2):59–62.

Davies JH, Shaw NJ. Investigation and management of hypercalcaemia in children. *Arch Dis Child*. 2012;97(6):533–538.

Di Iorgi N, Napoli F, Allegri AE, et al. Diabetes insipidus: diagnosis and management. *Horm Res Paediatr*. 2012;77(2):69–84.

Einaudi S, Bondone C. The effects of head trauma on hypothalamic–pituitary function in children and adolescents. *Curr Opin Pediatr*. 2007;19(4):465–470.

Foley TPJr. Thyrotoxicosis in childhood. *Pediatr Ann*. 1992;21(1):43–46, 48–49.

Lipiner-Friedman D, Sprung CL, Laterre PF, et al. Adrenal function in sepsis: the retrospective corticus cohort study. *Crit Care Med*. 2007;35(4):1012–1018.

Nallasamy K, Jayashree M, Singhi S, Bansal A. Low-dose vs standard-dose insulin in pediatric diabetic ketoacidosis: a randomized clinical trial. *JAMA Pediatr*. 2014;168(11):999–1005.

Neary N, Nieman L. Adrenal insufficiency: etiology, diagnosis and treatment. *Curr Opin Endocrinol Diabetes Obes*. 2010;17(3):217–223.

Ranadive SA, Rosenthal SM. Pediatric disorders of water balance. *Endocrinol Metab Clin North Am*. 2009;38(4):663–672.

Rivkees SA. Pediatric Graves' disease: controversies in management. *Horm Res Paediatr*. 2010;74(5):305–311.

Segni M, Gorman CA. The aftermath of childhood hyperthyroidism. *J Pediatr Endocrinol Metab*. 2001;14(suppl 5):1277–1282; discussion, 1297–1298.

Taylor SC, et al. Hypoparathyroidism and 22Q11 deletion syndrome. *Arch Dis Child*. 2003;88(6)520–522.

Wolfsdorf JI, Allgrove J, Craig ME, et al.; and International Society for Pediatric and Adolescent Diabetes. ISPAD clinical practice consensus guidelines 2014: diabetic ketoacidosis and hyperglycemic hyperosmolar state. *Pediatr Diabetes*. 2014;15(suppl 20):154–179.

Chapter 17

Toxicological Emergencies

Sandra D. W. Buttram and Anne-Michelle Ruha

Children are exposed to toxic substances more frequently than adults. In 2011, according to the American Association of Poison Control Centers National Poison Data System there were more than 3.6 million calls to poison centers in the United States, with almost half of all human exposures (48.9%) reported in children younger than 6 years. Toxicological emergencies in the pediatric population usually occur in a bimodal age distribution. Accidental or unintentional exposures typically involve children 0 to 5 years whereas intentional exposures more commonly involve the adolescent population. From 2000 to 2010, there was an increase in pharmaceutical-related exposures, hospital management of exposures, and serious medical outcomes resulting from exposures in young children.

Care of the poisoned patient should always begin with the ABCs per the Pediatric Advanced Life Support (PALS) guidelines.

Specific *historical facts* about the exposure are beneficial, if known:

- Timing
- Immediate versus extended-release formulation
- Dose

A thorough *physical examination* may identify specific toxidromes. Often, by time of admission to the pediatric intensive care unit, the window of opportunity for decontamination has passed. Clinical management and specific therapies should be instituted as soon as possible based on patient presentation and laboratory investigations.

Analgesics

Analgesics are responsible for almost 10% of exposures and 21% of fatalities in patients younger than 6 years.

Acetaminophen

Acetaminophen is one of the most commonly used mild analgesics. It can be purchased as a single ingredient, nonprescription preparation, in cough and cold formulations, and in prescription combinations usually with opioids. It is associated with significant accidental and intentional exposure and is the leading cause of acute liver failure in the United States. In appropriate dosing, oral acetaminophen is absorbed primarily in the small intestine and is metabolized hepatically by sulfate and glucuronide conjugation to water-soluble metabolites that are excreted renally. Toxic doses of more than 120 to 150 mg/kg can result in accumulation of the highly reactive intermediate N-acetyl-p-benzoquinone imine (NAPQI) resulting from saturation of the CYP2E1 glutathione-dependent conjugation pathway. NAPQI binds to hepatocytes and causes cellular necrosis, which can lead to acute liver failure.

Presentation

Symptoms of acetaminophen toxicity may not occur for 12 to 24 hours after an acute ingestion. They consist of anorexia, abdominal pain, nausea, and vomiting. Patients who present more than 36 hours after an acute ingestion may have fulminant hepatic failure with jaundice, metabolic acidosis, encephalopathy, and coagulopathy (Table 17.1). Evaluation for suspected acetaminophen toxicity should include a serum acetaminophen level, electrolytes, renal function, serum transaminase levels, and a coagulation profile to assess for altered hepatic function.

Management

N-acetylcysteine (NAC) is the treatment for acetaminophen toxicity (Table 17.2). NAC restores the glutathione required to conjugate the toxic NAPQI metabolite and enhances sulfate conjugation of acetaminophen. Optimally, treatment with NAC should begin immediately for patients with acetaminophen levels that are on or above the potential toxicity line on the Rumack-Matthew nomogram. If levels are unavailable or the time of ingestion Is unknown, then NAC therapy should be initiated empirically. Undetectable acetaminophen does not rule out toxicity in patients who present more than 24 hours after suspected exposure with elevated serum transaminase levels. Patients with fulminant hepatic failure may also require supportive care: airway management and mechanical ventilation for encephalopathy, fluid resuscitation and vasopressors for shock, transfusion for bleeding secondary to coagulopathy, and renal replacement therapy for renal failure. Patients with acidosis, encephalopathy, or coagulopathy (INR >5) should be evaluated for liver transplant.

Opiates and Opioids

Abuse of prescription drugs, primarily opioids, is the fastest growing drug problem in the United States and contributed to more than 29,000 unintentional pediatric opioid ingestions requiring medical evaluation from 2001 to 2008. Opiates are derived from the poppy plant (*Papaver somniferum*), whereas opioids are synthetic and semisynthetic chemicals that, like opiates, bind to mu opioid receptors. Collectively they comprise the opioid class of drugs that include, but are not limited to, morphine, fentanyl, codeine, hydrocodone, oxycodone, methadone, and heroin. Varied pharmacokinetics and

Table 17.1 Clinical Signs Associated with Toxin Exposure

Toxin	Neurological	Pupils	CV	Respiratory	GI/GU	Skin	Other
Acetaminophen	ALOC				Vomiting	Jaundice	
β-adrenergic blockers	ALOC		↓ HR AV block ↓ BP	Bronchospasm			
Calcium channel antagonists	ALOC		↓ HR AV block ↓ BP				
Carbon monoxide	ALOC Weakness Upgoing Babinski Ataxia Seizure		Myocardial ischemia	↑ RR			
Cyclic antidepressants	Hallucinations ALOC Seizure	Mydriasis	↑ HR Prolonged QRS ↓ BP	↓ RR	Urinary retention	Warm, dry	
Opiates	ALOC	Miosis	↓ HR ↓ BP	↓ RR			
Salicylates	ALOC Seizure		↑ HR	↑ RR	Vomiting	Diaphoresis	↑ Temp
Sulfonylurea[a]	ALOC Seizure		↑ HR			Diaphoresis	
Toxic alcohols	ALOC Seizure	Mydriasis ↓ Visual acuity (methanol)	↑ HR	↑ RR			

ALOC, altered level of consciousness; AV, atrioventricular; BP, blood pressure; CV, cardiovascular; GI, gastrointestinal; GU, genitourinary; HR, heart rate; RR, respiratory rate; Temp, temperature.

[a] Signs are a result of hypoglycemia, not direct medication effects.

Table 17.2 Treatment for Common Toxins

Toxin	Treatment	Route	Dose
Acetaminophen	N-acetylcysteine	PO	Loading dose: 140 mg/kg
			Maintenance dose: 70 mg/kg every 4 h × 17 doses[a]
		IV	Loading dose: 150 mg/kg (maximum, 15 g) over 1 h
			Second dose: 50 mg/kg (maximum, 5 g) over 4 h
			Maintenance dose: 6.25 mg/kg/h over 16 h[a]
β-adrenergic blockers	Atropine	IV	0.02 mg/kg (minimum, 0.1 mg; maximum, 0.5 mg)
	10% Calcium chloride	IV (central line)	20 mg/kg over 5–10 min
			Continuous infusion: 20–50 mg/kg/h
	Glucagon	IV	50 µg/kg over 1–2 min
			Continuous infusion: 50–100 µg/kg/h, titrate as needed
	Insulin	IV	1 IU/kg
			Continuous infusion: 0.5 IU/kg/h, titrate as needed
	Vasopressors	IV	
	Epinephrine		0.05 µg/kg/min, titrate to effect
	Norepinephrine		0.05 µg/kg/min, titrate to effect
Calcium channel antagonist	10% Calcium chloride	IV (central line)	20 mg/kg over 5–10 min
			Continuous infusion: 20–50 mg/kg/h
	Atropine	IV	0.02 mg/kg (minimum, 0.1 mg; maximum, 0.5 mg)
	Glucagon	IV	50 µg/kg over 1–2 min
			Continuous infusion: 50–100 µg/kg/h, titrate as needed
	Insulin	IV	1 IU/kg
			Continuous infusion: 0.5 IU/kg/h, titrate as needed
	Vasopressors	IV	
	Epinephrine		0.05 µg/kg/min, titrate to effect
	Norepinephrine		0.05 µg/kg/min, titrate to effect
Carbon monoxide	Oxygen	Inhaled	100%
Cyclic antidepressants	Sodium bicarbonate	IV	1–2 mEq/kg
			Continuous infusion: 150 mEq/L in D5W with 40 mEq potassium chloride added per liter, titrate as needed

Table 17.2 Continued

Toxin	Treatment	Route	Dose
Opiates	Naloxone	IV (alternate routes: IO, IM, SubQ, ET)	Nonlife threatening ≤5 y, 0.01 mg/kg >5 y, 0.4 mg Life threatening ≤5 y, 0.1 mg/kg (maximum, 2 mg) >5 y, 2 mg Continuous infusion: 25–40 µg/kg/h, titrate as needed
Salicylates	Sodium bicarbonate	IV	1–2 mEq/kg Continuous infusion: 150 mEq/L in D5W with 40 mEq potassium chloride added per liter, at 2–3 mL/kg/h
	Hemodialysis		
Sulfonylurea	25% Dextrose	IV	0.5–1 g/kg (2–4 mL/kg)
	Octreotide	SubQ	1 µg/kg every 6–12 h
Toxic alcohols	Fomepizole	IV	Loading dose: 15 mg/kg Subsequent dose: 10 mg/kg every 12 h × 4 doses, then 15 mg/kg every 12 h until level <20 mg/dL
	10% Ethanol	IV	Loading dose: 8–10 mL/kg (maximum, 200 mL)
	Folic acid	IV	Maintenance dose: 0.8 mL/kg/h
	Hemodialysis		1 mg/kg every 4 h

D5W, 5% dextrose solution; ET, endotracheal; IM, intramuscular; IO, intraosseous; IV, intravenous; PO, orally; SubQ, subcutaneous.

a Continue maintenance dosing until serum transaminase levels are decreasing, and coagulopathy is resolving.

pharmacodynamics exist for the numerous drugs in this category. In general, they have variable gastrointestinal absorption and undergo hepatic metabolism to both active and inactive metabolites. Excretion is primarily through urine.

Presentation

Patients with opioid toxicity present with central nervous system (CNS) depression and pinpoint pupils. More severe exposure leads to respiratory depression, apnea, bradycardia, hypotension, coma, and death (Table 17.1). Evaluation of the patient with suspected opioid ingestion should include acetaminophen and salicylate levels because of the risk of exposure to combination products. Routine laboratory studies for isolated opioid toxicity are neither indicated nor helpful in guiding therapy.

Management

Patients with respiratory depression or acute respiratory failure secondary to opioid toxicity should be treated with naloxone. Naloxone is a competitive antagonist that displaces opioids at the opioid receptor. When administered intravenously (IV), its onset of action is within 2 minutes, and its duration is 20 to 60 minutes. This is often shorter than the duration of the offending agent; therefore, the naloxone dose may need to be repeated or a continuous infusion initiated (Table 17.2). In addition, patients may require supportive care, including airway management and mechanical ventilation, fluid resuscitation, and vasopressors for shock.

Salicylates

Salicylates are used for mild analgesia, anti-inflammation, antipyresis, and platelet inhibition. They are available as a nonprescription, single-agent preparation (aspirin), combination products with opioids and caffeine, in topical preparations for treatment of myalgias, and as oil of wintergreen (methyl salicylate). Salicylates acetylate cyclooxygenase (COX)-1 irreversibly, which prevents platelet production of thromboxane A_2 at low doses. At intermediate doses, salicylates inhibit COX-1 and COX-2, which blocks prostaglandin production, resulting in antipyretic and analgesic effects. Aspirin is absorbed in the stomach and small intestine, metabolized in the liver (enzymes are saturable), and eliminated in the urine. With toxicity, salicylates cause direct stimulation of the CNS respiratory center, resulting in tachypnea, hyperpnea, and respiratory alkalosis. They also uncouple oxidative phosphorylation, inhibit the Krebs cycle and amino acid metabolism, and stimulate lipid metabolism (forming ketones), which results in metabolic acidosis. Impaired glucose metabolism can cause early hyperglycemia, which progresses to hypoglycemia.

Presentation

Mild salicylate toxicity can present with tinnitus, tachypnea, tachycardia, and vomiting. As toxicity progresses, a mixed respiratory alkalosis and metabolic acidosis occurs. Severe toxicity can cause seizures, coma resulting from cerebral edema, anion gap metabolic acidosis, and pulmonary edema (Table 17.1). Patients may be hypovolemic as a result of volume loss from the following sources: gastrointestinal (vomiting), respiratory (tachypnea), skin (diaphoresis), and renal. Evaluation of patients with toxicity should include serial salicylate levels until they have peaked and are declining. Serum electrolytes, renal function, liver transaminases, complete blood count, and coagulation profile should be obtained. Blood gases (arterial or venous) should be monitored serially for patients receiving alkalinization.

Management

Hypovolemia should be corrected with isotonic IV fluid volume expansion. Patients with salicylate levels more than 30 mg/dL should be treated aggressively, because levels may increase rapidly after initial presentation.

Alkalinization with sodium bicarbonate decreases CNS penetration and increases elimination of salicylates in the urine (Table 17.2). Serial blood gases and urine pH should be monitored with a goal serum pH of 7.55 and a urine pH of 7.5 to 8. Alkalinization may cause hypokalemia, and potassium should be repleted as needed. Hemodialysis should be instituted for patients with severe toxicity marked by salicylate levels greater than 90 mg/dL, refractory acidosis, encephalopathy, or renal failure.

Carbon Monoxide

Carbon monoxide (CO) poisoning is the leading cause of unintentional poisoning death in the United States, and pediatric patients are the age group most commonly exposed (25.7 children/million/y). CO is a gas produced from the incomplete combustion of carbon-containing fuels such as gasoline, natural gas, wood, and coal. CO accumulates when such fuels are burned (appliances, generators, motor vehicles, and so on) in poorly ventilated spaces. Fire with smoke inhalation can also result in CO toxicity. CO diffuses readily across the alveoli and has an affinity 250 times greater for hemoglobin than oxygen. This results in tissue hypoxia and end-organ damage most common in the brain, myocardium, and skeletal muscle.

Presentation

Symptoms of CO poisoning can be nonspecific and include headache, dizziness, nausea, and vomiting. Prolonged or severe exposure to CO can result in altered mental status, syncope, loss of consciousness, seizure, and death (Table 17.1). Carboxyhemoglobin levels measured by an arterial or venous blood gas greater than 2% are abnormal in nonsmokers and are indicative of exposure. Other diagnostic studies should include creatine phosphokinase to evaluate for rhabdomyolysis, electrocardiogram (ECG), creatine kinase with muscle–brain subunits, and troponin to evaluate for myocardial ischemia. Neuroimaging including computed tomography and/or magnetic resonance imaging should be performed if alterations in neurological examination persist after normalization of carboxyhemoglobin levels.

Management

The treatment for CO poisoning is 100% oxygen, which induces a fivefold decrease in the half-life of carboxyhemoglobin (room air $t_{1/2}$ 4–6 hours vs. 100% oxygen $t_{1/2}$ 60–75 minutes). Oxygen can be administered via a nonrebreather mask or an endotracheal tube. Therapy should be continued until carboxyhemoglobin levels are less than 5% and symptoms have resolved. Hyperbaric oxygen therapy is controversial. It may be recommended for patients with acute, severe poisoning; carboxyhemoglobin levels greater than 20%; and/or abnormal neurological examination. Theoretical advantages to hyperbaric oxygen therapy compared with normobaric oxygen therapy include increased dissolved oxygen content in blood and accelerated elimination of CO ($t_{1/2}$ 20 minutes).

Cardiovascular Medications

Accidental and intentional exposure to cardiovascular agents has been increasing rapidly during the past decade. They are responsible for the second largest number of fatalities resulting from poisonings in the United States.

Calcium Channel Antagonists

Calcium channel antagonists are used therapeutically to treat hypertension, angina, and arrhythmias. There are three classes of calcium channel antagonists: (1) dihydropyridines, (2) phenylalkylamines, and (3) benzothiazepines. These agents bind to L-type calcium channels and block the intracellular influx of calcium to myocytes primarily in the peripheral vasculature and myocardium. They also inhibit insulin release in pancreatic β cells. In general, calcium channel antagonists are well absorbed after oral ingestion, have a large volume of distribution, and are highly protein bound. They undergo first-pass hepatic metabolism and are excreted in the urine and feces. These medications are available in immediate and extended-release formulations, the latter of which can prolong symptoms after exposure. The dihydropyridines (e.g., amlodipine, isradipine, nicardipine, nifedipine) have greater effect in the vasculature and cause arterial vasodilation, whereas the nondihydropyridines (diltiazem, verapamil) primarily affect myocardial contractility and conduction, resulting in hypotension and bradycardia.

Presentation

With mild toxicity, calcium channel antagonist exposure leads to dizziness and fatigue, which are manifestations of mild bradycardia and hypotension. With significant exposure, clinical signs can include bradycardia, dysrhythmias (atrioventricular conduction block), cardiogenic shock, and complete cardiovascular collapse with cardiac arrest (Table 17.1). A prolonged shock state can lead to metabolic acidosis and multiorgan dysfunction. Evaluation should include serum electrolytes, glucose, renal function, blood gas (venous or arterial), lactic acid, and an ECG. Cardiac enzymes including creatine kinase with muscle–brain subunits and troponin should be monitored serially for concerns of myocardial ischemia.

Management

Patients with significant hemodynamic instability and/or altered mental status may require mechanical ventilatory support and access with central venous and arterial lines. Initial treatment of calcium channel antagonist exposure is IV calcium (Table 17.2). If there is a beneficial effect, a continuous infusion can be initiated. Ionized calcium levels should be monitored serially to prevent hypercalcemia. Atropine should be administered per PALS guidelines for severe bradycardia, although its effectiveness is variable (Table 17.2).

Persistent hypotension should be treated with isotonic IV fluid resuscitation to correct hypovolemia, followed by vasopressors. Unfortunately, no single adrenergic agent has been shown to be more efficacious in this setting. Thus, norepinephrine is a reasonable choice for patients with low systemic vascular resistance. However, for patients with decreased contractility and low systemic vascular resistance, epinephrine may be beneficial because of its α- and β-receptor agonist effects. In adults, a median of two (range, 1–5) vasopressors were required, and very large doses may be necessary.

Glucagon stimulates adenyl cyclase on cardiac myocytes, which theoretically results in positive inotropic and chronotropic effects and should be considered with refractory hemodynamic instability. It can be delivered IV and has a rapid onset (1 minute) with a short duration of action (20 minutes). If effective, an infusion can be initiated (Table 17.2). Hyperinsulinemia/euglycemia therapy has also been reported to be efficacious. This therapy counters the hypoinsulinemic effects of calcium channel antagonist exposure, which leads to hyperglycemia and inability of the myocardium to use glucose as an energy source. Concomitant dextrose infusions may be necessary to maintain euglycemia and should be titrated based on serial serum glucose levels. Lipid emulsion therapy (intralipid 20%: IV 1.5 mL/kg bolus, 0.25 mL/kg over 1 hour) has been reported beneficial in one pediatric case report. The mechanism of action is theorized to be a myocardial energy source and activation of the L-type calcium channel.

In extremely symptomatic patients, external pacing can be considered for refractory bradycardia and atrioventricular block. Extracorporeal life support (ECLS) should be considered for hemodynamic instability refractory to the measures described previously and has been beneficial in pediatric case reports.

β-Adrenergic Blockers

Therapeutic indications for treatment of ingestion of β-adrenergic blockers are similar to calcium channel antagonists. These drugs competitively inhibit catecholamines from binding to the β_1 and β_2 adrenoreceptors, which prevents activation of adenyl cyclase and subsequent phosphorylation of L-type calcium channels. Calcium channels remain closed, preventing calcium influx, which results in bradycardia, hypotension, and conduction abnormalities. In general, β-adrenergic blockers are well absorbed, undergo first-pass hepatic metabolism, and are excreted in the urine. They are available in immediate and extended-release formulations, which can affect both the onset and duration of toxicity.

Presentation

The presentation and evaluation of β-adrenergic blocker toxicity is similar to calcium channel antagonists. In addition to bradycardia and hypotension, patients can also have bronchospasm and respiratory distress (Table 17.1).

Management

The management of β-adrenergic blocker toxicity is also similar to calcium channel antagonists, including atropine for bradycardia and isotonic IV fluids/vasopressors for hypotension. In addition, calcium, glucagon, hyperinsulinemia/euglycemia therapy, and lipid emulsion therapy may be beneficial. Nonpharmacological support such as external pacing and ECLS should be considered for cases refractory to other therapies.

Cyclic Antidepressants

Cyclic antidepressants are used to treat major depression, chronic pain, and migraine headaches. They inhibit the reuptake of norepinephrine and serotonin by presynaptic neurons. Tricyclic antidepressants (e.g., amitriptyline, desipramine, doxepin, imipramine) also inhibit histamine, dopamine, muscarinic, γ-aminobutyric acid, α_1-adrenergic receptors, and fast sodium channels in the myocardium. This results in symptoms of CNS depression (histamine), anticholinergic effects including tachycardia (muscarinic), hypotension (α_1), and cardiac conduction (sodium channel) abnormalities. Cyclic antidepressants are well absorbed, highly protein bound, hepatically metabolized, and renally excreted. Toxicity generally occurs within 2 hours of ingestion.

Presentation

Patients with mild toxicity present with sedation, hallucinations, tachycardia, and other anticholinergic effects including dry mouth, blurred vision, and urinary retention. Significant toxicity can present with seizures, coma, acute respiratory failure, hypotension, and ventricular dysrhythmias with wide-complex tachycardia and torsades de pointes (Table 17.1). Evaluation should include serum electrolytes, renal function, hepatic transaminases, creatine phosphokinase, and urinalysis to evaluate for rhabdomyolysis. In severe toxicity, serial ECGs should be monitored to evaluate conduction intervals and blood gases to follow the acid–base status.

Management

Patients with significant cyclic antidepressant exposure frequently require intubation and mechanical ventilation resulting from mental status changes and hemodynamic instability. Central venous and arterial lines should be placed for patients with dysrhythmias or shock. Cardiac conduction disturbances should be treated with IV sodium bicarbonate (Table 17.2). Alkalinization with serum pH goals of 7.45 to 7.55 should be followed with serial blood gases. Severe ventricular dysrhythmias refractory to bicarbonate boluses may require treatment per the PALS guidelines. Hypotension should be treated with isotonic IV fluids to correct hypovolemia, followed by direct-acting vasopressors (e.g., norepinephrine). Lipid emulsion therapy (IV intralipid 20%: 1–1.5 mL/kg, 0.25 mL/kg/min) has been reported in two pediatric patients with resolution of wide-complex dysrhythmias. ECLS can be considered for refractory dys-rhythmias or shock. Seizures should be treated with benzodiazepines and may require continuous electroencephalographic monitoring.

Sulfonylureas

Sulfonylureas are the most widely used class of drugs for the treatment of type 2 diabetes mellitus. Second-generation sulfonylureas (e.g., gliclazide, glimepiride, glipizide, glyburide) are available in immediate and extended-release formulations. Oral doses are absorbed rapidly, metabolized in the liver to active and inactive metabolites, and excreted in the urine. The sulfonyl-urea receptor antagonizes the adenosine triphosphate-dependent potassium channel, which leads to membrane depolarization, calcium influx to pancre-atic β cells, and insulin secretion independent of circulating glucose levels. Sulfonylureas also increase insulin sensitivity in peripheral tissue.

Presentation

Sulfonylurea toxicity typically presents within 8 hours of ingestion with symp-toms of hypoglycemia such as tremor, irritability, diaphoresis, and nausea. Infants may have difficulty feeding. With severe hypoglycemia, progressive CNS depression manifests with lethargy, seizure, and coma (Table 17.1). Evaluation for suspected sulfonylurea toxicity should include serum glucose and electrolytes. Neuroimaging (computed tomography or magnetic reso-nance imaging) should be performed if alterations in neurological examination persist after normalization of glucose levels.

Management

Asymptomatic patients should be allowed a regular diet and should not be given glucose containing IV fluids. They should be monitored with serial blood glucose levels (every 2 hours while awake, hourly while sleeping) for 24 hours. The initial treatment for patients with glucose less than 60 mg/dL is IV dextrose (Table 17.2). Dextrose administration restores euglycemia but potentiates pancreatic insulin release, which can result in recurrent episodes of hypoglycemia. For patients with repeated episodes (two or more) of hypo-glycemia, octreotide is an adjunctive therapy (Table 17.2). Octreotide binds to the somatostatin receptor attached to the voltage-gated calcium channel on pancreatic β cells, which reduces the calcium influx and thus inhibits insulin release.

Toxic Alcohols

Although alcohols were responsible for only 1% of pediatric exposures (<6 years) in 2011, they were responsible for almost 4% of deaths. Toxic alcohols include methanol, ethylene glycol, and isopropanol. They are found in household substances such as windshield washer fluid (methanol), antifreeze (ethylene glycol), and rubbing alcohol (isopropanol). The toxic alcohols are metabolized in the liver by alcohol dehydrogenase and form toxic metabolites. Methanol is metabolized to formic acid, which can lead to blindness. Oxalic acid is the toxic metabolite of ethylene glycol that combines with calcium to form calcium oxalate crystals in the renal tubules, which can lead to acute renal failure. Isopropranol is metabolized to acetone, which does not result in a metabolic acidosis.

Presentation

Patients with toxic alcohol exposures may be asymptomatic or exhibit CNS depression, nausea, and vomiting. More severe exposure presents with seizure, coma, tachycardia, hypotension, and multiorgan dysfunction (Table 17.1). Methanol and ethylene glycol toxicity presents with an osmol and anion gap metabolic acidosis:

- Osmol gap = Measured osmolality – Calculated osmolality
- Calculated osmolality = 2 × (Serum sodium [mEq/L]) + (Serum glucose [mg/dL])/18 + (Serum BUN [mg/dL])/2.8 + (Serum ethanol [mg/dL])/3.7
- Normal osmol gap less than 10 mOsm/kg

Evaluation should include serum electrolytes (including calcium), renal function, blood gas (arterial or venous), and osmolality. Serum ethanol levels should be obtained to evaluate for co-ingestion. Quantitative methanol and ethylene glycol levels can be measured if available.

Management

Treatment of patients with toxic alcohol exposure is based on clinical signs, including depressed level of consciousness and/or metabolic acidosis. Supportive care with airway management and mechanical ventilation, isotonic fluid resuscitation, vasopressors for hypotension, and benzodiazepines for seizures may be required.

The treatment for toxic alcohol exposure is fomepizole or ethanol. Both produce competitive inhibition of alcohol dehydrogenase, which prevents formation of toxic metabolites (Table 17.2). If levels are available, methanol or ethylene glycol >20 mg/dL are indications for therapy. Therapy should be continued until levels are undetectable and acidosis has resolved. In an adult study, fomepizole was associated with fewer adverse events (0.13 vs. 0.92 events per treatment day) than ethanol. If fomepizole is unavailable, ethanol infusion should be titrated to goal levels of 100 to 150 mg/dL. Patients require close glucose monitoring to prevent hypoglycemia during ethanol infusion. Folic acid should also be administered to patients with methanol toxicity because it has been shown to enhance metabolism of formic acid in an animal model (Table 17.2). Hemodialysis should be initiated in patients with refractory metabolic acidosis, renal failure, or multiorgan dysfunction.

Conclusion

Pediatric toxic exposures occur more frequently than any other age group and are often unintentional in the young child (<6 years). Unfortunately, exposures that require medical intervention and result in adverse outcomes are increasing. Critical illness with organ dysfunction requiring invasive monitoring and interventions can result from many poisonings. Supportive care and specific therapies unique to the pediatric intensive care unit are crucial to the management of poisoned patients. Intensivists should be familiar with toxins that can result in critical illness and their therapies.

Further Reading

Spiller HA, Beuhler MC, Ryan ML, et al. Evaluation of changes in poisoning in young children: 2000 to 2010. *Pediatr Emerg Care.* 2013;29(5):635–640.

Kerns W 2nd. Management of beta-adrenergic blocker and calcium channel antagonist toxicity. *Emerg Med Clin North Am.* 2007;25(2):309–331.

Presley JD, Chyka PA. Intravenous lipid emulsion to reverse acute drug toxicity in pediatric patients. *Ann Pharmacother.* 2013;47(5):735–743.

Masson R, Colas V, Parienti JJ, et al. A comparison of survival with and without extracorporeal life support treatment for severe poisoning due to drug intoxication. *Resuscitation.* 2012;83(11):1413–1417.

Brooks DE, Levine M, O'Connor AD, French RN, Curry SC. Toxicology in the ICU: part 2: specific toxins. *Chest.* 2011;140(4):1072–1085.

Spiller HA, Sawyer TS. Toxicology of oral antidiabetic medications. *Am J Health-Syst Pharm.* 2006;63(10):929–938.

Chapter 18

Pediatric Critical Care Pharmacology

Athena Zuppa

Pharmacology is essential to our understanding of how drugs are handled by the body and how they interact with one another, and to help guide their administration. Pediatric pharmacotherapy is especially challenging because of developmental changes that may alter drug kinetics, pathophysiological differences that may alter pharmacodynamics, disease etiologies that may differ from adults, and other factors that may result in great variation in safety and efficacy. The situation becomes more difficult when one considers critically ill children, organ dysfunction, and polypharmacy, with the paucity of well-controlled pediatric clinical trials in this population. Prescribing caregivers of critically ill children must have some understanding of the basic processes that govern the current dosing recommendations for their patients. This chapter provides a review of the pharmacological principles that guide pharmacotherapy in general, with a focus on pharmacotherapy used frequently in the pediatric critical care setting.

Fundamentals of Pharmacology

Pharmacokinetics is often summarized as *what the body does to the drug*, and it includes absorption, distribution, metabolism, and excretion. *Pharmacodynamics* is the physiological *effects of the drug on the body*, focusing largely on mechanisms of drug action and the relationship between concentration and effect (Figure 18.1).

Absorption

Absorption is the transfer of a drug from its site of administration to the blood stream. The rate and efficiency of absorption depend on the route of administration. For intravenous administration, absorption is complete; the total dose reaches the systemic circulation. Drugs administered enterally may be absorbed either by passive diffusion or active transport.

The bioavailability (F) of a drug is defined by the extent of absorption following administration by any route other than intravenous injection. If a drug is administered intravenously, then the bioavailability is 100% and F = 1.0. When drugs are administered by routes other than intravenous, the bioavailability is less.

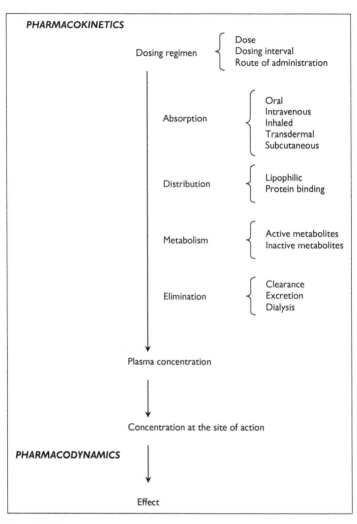

Figure 18.1 Fundamentals of pharmacology.

Distribution

The volume of distribution (Vd) is a hypothetical volume of fluid through which a drug is dispersed. A drug rarely disperses solely into the water compartments of the body. Instead, most drugs disperse to several compartments, including adipose tissue and plasma proteins. The total volume into which a drug disperses is called the *apparent volume of distribution*. This volume is not a physiological space, but instead is a derived parameter. It relates the total amount of drug (Drug) in the body to the concentration of drug (C_p) in the blood or plasma:

$$Vd = \frac{Drug}{C_p}.$$

Figure 18.2 represents the fate of a drug after intravenous administration. After administration, a maximal plasma concentration is achieved, and the drug is immediately distributed. The plasma concentration then decreases over time. This initial phase is called the *alpha* (α) *phase* of drug distribution, during which the decline in plasma concentration is a result of the distribution of the drug. When a drug is distributed, it may undergo metabolism and is excreted. The second phase is called the *beta* (β) *phase*, when the decline in plasma concentration is a result of drug metabolism and excretion. The distribution half-life and elimination half-life can be determined, respectively, by

$$t_{1/2\alpha} = \frac{0.693}{\alpha} \quad \text{and} \quad t_{1/2\beta} = \frac{0.693}{\beta}.$$

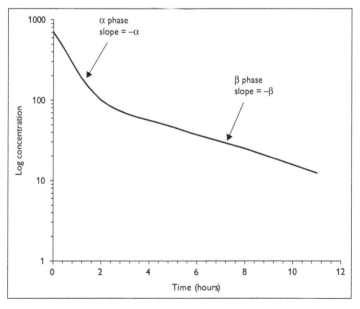

Figure 18.2 Semilogarithmic plot of concentration versus time after an intravenous administration of a drug that follows two-compartment pharmacokinetics.

Metabolism

The liver is the principal organ of drug metabolism. Other tissues that display considerable metabolic activity include the gastrointestinal tract, the lungs, the skin, and the kidneys. Following oral administration, many drugs are absorbed intact from the small intestine and transported to the liver via the portal system, where they are metabolized. This process is called *first-pass metabolism* and may greatly limit the bioavailability of orally administered drugs.

In general, all metabolic reactions can be classified as either phase I or phase II biotransformation. Phase I reactions usually convert the parent drug to a polar metabolite by introducing or unmasking a more polar site (–OH, –NH$_2$). If phase I metabolites are sufficiently polar, they may be excreted readily. However, many phase I metabolites undergo a subsequent reaction (phase II biotransformation) during which endogenous substances such as glucoronic acid, sulfuric acid, or an amino acid combine with the metabolite to form a highly polar conjugate. However, phase II reactions may precede phase I reactions, as in the case of isoniazid.

Phase I reactions are usually catalyzed by enzymes of the cytochrome P450 system. These drug-metabolizing enzymes are located in the lipophilic membranes of the endoplasmic reticulum of the liver and other tissues. Three families—CYP1, CYP2, and CYP3—are responsible for most drug biotransformations. The CYP3A subfamily accounts for greater than 50% of phase I drug metabolism, predominantly by the CYP3A4 subtype. *CYP3A4 is responsible for the metabolism of drugs commonly used in the intensive care setting*, including acetaminophen, cyclosporine, diazepam, methadone, midazolam, spironolactone, and tacrolimus. Most other drug biotransformations are performed by CYP2D6 (e.g., clozapine, codeine, flecainide, haloperidol, oxycodone), CYP2C9 (e.g., phenytoin, S-warfarin), CYP2C19 (e.g., diazepam, omeprazole, propanolol), CYP2E1 (e.g., acetaminophen, enflurane, halothane), and CYP1A2 (e.g., acetaminophen, caffeine, theophylline, warfarin). Drug biotransformation reactions may be enhanced or impaired by multiple factors, including age, enzyme induction or inhibition, pharmacogenetics, and the effects of other disease states.

The metabolic transformation of dugs is catalyzed by enzymes, and most reactions follow Michaelis Menten kinetics:

$$V(\text{rate of drug metabolism}) = \frac{(V_{max})(C)}{(Km+C)},$$

where C is the drug concentration and Km is the Michaelis Menten constant. In most situations, the drug concentration is much less than Km, and the equation simplifies to

$$V(\text{rate of drug metabolism}) = \frac{(V_{max})(C)}{Km}.$$

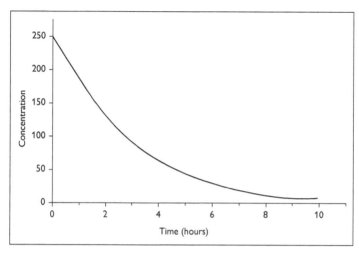

Figure 18.3 Concentration-versus-time profile of a drug demonstrating first-order elimination.

In this case, the rate of drug metabolism is directly proportional to the concentration of free drug and follows *first-order kinetics*. A constant percentage of the drug is metabolized over time, and the rate of elimination is proportional to the amount of drug in the body. Most drugs used in the clinical setting are eliminated in this manner. Figure 18.3 represents the concentration–time curve of drug that follows first-order elimination. A semilogarithmic plot results in a straight line, as represented in Figure 18.4.

A few drugs, such as aspirin, ethanol, and phenytoin, are used in higher doses, resulting in greater plasma concentrations. In these situations, C is much greater than Km, and the equation reduces to

$$V(\text{rate of drug metabolism}) = \frac{(V_{max})(C)}{(C)} = V_{max}.$$

The enzyme system becomes saturated by a high free-drug concentration, and the rate of metabolism is constant over time. This is called *zero-order kinetics*, and a constant amount of drug is metabolized per unit time. A large increase in serum concentration can result from a small increase in dose for drugs that follow zero-order elimination. A plot of concentration versus time results in a straight line, as represented in Figure 18.5. A semilogarithmic plot of concentration versus time demonstrates a convex line, as seen in Figure 18.6.

Excretion

Clearance is usually referred to as the amount of blood from which all drug is removed per unit time (volume/time). The main organs responsible for drug

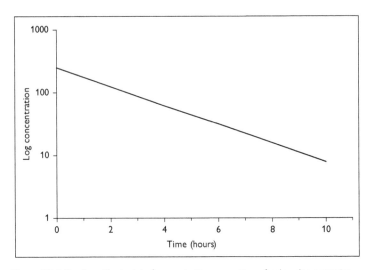

Figure 18.4 Semilogarithmic plot of concentration versus time of a drug demonstrating first-order elimination.

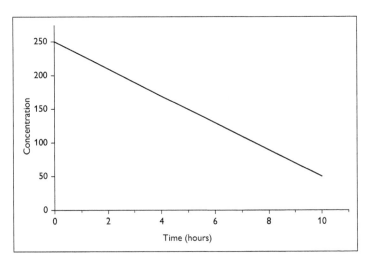

Figure 18.5 Concentration-versus-time profile of a drug demonstrating zero-order elimination.

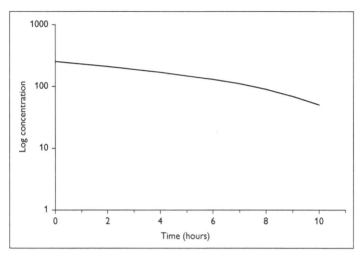

Figure 18.6 Semilogarithmic plot of concentration versus time of a drug demonstrating zero-order elimination.

clearance are the kidneys and the liver. The total body clearance of a drug is equal to the sum of the clearances from all mechanisms. Most elimination by the kidneys is accomplished by glomerular filtration. Therefore, an attempt to estimate the glomerular filtration rate is crucial to the proper dosing of drugs eliminated renally. Glomerular integrity, the size and charge of the drug, water solubility, and the extent of protein binding determine the amount of drug filtered. Highly protein-bound drugs are not filtered readily. In addition to glomerular filtration, drugs may be eliminated from the kidneys via active secretion. Secretion occurs predominantly at the proximal tubule, where energy-requiring active transport systems secrete primarily organic acids and bases. Organic acids include most cephalosporins, loop diuretics, methotrexate, nonsteroidal anti-inflammatories, penicillins, and thiazide diuretics. Organic bases include ranitidine and morphine. As drugs move toward the distal convoluted tubule, the concentration increases. High urine flow rates decrease the concentration of drug in the distal tubule, decreasing the likelihood that a drug diffuses from the lumen. For both weak acids and bases, the nonionized form of the drug is reabsorbed more readily. Altering the pH of the urine (ion trapping) can minimize this process by placing a charge on the drug and preventing its diffusion. For example, salicylate is a weak acid. In case of salicylate toxicity, urine alkalinization places a charge on the molecule and thus increases its elimination. The liver also contributes to elimination through metabolism or excretion into the bile. After a drug is secreted in the bile, it may then be either excreted into the feces or reabsorbed via enterohepatic recirculation.

Achieving steady state

The time to reach steady state is defined by the elimination half-life of the drug. After 1 half-life, 50% of the steady state concentration will be achieved. After 2 half-lives, 75% of steady state is reached, and after 3 half-lives about 87.5% of steady state is achieved, with final steady state achieved after 5 half-lives (97% of steady state achieved). For drugs with long half lives, target steady state concentrations can be achieved more quickly by using a loading dose.

Pediatric Implications

Absorption

Overall, the rate at which most drugs are absorbed is slower in neonates and young infants than in older children. As a result, the time required to achieve maximal plasma levels is longer in the very young. The effect of age on enteral absorption is not uniform and is difficult to predict. Gastric emptying and intestinal motility are the primary determinants of the rate at which drugs are presented to and dispersed along the mucosal surface of the small intestine. At birth, the coordination of antral contractions improves, resulting in a marked increase in gastric emptying during the first week of life. Similarly, intestinal motor activity matures throughout early infancy, with consequent increases in the frequency, amplitude, and duration of propagating contractions. Changes in the intraluminal pH in different segments of the gastrointestinal tract can affect directly both the stability and the degree of ionization of a drug, thus influencing the relative amount of drug available for absorption. During the neonatal period, intragastric pH is relatively elevated (pH >4). Thus, oral administration of acid-labile compounds such as penicillin G produces greater bioavailability in neonates than in older infants and children. In contrast, drugs that are weak acids, such as phenobarbital, may require larger oral doses in the very young to achieve therapeutic plasma levels. Other factors that impact the rate of absorption include age-associated development of villi, splanchnic blood flow, changes in intestinal microflora, and intestinal surface area.

Distribution

As children develop and grow, changes in body composition, development of metabolizing enzymes, and maturation of renal and liver function all impact drug disposition. The effect of age on enteral absorption is not uniform and is difficult to predict. The percent of total body water drops from about 85% in premature infants to 75% in full-term infants to 60% in the adult. Extracellular water decreases from 45% in the infant to 25% in the adult. Total body fat in the premature infant can be as low as 1%, compared with 15% in the normal, term infant. Many drugs are less bound to plasma proteins in the neonate and infant than in the older child.

Metabolism

Hepatic biotransformation reactions are reduced substantially during the neonatal period. At birth, the cytochrome P450 system is 28% that of the adult. The expression of phase I enzymes such as the P450 cytochromes changes markedly during development. CYP3A7, the predominant CYP isoform expressed in fetal liver, peaks shortly after birth and then declines rapidly to levels that are undetectable in most adults. Within hours after birth, CYP2E1 activity surges, and CYP2D6 becomes detectable soon thereafter. CYP3A4 and CYP2C (CYP2C9 and CYP2C19) appear during the first week of life, whereas CYP1A2 is the last hepatic CYP to appear, at 1 to 3 months of life. The ontogeny of phase II enzymes is less well established than the ontogeny of reactions involving phase I enzymes. Available data indicate the individual isoforms of glucuronosyltransferase (UGT) have unique maturational profiles with pharmacokinetic consequences. For example, the glucuronidation of acetaminophen (a substrate for UGT1A6 and, to a lesser extent, UGT1A9) is decreased in newborns and young children compared with adolescents and adults. Glucuronidation of morphine (a UGT2B7 substrate) can be detected in premature infants as young as 24 weeks of gestational age.

Excretion

Renal function in the premature and full-term neonate, both glomerular filtration and tubular secretion, is reduced significantly compared with older children. Maturation of renal function is a dynamic process that begins during fetal life and is complete by early childhood. Maturation of tubular function is slower than that of glomerular filtration. The glomerular filtration rate is approximately 2 to 4 mL/min/1.73 m² in term neonates, but it may be as low as 0.6 to 0.8 mL/min/1.73 m² in preterm neonates. The glomerular filtration rate increases rapidly during the first 2 weeks of life and continues to increase until adult values are reached at 8 to 12 months of age. For drugs that are renally eliminated, impaired renal function decreases clearance, increasing the elimination half-life. Therefore, for drugs that are eliminated primarily by the kidney, such as vancomycin, dosing should be performed in an age-appropriate fashion that takes into account both maturational and disease-related changes in kidney function.

Critical Illness

Renal Dysfunction

Renal failure can impact the pharmacokinetics of drugs. In renal failure, the binding of acidic drugs to albumin is decreased because of competition with accumulated organic acids and uremia-induced structural changes in albumin that decrease drug-binding affinity, altering Vd. Drugs that are more than 30% eliminated unchanged in the urine are likely to have significantly diminished clearance in the presence of renal insufficiency.

Hepatic Dysfunction

Drugs that undergo extensive first-pass metabolism may have a significantly greater oral bioavailability in patients with liver failure than in normal subjects. Gut hypomotility may delay the peak response to enterally administered drugs in these patients. Hypoalbuminemia may affect the fractional protein binding of acidic or basic drugs. Altered plasma protein concentrations may affect the extent of tissue distribution of drugs that are normally highly protein bound. The presence of significant edema and ascites may alter the Vd of highly water-soluble agents, such as aminoglycoside antibiotics. The capacity of the liver to metabolize drugs depends on hepatic blood flow and liver enzyme activity, both of which can be affected by liver disease. In addition, some P450 isoforms are more susceptible than others to liver disease, impairing drug metabolism.

Cardiac Dysfunction

Circulatory failure, or shock, can alter the pharmacokinetics of drugs used frequently in the intensive care setting. Drug absorption may be impaired because of bowel wall edema. Passive hepatic congestion may impede first-pass metabolism, resulting in greater plasma concentrations. In addition, liver hypoperfusion may alter the drug-metabolizing enzyme function, especially flow-dependent drugs such as lidocaine. Peripheral edema inhibits absorption by intramuscular parenteral routes. The balance of tissue hypoperfusion versus increased total body water with edema may alter Vd unpredictably.

Important Drug Interactions

The patients cared for in the intensive care setting are treated with many drugs, increasing the chance of a drug–drug interaction. These interactions can alter absorption, distribution metabolism, and clearance. Drug interactions that affect absorption include formation of drug–drug complexes, alterations in gastric pH, and changes in gastrointestinal motility. This can have a significant impact on the bioavailability of enterally administered agents. The volume of distribution may be altered with competitive plasma protein binding and subsequent changes in free drug concentrations.

Drug biotransformation reactions vary greatly among individuals and are susceptible to drug–drug interactions. *Induction* is the process by which enzyme activity is increased by exposure to a certain drug, resulting in an increase in metabolism of other drugs, and *lower plasma concentrations*. Common inducers include barbiturates, carbamezapine, isonizaid, and rifampin. On the contrary, *inhibition* is the process by which enzyme activity is decreased by exposure to a certain drug, resulting in a decrease in metabolism of other drugs, and subsequent *higher plasma concentrations*. Common enzyme inhibitors include ciprofloxacin, fluconazole, metronidazole, quinidine, and valproic acid.[1] Inducers and inhibitors of phase II enzymes have been characterized less extensively, but some clinical applications of this information have emerged, including the use of phenobarbital to induce glucuronyl transferase activity in icteric neonates. The clearance of drugs excreted entirely by glomerular filtration is unlikely to be affected by other drugs. In contrast, organic acids and bases are secreted renally and can compete with one another for elimination, resulting in unpredictable drug disposition.

Conclusion

An understanding of pharmacokinetics and pharmacodynamics can allow for a rational approach toward prescribing medications for critically ill children. Absorption, distribution, metabolism, elimination, and the response to medications are affected by age and disease state. One should consult a pediatric formulary for guidelines regarding drug dosing, dosing intervals, and therapeutic drug monitoring in pediatric patients. Medications administered inappropriately may not allow patients to receive the optimal therapeutic potential and may expose them to unnecessary drug toxicity. Consultation with reference books and clinical pharmacists is strongly recommended.

Reference

1. Carruthers SG, Hoffman BB , Melmon KL, et al., eds. *Clinical Pharmacology Basic Principles in Therapeutics.* 4th ed. New York: McGraw-Hill. 2000:1433.

Further Reading

Chernow B, ed. *The Pharmacologic Approach to the Critically Ill Patient.* 3rd ed. Baltimore: Williams and Wilkins; 1994:1220.

Katzung BG, ed. *Basic and Clinical Pharmacology.* 8th ed. McGraw Hill; 2001.

Kearns GL, Abdel-Rahman SM, Alander SW, et al. Developmental pharmacology: drug disposition, action, and therapy in infants and children. *N Engl J Med.* 2003;349(12):1157–1167.

Krishnan V, Murray P. Pharmacologic issues in the critically ill. *Clin Chest Med.* 2003;24(4):671–688.

Rodighiero V. Effects of liver disease on pharmacokinetics: an update. *Clin Pharmacokinet.* 1999;37(5):399–431.

Chapter 19

Pediatric Trauma

Joanna C. Lim, Catherine Goodhue, Elizabeth Cleek,
Erik R. Barthel, Barbara Gaines, and Jeffrey S. Upperman

In the United States, injury is the leading cause of death for children ages 1 through 14 years. More children are killed as the result of unintentional injuries than the next eight leading causes of death combined. Even when children survive, thousands each year are left with temporary and permanent disability secondary to their injuries.

Pediatric injuries are categorized by mechanism: blunt, penetrating, thermal, and anoxic. Overwhelmingly, blunt trauma is the leading mechanism (e.g., falls, motor vehicle crashes, sports injuries). Although half of all blunt pediatric injuries are secondary to falls, the leading mechanism resulting in pediatric death is motor vehicle collision.

Comprehensive, safe, and effective trauma care is provided through a systematic approach. To do this, a trauma system must include all components required for optimal trauma care, including prevention, open access to care, prehospital care, acute care, rehabilitation, and research.

The leading, verifying body for trauma centers is the American College of Surgeons' criteria, which are outlined in the *Resources for Optimal Care of the Injured Patient*. In addition, trauma centers may be designated by county or state jurisdictions. Trauma centers must have all the needed surgical and medical services required for care—from arrival through discharge. This includes the emergency department, operating room, pediatric intensive care unit and acute care units, and rehabilitation, as well as all the ancillary services needed to care for children and their families. Providers caring for acutely injured children must be familiar with their institution's designated level of trauma care as well as the indications and logistics of timely transfer to higher level trauma centers.

Pathophysiology

The overall pathophysiology of trauma is known as the "bloody vicious cycle" (Figure 19.1). The theory is that trauma-induced tissue ischemia results in coagulopathy, which is exacerbated by hypothermia and metabolic acidosis. If a patient enters the cycle, clinical deterioration ensues unless the team works actively to correct these factors.

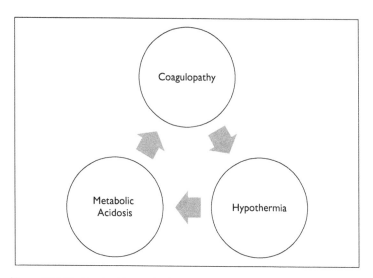

Figure 19.1 The bloody, vicious cycle of trauma.

Initial Management

Initial management of a critically injured child requires prompt identification and treatment of life-threatening injuries. Ideally, initial management is done with a multidisciplinary team experienced in pediatric trauma care, including emergency room physicians, surgeons, critical care specialists, nurses, and allied health providers experienced in pediatric trauma care. Advanced Trauma Life Support guides providers to evaluate the injured child through the *A, B, C, D, and Es of trauma care*, first addressing life-threatening injuries in the primary survey before focusing on distracting injuries. Every patient should undergo primary survey and then secondary survey to ensure a complete and thorough examination that is not distracted by obvious injuries.

Airway

While maintaining cervical spine (c-spine) precautions, the team evaluates for a patent and protected airway. A child may not be able to protect his or her airway secondary to a brain injury and a diminished Glasgow Coma Scale (GCS) score. In addition, an airway may be obstructed from facial trauma or impaired by inhalation injury.

When necessary, a child is intubated per the Pediatric Advanced Life Support protocol while c-spine precautions are maintained. When an endotracheal tube cannot be inserted orally or nasally, a surgical airway may be required, such as a tracheostomy, but this is rare. If possible, a cricothyroidotomy should be avoided in young children because it can lead to subglottic stenosis.

Breathing

When an airway is secured, the examination focuses on breathing, including respiratory rate, work of breathing, and breath sounds. Sequelae from blunt or penetrating trauma may include hemo- or pneumothorax, pulmonary contusions, or rib fractures. Because children are quite pliable and high forces are required to break bones, fractures should raise the suspicion for major intrathoracic injury. Burn inhalation injuries and anoxic injuries often lead to pulmonary edema.

Interventions may include chest tube insertion for a hemo- or pneumothorax. A tension pneumothorax is a life-threatening emergency, commonly presenting with tracheal deviation away from the affected side, absent breath sounds on the affected side, and difficult ventilation. This emergency must be treated promptly with placement of a large-bore intravenous (IV) catheter in the second intercostal space in the midclavicular line on the affected side followed by chest tube insertion.

Circulation

In trauma, impaired circulation is related directly to blood loss. It is essential to ask prehospital personnel about blood loss in the field and en route to the hospital. In addition to palpating pulses and measuring blood pressure to assess circulation, large-bore IV access should be placed at this time for resuscitation. If prompt peripheral access cannot be obtained, intraosseous infusion in an uninjured long bone (that is not distal to a more proximal extremity vascular injury) is the next choice for pediatric infusion.

In trauma patients, shock is presumed to be hemorrhagic until proved otherwise. Differential diagnosis for shock in the trauma patient should also include consideration of tension pneumothorax; cardiac shock such as tamponade, contusion, or aortic dissection; or neurological shock. One significant difference in hypovolemic shock between adults and children is that hypotension is a very late finding in children whereas it is an early sign in adults.

Reestablishing circulating volume is accomplished with both isotonic fluids and blood products when indicated. Pediatric resuscitation is guided by weight, starting with boluses of isotonic fluid at 20 mL/kg. If the patient does not respond appropriately after three boluses of isotonic fluid, the following bolus should be packed red blood cells at 10 mL/kg. If multiple packed red blood cell transfusions are indicated to maintain perfusion, plasma (20 mL/kg) and platelets (10–15 mL/kg or 1 U/10 kg) should be administered and a massive blood transfusion protocol activated. Ultimately, operative intervention may be required to stop the hemorrhage after initial resuscitation.

Hemodynamic stability can be gauged by hemostasis, capillary refill, skin warmth, normal blood pressure, pulse rate, and respiratory rate for age, and adequate urine output.

Next Steps – Secondary Survey

When the primary survey is complete and the patient is stabilized, a *secondary survey* is initiated—a thorough and comprehensive head-to-toe examination evaluating for any remaining injuries. It repeats the ABCs of the primary survey to reassess for any changes in hemodynamics before proceeding with D and E.

Disability

Next, the neurological examination is assessed by GCS score (Box 19.1). For young, nonverbal children, the infant GCS can be used.

Exposure

The final component of the primary survey is exposure and environmental control, removing any extra clothing while avoiding hypothermia. It is important to maintain normothermia as much as possible, because children are more prone to heat loss as a result of the larger surface-to-volume ratio. The child is rolled while maintaining c-spine and full spine precautions to inspect for further injuries and to palpate the entire spine for step-offs or abnormalities. A digital rectal examination is completed as indicated to evaluate for spinal cord and rectal injury. Trauma patients should receive a chest X-ray before leaving the trauma bay.

As with all patients, comprehensive care requires a medical history. On arrival, emergency medical service personnel give a pertinent history of the trauma events, including mechanism, field examination, vital signs, blood loss, and interventions in the field. In addition, they may be able to provide an *AMPLE history—Allergies, Medications, Past illnesses/Pregnancy, Last meal, Events/Environment*—related to the injury. In pediatric trauma, this history may

Box 19.1 Infant Glasgow Coma Scale		
Eyes	**Verbal**	**Motor**
4: Spontaneous 3: To verbal 2: To pain 1: No response	5: Smiles, oriented to sounds, coos, babbles 4: Cries but consolable, inappropriate interactions 3: Inconsistently inconsolable, moaning 2: Inconsolable, agitated 1: No response	6: Moves spontaneously 5: Withdraws from touch 4: Withdraws from pain 3: Flexion to pain 2: Extension to pain 1: No response

be delayed until a parent arrives. In adolescents, a HEADSS—*Home, Education and Employment, Activity, Drugs, Sexuality, and Suicidality/Safety*—assessment should be obtained because trauma may be the direct result of intentional high-risk behaviors.

Injury By System

Head Trauma

Head trauma is a leading cause of injury in childhood; falls and traffic crashes are common mechanisms of injury. Management principles include rapid identification and treatment of the primary injury and minimizing the secondary injuries resulting from diminished cerebral perfusion.

As the patient is undergoing the primary survey, spine precautions should be maintained with a cervical collar and logroll motion. An incorrectly sized cervical collar can impair the airway. The child's neurological status should be assessed by *AVPU—Alert, Verbal, Pain, Unresponsive.* Level of consciousness should be recorded using the GCS, comparing the score with prehospital assessment while factoring history of any loss of consciousness and its duration at the scene or during transport. Children with a GCS score of 8 points or less require immediate intubation. Increased intracranial pressure may manifest through signs and symptoms (Box 19.2).

Patients with neurological impairment or concerning mechanisms should be imaged by a brain CT and cervical spine radiographs. If any head or neck injuries are detected, neurosurgery should be involved promptly. If the c-spine X-ray is negative, the collar can be removed while assessing for pain, sensation, and mobility. If an injury is suspected, the child should stay in strict c-spine immobility and neurosurgery should be notified. Magnetic resonance imaging is sensitive to ligamentous injury. If seizures occur, anticonvulsant therapy should be administered.

Skull fractures and intracranial injury should be suspected in the presence of a scalp hematoma, and fractures may require surgical intervention if depressed

Box 19.2 Neurological Signs and Symptoms of Intracranial Hypertension	
Signs	**Symptoms**
• Alteration in consciousness	• Irritability
• Abnormal posturing	• Vomiting
• Changes in pupillary size, symmetry, and/or reaction	• Headache
• Bulging anterior fontanelle in infants	• Seizures
• Sunsetting (restricted upward gaze)	

or comminuted. Basilar skull fractures typically present with Battle sign (mastoid ecchymosis), hemotympanum, or cerebrospinal fluid leakage from the nose or ear. Historically, antibiotics have been given to prevent ascending meningitis from cerebrospinal fluid leaks, but recent evidence does not support this practice. A fracture involving the temporal bone requires evaluation by otolaryngology. The child will require an audiogram and otolaryngological follow up 4 to 6 weeks after discharge. Orbital fractures require evaluation by an ophthalmologist to assess for entrapment and evaluation by a surgeon who specializes with facial fractures, such as a plastic surgeon. Most children with a skull fracture are admitted for observation and frequent assessment of their neurological status. Initially, on admission, the child is given nothing by mouth for 12 to 24 hours, then the diet is advanced slowly. The fracture often heals on its own in 6 to 8 weeks if no surgical intervention is indicated, and, in the interim, the child should avoid activities that could result in another head trauma.

Intracranial hemorrhage is diagnosed with CT. Epidural hematomas are typically a result of tears in the middle meningeal artery. The usual presentation is loss of consciousness at the scene and a lucid period followed by deterioration. Subdural hematomas are the result of tears in the bridging veins. Hematomas causing significant midline shift require neurosurgical evacuation; children with smaller hematomas are admitted for close observation. Patients with intracranial hemorrhage are admitted for observation but may require decompression, depending on size and location.

Thoracic Trauma

Blunt thoracic trauma is suspected in children who fall from a great height or who are involved in high-velocity motor vehicle collisions. Penetrating chest trauma is seen in stabbings and gunshot injuries. Clinicians should assess for signs and symptoms of hypovolemic shock. Prehospital providers and others *should not* remove any penetrating objects from the patient until surgeons, in a controlled setting, evaluate the patient. Clinicians must stabilize the object until it can be removed safely in the operating room. Providers should obtain a chest radiograph.

Cardiac tamponade is a life-threatening condition and is suspected by muffled heart tones, jugular venous distention, and hypotension, and should be treated promptly with the administration of isotonic fluids and pericardiocentesis. Although drainage procedures can be sufficient, one should anticipate that definitive management may require thoracotomy, whether in the trauma bay or in the operating room. Tension pneumothorax can often present similarly with jugular venous distention and hypotension, but with tracheal deviation—often a late sign. As described previously, emergent management is needle decompression followed by insertion of a chest tube.

Ribs in infants and young children are cartilaginous and rarely sustain fractures; if fractures are found, one should suspect high-energy injury or, in cases when an insignificant mechanism is reported, nonaccidental trauma. Older children may sustain rib fractures, so examine the child carefully for underlying injury to the lungs and heart. Rib fractures are painful. Adequate analgesia is the most crucial part of management, because pain-limited inspiration puts the patient at risk for pneumonia. Pulmonary contusion may be diagnosed on chest radiography; however, a spiral CT scan may be necessary for diagnosis. Monitor the child's respiratory status and ensure adequate ventilation. If cardiac contusion is suspected, obtain an electrocardiogram. Cardiology consult is warranted for an abnormal electrocardiogram, and an echocardiogram may be obtained. The child should be admitted for telemetry.

Abdominal Trauma

Blunt abdominal trauma is common in injured children, and multiorgan injury should be suspected because of the close proximity of the viscera in the pediatric population. During the secondary survey, the abdomen should be examined by visualization, auscultation, percussion, and palpation.

Diagnostic workup for the child with a potential intra-abdominal injury includes laboratory and imaging studies. Clinicians should obtain a hematocrit, alanine aminotransferase (aka ALT or SGPT), aspartate aminotransferase (aka AST or SGOT), lipase, and amylase as well as a urinalysis. A CT scan is the gold standard for diagnosing solid abdominal organ injury; however, it involves risks associated with radiation exposure. Clinical prediction models for determining which patients should undergo abdominal CT are under development. Focused Assessment with Sonography for Trauma (FAST) may be a useful adjunct in diagnosing injury.

Identification of solid-organ injury (liver, spleen, and kidney) is crucial, especially in hemodynamically unstable patients without visible hemorrhage. Prompt surgical evaluation may be the safest maneuver in diagnosing and treating the problem. In most stable patients, CT scan evaluation is the best choice for detecting and staging these injuries. Solid-organ injuries are graded on a scale developed by the American Association for the Surgery of Trauma (Table 19.1).

Most injuries are managed nonoperatively, with serial examinations assessing for hemodynamic instability. The American Pediatric Surgical Association has proposed management guidelines for isolated liver and spleen injuries (Table 19.2). Hemodynamic instability or high-grade solid-organ injury require exploratory laparotomy.

Penetrating abdominal trauma, including stabbing, gunshot, or impalement with a foreign object, requires thorough exposure and inspection to determine entrance and exit wounds. Do not remove impaled objects until the child is in a controlled setting.

Genitourinary Trauma

The most common genitourinary trauma is the result of a straddle injury. Providers must obtain a thorough history and be vigilant for nonaccidental

Table 19.1 Grading of Splenic and Liver Injuries

Grade[a]	Injury Type	Splenic Injury	Hepatic Injury
I	Hematoma	Subcapsular: <10% SA	Same as splenic
	Laceration	Capsular: <1 cm parenchymal depth	Same as splenic
II	Hematoma	Subcapsular: 10%–50% SA Intraparenchymal: <5-cm diameter	Subcapsular: 10%–50% SA Intraparenchymal: <10-cm diameter
	Laceration	1–3 cm parenchymal depth, does not involve trabecular vessel	1–3 cm parenchymal depth, <10 cm in length
III	Hematoma	Subcapsular: >50% SA or expanding Ruptured hematoma Intraparenchymal: >5 cm or expanding	Subcapsular: >50% SA or expanding Intraparenchymal: >10 cm or expanding Ruptured hematoma
	Laceration	>3 cm parenchymal depth or involving trabecular vessels	>3 cm parenchymal depth
IV	Laceration	Involving segmental or hilar vessels producing major devascularization (>25% of spleen)	Parenchymal disruption involving 25%–75% of hepatic lobe or one to three Couinaud's segments within a single lobe
V	Laceration	Completely shattered	Parenchymal disruption involving >75% of hepatic lobe or more than three Couinaud's segments within a single lobe
	Vascular	Hilar vascular injury with devascularized spleen	Juxtahepatic venous injuries (retrohepatic vena cava or major hepatic veins)

NA, not applicable; SA, surface area.

[a] Advance one grade for multiple injuries, up to grade 3.

Modified from Moore EE, Cogbill TH, Jurkovich GJ, Shackford SR, Malangoni MA, Champion HR. Organ injury scaling: spleen and liver (1994 revision). *J Trauma.* 1995;38(3):323–324.

trauma in an infant or young child with a perineal injury. Examine the genitalia carefully, noting the Tanner stage; if a child is extremely uncooperative or more extensive trauma is suspected, examination under anesthesia may be necessary.

Males who present with blood at the urethral meatus require a retrograde urethrogram to determine the integrity of the urethra. Clinicians should not attempt to pass a urinary catheter. Instead, keep the child in nothing-by-mouth status and obtain a urology consult.

Table 19.2 Management Guidelines for Isolated Liver and Spleen Injuries

	Computed tomography (CT) Grade			
	I	II	III	IV
Intensive care unit stay, d	None	None	None	1
Hospital stay, d	2	3	4	5
Predischarge imaging	None	None	None	None
Postdischarge imaging	None	None	None	None
Activity restriction for normal, age-appropriate activity, wk[a]	3	4	5	6

[a] Return to full-contact, competitive sports should be at the discretion of the individual pediatric trauma surgeon.

Modified from Stylianos S; and the APSA Trauma Committee. Evidence-based guidelines for resource utilization in children with isolated spleen or liver injury. *J Pediatr Surg*. 2000;35(2):164–169.

Orthopedic Trauma

Orthopedic injuries may be a stand-alone injury or part of the injury complex in a polytrauma patient. As usual, clinicians should obtain a detailed history of the event and be aware of the child's developmental level because the history of the trauma may not be congruent with the child's age. Consider nonaccidental trauma in spiral fractures of the long bones in an infant or nonmobile child. An orthopedic consult should be obtained after physical examination and X-rays of the injured extremity are acquired. Assess the entire injured extremity for deformity, pulses, capillary refill, color, sensation, mobility, pain, and edema.

Any open fracture requires intravenous antibiotics, typically a first-generation cephalosporin, but vancomycin should also be considered if the patient is at risk of community- or hospital-acquired methicillin-resistant *Staphylococcus aureus*. When stable, the child requires irrigation, debridement, and reduction/fixation of the fracture in the operating room.

Some fractures can be reduced in the emergency department whereas more complex injuries require surgical repair. All staff should reevaluate the extremity for pain, sensation, mobility, pallor, pulses, and capillary refill after reduction and/or casting/splinting for timely identification of compartment syndrome.

Burns

The modern approach to management of burns with high-volume fluid resuscitation was inaugurated after the 1942 Cocoanut Grove fire in Boston, when the relation between body surface area burned and fluid resuscitation

requirements was first postulated. Burn care has now progressed to a sophisticated subset of critical care with unique challenges and considerations.

Initial management begins with the Advanced Trauma Life Support primary
survey, but special considerations should be made at each step.

Airway

Immediate attention must be paid to the airway; burn injury can cause severe
airway edema that can progress over a short period of time. A history of a
fire in an enclosed space should raise suspicion of serious airway injury. The
assessment of the external airway should focus on facial burns, singed nose
hairs, and a thorough oropharyngeal examination, noting any internal burns,
edema, and any carbonaceous sputum. These findings are indicative of injury
that may be more severe than external findings suggest, and immediate intubation should be considered to avoid a more difficult airway after a short period
of time secondary to evolving edema. A carboxyhemoglobin level and arterial
blood gas must be obtained routinely.

Breathing

On inspection of the chest as part of the breathing assessment, careful note
should be taken of any circumferential torso burns. If present, these can
result in acute, restrictive lung physiology that can limit tidal volumes severely.
Circumferential torso burns may require escharotomy by a surgeon to permit
normal chest mechanics.

Circulation

Burn patients should have two large-bore IV catheters placed immediately. If
central venous catheterization is required, lines may be placed through burn
eschar if no other access sites are available. The fluid management strategy
for burns is one of high-volume crystalloid resuscitation to replace insensible
losses from the burn surfaces as well as third spacing and capillary leak from
the inflammatory response, which is activated for burns of more than 25%
total body surface area (TBSA).

Specifically, the initial estimate of required fluid resuscitation for deep
partial-thickness or full-thickness burns can be computed using the Parkland
formula:

$$\text{Total fluid required} = \frac{4 \text{ cc}}{\text{kg}} \times (\% \text{ TBSA burn}) \times (\text{Weight in kg}).$$

Half of this volume is given during the first 8 hours, with the other half
administered the following 16 hours. This is only an estimate because the fluid
resuscitation rate is titrated for a urine output of 2 to 3 mL/kg/h in children.
Beware of underresuscitation if the burn area is underestimated or urine output is not monitored.

The remainder of the trauma assessment should finish with rapid neurological examination and complete exposure to evaluate for other injuries or burns

hidden by clothing, or in the presence of chemical burns. Narcotics should be administered liberally to minimize pain. Warm blankets should be placed to minimize heat loss.

The TBSA must be estimated when the patient is completely exposed. A useful mnemonic is the "rule of 9s," which must be modified in children, because the head and neck area of the child is disproportionately large compared with adults:

In adults, each arm and the head make each up approximately 9% of the TBSA. Each leg and the anterior and posterior thorax each make up approximately 18%. The remaining 1% is from the genitourinary area. In children, the head makes up 18%, and each leg makes up 14%. The genitourinary area is not counted separately.

Another approach is to use the size of the patient's palm to estimate 1% body surface area. Initially, burns should be covered with clean, dry gauze dressings. A trauma surgeon can then determine the type of dressing or topical agents after assessing the burns.

Additional considerations in pediatric burns are nonaccidental trauma and the decision to transfer to a burn center. In the case of pediatric burns, circumferential burns of limbs, burns that suggest abuse with a heated object, or caregiver histories that do not match with examination findings should prompt suspicion of a nonaccidental mechanism. When the patient is stabilized, a decision must be made as to whether the child should be transferred to a burn center. Burn centers are accredited by the American College of Surgeons and American Burn Association and offer specialized surgical, nursing, and wound care as well as long-term follow-up. Current recommendations are for *all* children younger than 10 years of age with more than 10% TBSA second- and third-degree burns to be transferred, as well as burns involving joints, hands, face, feet, genitalia, or the perineum; electrical or chemical burns; or inhalation injury; and all cases in which child abuse or neglect is suspected.

Nonaccidental Trauma

Nonaccidental trauma is an unfortunate reality of pediatric care, with recent estimates showing 6.2 severely abused children per 100,000 in the United States. The three most important aspects of nonaccidental trauma care are a high index of suspicion, careful documentation and reporting, and multidisciplinary care.

Regardless of socioeconomic status or perceived caretaker concern, history and physical discordance should trigger suspicion, as well as certain injury patterns such as intracranial bleeds or multiple fractures (especially clavicle, sternum, rib, or spiral long bone). Although children may have abrasions or contusions from baseline activity, infants are too stationary to acquire these injuries: *If you don't cruise, you don't bruise.*

When documenting the history, one must record the source, the unfolding of events, the location, and the witnesses present. If assessment has already taken place, it is crucial to allow the caretaker to describe the mechanism and not to provide one for them.

Lastly, we strongly advocate a multidisciplinary team approach. All trauma should receive a social work evaluation routinely; but, if nonaccidental trauma is suspected, a separate specialized forensics team should also be consulted that examines the case separately and investigates the child's safety outside the hospital. Additional workup may include skeletal survey for occult fractures, head CT for past bleeds, ophthalmological examination for retinal hemorrhage, and lab work to rule out medical etiology (complete blood count, prothrombin time/partial thromboplastin time).

Further Reading

American College of Surgeons Committee on Trauma. Resources for optimal care of the injured patient. 6th ed. https://www.facs.org/~/media/files/quality%20programs/trauma/vrcresources.ashx Published 2014. Accessed October 12, 2016.

Reed JL, Pomerantz WJ. Emergency management of pediatric burns. *Pediatr Emerg Care.* 2005;21(2):118–129.

Schonfeld D, Lee LK. Blunt abdominal trauma in children. *Curr Opin Pediatr.* 2012;24(3):314–318.

Stylianos S. Evidence-based guidelines for resource utilization in children with isolated spleen or liver injury. The APSA Trauma Committee. *J Pediatr Surg.* 2000;35(2):164–167; discussion 7–9.

American College of Surgeons Committee on Trauma. *ATLS: Advanced Trauma Life Support for Doctors.* 8th ed. 2008. [student course manual]. American College of Surgeons: Chicago, IL.

Chapter 20

Supportive and End-of-Life Care in the Pediatric Intensive Care Unit

Kelly N. Michelson and Joel E. Frader

Although pediatric intensive care units (PICUs) generally enjoy good outcomes, 2% to 7% of PICU patients in developed countries die. As a result, PICU clinicians need to develop competence and confidence in helping families deal with difficult matters, such as the likelihood of imminent death, clarifying and setting the goals of treatment, and the realities of end-of-life care. In addition, children receiving care in the PICU may experience unpleasant and unsettling symptoms that deserve treatment. This chapter contains some basic elements of pediatric palliative and end-of-life care relevant to the PICU.

Limiting and Withdrawing Life Support

Some deaths in the PICU occur after failed resuscitation, although many more deaths follow decisions to limit life-supportive therapies, including, but not limited to, mechanical ventilation, vasoactive drug support, renal replacement therapies, and antibiotics. Although withdrawing treatment sometimes feels more difficult than withholding it, both contemporary medical ethics and law regard the two as equivalent. In addition, sometimes a time-limited trial of aggressive support may help a family to come to terms with the inability of advanced life support to restore their child to an adequate level of well-being. Such trials may also help clinicians feel confident that treatment will no longer provide a benefit. In pediatrics, intensivists make decisions with the participation and consent of parents (or other guardians) after careful discussion about the child's condition and the benefits versus burdens of further intervention. Intensivists need excellent communication skills to elicit effectively the values and goals families have for their children and to provide understandable information and support so that families can share in decision making. Ideally, discussions about withdrawing or withholding life support should not occur the first time the intensivist engages in substantive interaction with a family, or the first time the parents learn of the child's precarious state.

These discussions require compassion and empathy and, although some controversy remains, most families want the clinical recommendations of the intensivist (as well as physicians with whom they and their child have had long-term relationships). Questions intensivists should strive to answer include the following:

- How well does the family understand the child's condition? What more do family members need to know and what methods will most likely help them comprehend the situation?
- Are the family members ready and willing to receive new information?
- Do the parents understand the options facing them and the clinical team? Have they been given sufficient time to consider these options?
- What are the family's goals for the child? Do they value an additional short time with the child after successful treatment of sepsis, even if that time will include difficult-to-tolerate chemotherapy? Or do they feel the child has already suffered enough and they prefer to concentrate on comfort care? Do they feel this episode of pneumonia and respiratory failure in their child with severe static encephalopathy signals a tipping point? Or do they value the child's responses to them and the environment sufficiently to justify continued mechanical ventilation without hope of cure?
- Who can best help the parents think about next steps (e.g., family, friends, pastors or other religious advisors)? Do they want these people present for decision-making discussions?
- If all parties agree to limit support, what do the new goals of care mean in practical terms?
- If support is to be limited or withdrawn, and death is expected to follow, who should attend at the time of discontinuing mechanical ventilation or vasoactive support? Are there special considerations regarding timing (e.g., time for a relative to arrive, avoiding a birthday)?

After clinicians and the family decide to limit or withdraw treatment, children must receive care that prioritizes maximizing their comfort. The specific goals of this care should be explicit, especially with respect to the use of analgesics and sedatives, and well-monitored by the family and the entire clinical team, including bedside personnel. If the plan includes withdrawing mechanical ventilation, intensivists should explain the plan to involved respiratory therapists as well as nurses. As the intensive care unit course proceeds, the goals of care may change depending on the evolving clinical situation. In some cases, time to death may extend beyond the expectations of even experienced clinicians, and families need to know about the difficulty of making accurate predictions.

Symptom Management

Pain Control Principles

Most pediatric intensivists have considerable experience treating pain, be it postoperative, a result of trauma, or secondary to an underlying medical condition, such as cancer, sickle cell disease, or autoimmune disorders. Nevertheless, when the focus of care shifts from restoration of health or the patient's baseline condition to comfort as death approaches, pain management changes as well. Some general issues should be addressed for all patients.

General Notions

- Weak analgesics (nonsteroidal anti-inflammatory drugs [NSAIDs], acetaminophen) have minor, if any, role in end-of-life care as stand-alone agents.
  - NSAIDs may help for rheumatological diseases or bone lesions (Table 20.1).
  - Patients experiencing discomfort from fever may benefit from NSAIDs and acetaminophen.
- Some criticize using multiple analgesics simultaneously as unnecessary polypharmacy; however,
  - Different types of pain medication work at different levels in the pathway between injured tissue/disordered neurons and the central nervous system (CNS)

Table 20.1 Primary Analgesics

Drug	Enteral Dose	Intravenous Dose	Initial Infusion Rate	Comments
Acetaminophen	10–15 mg/kg every 4–6 h	10–15 mg/kg every 4–6 h	NA	Do not exceed 75 mg/kg/24 h
Ibuprofen	5–10 mg/kg every 6 h	Rarely used	NA	May help for bony lesions
Morphine	0.3 mg/kg/dose every 2–4 h	0.1 mg/kg/dose every 2–4 h	0.04 mg/kg/h	Dose and interval needs vary considerably; may not need weight-based doses in patients weighing more than 70 kg
Hydromorphone	30–80 µg/kg/dose every 3 to 4 h	15–25 µg/kg/dose every 2–4 h	0.005 mg/kg/h	May be useful when morphine induces itching
Fentanyl	NA	1–3 µg/kg/dose every 10–60 minutes	1 µg/kg/h	Useful for procedures or with opioid-induced itching
Methadone	0.1–0.2 mg/kg/dose every 8 to 12 h	0.1 mg/kg/dose every 8 to 12 h	NA	Dosing interval needs vary greatly

NA, not applicable

- Combinations of analgesics may have additive or synergistic effects, improving patient comfort
- Interest in nonopioid pain treatment is growing.
- The term *adjunctive* should be abandoned for *coanalgesics*.
  - Steroids and NSAIDs inhibit tissue phospholipid breakdown into pain-pathway-inciting prostaglandins in response to insults, blocking *transduction* of painful impulses.
  - Ion channel stabilizers (e.g., gabapentin, pregabalin) inhibit pain *conduction* in disordered neurons, having special value in treating neuropathic pain. Action may take weeks of slow-dose escalation to become effective.
  - Anesthetics (e.g., lidocaine) administered locally or systemically have similar effects.
  - Tricyclic antidepressants and selective serotonin, norepinephrine, or mixed neurotransmitter reuptake inhibitors work in the neuronal junctions in the dorsal horns of the spinal cord, affecting pain *transmission*.
  - Other agents working at this level include methadone (with opioid and N-methyl-D-aspartate [NMDA] antagonist properties) and ketamine (an NMDA blocker).
- PICU patients started on coanalgesics before switching to purely comfort-based care should generally remain on them.
- Some drugs may deserve the label *adjuvant*.
  - Patients with bone pain may benefit from bisphosphonates (may take days to work). Possible side effects include fever, chills, or myalgia after their administration, as well as hypocalcemia. Use with care in patients with severe renal impairment.
  - Patients with cortical brain injury or muscle cramping for other reasons may benefit from antispasmotics (e.g., baclofen or diazepam).
- Anxiolytics, especially benzodiazepines (BZDs), play an important role in palliative care in the PICU.
  - BZDs have no classic analgesic properties but *modulate* brain responses to transmitted pain signals, provide sedation, reduce anxiety, relax muscles, and often produce amnesia.
  - Different BZDs have different solubility, metabolism, and elimination properties.
    - This requires attention to drug interactions and the need for dose adjustment with renal or hepatic dysfunction.
    - Diazepam, midazolam, and lorazepam are commonly used as constant infusions and as part of a palliative "cocktail" to treat pain, agitation, and/or anxiety in critically ill and dying children.
      - Rare patients have paradoxical responses to BZDs and develop agitation or euphoria. Dose reductions may help. Mild symptoms typically dissipate in 24 to 48 hours.

- Regional and local anesthesia are valuable for palliation in the PICU and are likely underused.
  - Epidural catheters can administer opioids, α-2 agonists (e.g., clonidine), local anesthetics, and/or baclofen. The catheters can be tunneled and left in place for days to weeks with a low risk of CNS infection.
  - Epidurals may help for lower extremity and abdominal pain from metastatic disease, graft-versus-host disease, and so on.
  - Regional blocks, with local anesthetic agents or chemical neurolytics, may help with localized lesions, such as tumors or infection.
    - Many pediatric anesthesiologists place catheters for regional blockade with ultrasound guidance.
    - In some institutions, interventional radiologists use fluoroscopy or computed tomographic guidance to place catheters for local anesthetic infusion or needles/probes for neurolysis or for radiofrequency or cold ablation of nerve ganglia.
    - Transdermal patches with lidocaine or similar agents may help with localized pain syndromes.
- Nonpharmacological treatments have value as part of a comprehensive palliative care approach.
  - Music therapy may calm agitated patients (as well as family members and hospital staff in the patient's room).
  - Massage may relax patients and reduce pain.
  - Art therapy—for patients able to participate—provides distraction, reduces discomfort and distress, and may facilitate communication with family and staff.
  - Hypnosis and guided imagery may reduce pain and anxiety.
  - Acupuncture and acupressure have value for pain and nausea.
- Each of these measures may permit reduction in opioids and/or sedatives, allowing patients greater opportunities to interact with loved ones.

Pain Control

Adequate pain management must be a priority.

- Opioids are the mainstay of pain relief for palliative care patients in the PICU. Table 20.1 lists some useful opioids, with dosing and selected comments. Although additional opioids are available, clinicians should develop familiarity and comfort with a limited number. Tenets of end-of-life use of opioids are as follows.
  - Responses to opioids depend on
    - The specific medication, because they affect different (mu, delta, and kappa) opioid receptors
    - Individual differences in drug distribution, metabolism, and elimination
    - Differences in neuropsychiatric responses to pain

- Clinicians must
  - Choose a drug
  - Start at a reasonable dose
  - Administer the drug in a manner appropriate for the patient
  - Most important, *assess the effects of the drug carefully* with respect to
    - Time to clinical response
    - Adequacy of the dose
    - Duration of effect
    - Side effects
  - Assessment of effectiveness should include
    - Inquiry regarding the patient's level of pain reduction (e.g., using a verbal or visual analog scale)
    - Observation of changes in heart rate, blood pressure, sweating, and so on.

Important Clinical Notes

Individual responses to treatment are highly variable and merit close attention.

- For some patients, 0.1 mg/kg of intravenous morphine may control pain for 2 hours; others may have relief for 4 hours or more.
- Reliance on objectively measured vital signs makes most sense when dealing with acute pain.
- Autonomic responses to pain attenuate in patients who have lived with pain for days or weeks and may not be reflective of the level of discomfort.
  - Pain is a subjective phenomenon.
    - We have *no* tools to predict the adequacy or duration of pain relief.
    - *No matter which drugs one uses, there is no substitute for frequent clinical assessment until the clinician understands each patient's needs and responses to the agents used.*
    - Treat serious pain with *scheduled*, not on-demand (prn), opioids. This avoids patients experiencing peaks of discomfort and waiting times for drug administration, and then the effect of medications.
  - After establishing how much opioid the patient needs—and how often—convert from periodic dosing to a constant infusion (or a scheduled, long-acting opioid), with or without a patient-/parent-/nurse-controlled administration (so-called *patient-controlled analgesia* [PCA]), based on the amount needed for pain relief in the previous 12, 24, or 48 hours.
  - Approaches to PCA administration remain divided into two camps:
    - Reliance on the patient or caregiver to administer relatively frequent bolus doses of opioid with little or no continuous infusion
    - A constant infusion per hour roughly equal to the amount of drug required in the prior 24 hours divided by 24
      - Supplement this with bolus doses, especially for pain associated with movement or procedures.
      - No- or low-dose PCA approaches may prevent oversedation. However, palliative care focuses on overall comfort with the least effort required of patients or caregivers to achieve that goal.

- Most pediatric palliative care clinicians favor relatively high-dose constant infusions plus supplements. All opioids may produce troubling side effects.
- Common and unwelcome is itching. Morphine probably produces itching in a greater proportion of patients than other opioids, but any can produce this adverse reaction.
  - The mechanism of opioid-induced pruritus remains uncertain.
    - Opioid release of mast cell histamine
    - Direct opioid action on the CNS
  - Clinical studies show mixed benefit from antihistamines for the former and ondansetron for the latter.
    - Antihistamines can add sedation and make opioid-related constipation or urinary retention worse.
    - Serotonin antagonists such as ondansetron may also produce constipation.
    - Another approach involves a constant low-dose infusion of the opioid antagonist naloxone (0.25–1 μg/kg/h).
    - Naloxone in similar doses may also help with opioid-induced constipation, nausea, and urinary retention.
  - Opioids may also produce dysphoria (typically wanes in hours to days).
  - Opioids may also trigger myoclonus. Treat with muscle relaxants (baclofen or BZDs) and/or rotate to alternative opioids.
  - Respiratory depression of a threatening degree occurs much less commonly than believed. Tolerance to the respiratory depressant effects of opioids develops rapidly (24–72 hours) after starting regular dosing.
    - Although opioids may increase the risk of respiratory depression, this has no impact for patients on mechanical ventilation.
    - For dying patients, the goal of comfort should generally outweigh concerns about reducing respiratory effort.
    - Opioids can produce tachyphylaxis or tolerance. Clinicians may have difficulty knowing whether the apparent need to increase opioid doses to control pain stems from patient tolerance or escalating pain associated with one or more of the patient's conditions. Approaches include (1) responding to the need for higher and higher doses of an opioid to get the same effect by increasing the dose—typically in 20% to 30% increments until relief is achieved and (2) switching to an alternative opioid (so-called *rotation* or substitution).
    - Initiating coanalgesic medications, such a low-dose ketamine or propofol (using ~10% of the dose used for procedural sedation) (Table 20.2), may allow substantial reduction in the opioid doses needed for pain control.
  - Some palliative care programs routine rotate opioids every 1 to 2 weeks to try to avoid tolerance, although this practice is not well studied.

Table 20.2 Coanalgesics and Sedatives

Drug	Periodic Use Dose	Infusion Dose	Comments
Diazepam	0.1–0.8 PO mg/kg/24 h divided every 6 h		Accumulation and paradoxical responses
Lorazepam	25–50 µg/ kg PO or SQ every 2 h		
Midazolam	500 µg/kg IV, SQ, or intranasally	12.5–30 µg/kg/h	
Dexmedetomidine	NA	1 µg/kg loading dose over 10 min then, 0.2–0.7 µg/ kg/h	May decrease blood pressure or heart rate
Ketamine	1–2 mg/kg IV	0.1 mg/kg IV test dose, then 0.1 mg/kg/h; titrate to effect	May increase secretions; treat with glycopyrrolate or scopolamine patch. May cause hallucinations; treat with benzodiazepines or haloperidol.
Propofol		1 mg/kg/h IV; titrate in 0.5-mg/ kg/h steps every 30 min	Requires dedicated IV line; may decrease blood pressure or heart rate.
Pentobarbital		2 mg/kg IV loading dose over 30 min; titrate as needed in 1-mg/kg/h steps every 30–60 min	

IV, intravenous; PO, by mouth; SQ, subcutaneous.

Notes Regarding Methadone

Methadone has important value not only for managing opioid dependence, but as an important analgesic itself.

• Often used to treat opioid dependence, methadone—a potent analgesic— has particular value in palliative care.
• Its long half-life may allow oral administration only twice a day.
• Because it has NMDA antagonist properties, methadone has special value for neuropathic pain.
   • Individuals vary greatly in their elimination of the drug, making it necessary to observe patients closely for several days after initiating use

- Methadone may increase the QT interval in susceptible patients.
  - Some clinicians recommend routine electrocardiograms before and after starting methadone, especially when used with other drugs affecting cardiac conduction.
  - Whether this matters in end-of-life situations deserves consideration among clinicians and the family.

Nausea

Nausea is a common, profoundly disturbing symptom in the PICU, especially, but not exclusively, among patients at the end of life.

- Patients at the end-of-life experience nausea for many reasons:
  - Underlying condition, especially involving the CNS or gastrointestinal (GI) tract
  - Drug or radiation effects
  - Substances produced by tumors or malfunctioning organs
  - Anxiety and depression, especially in children
- Start treatment with measures to remove or mitigate inciting causes directly.
- Nausea is often multifactorial and treatment may require complementary therapies and multiple medications.
  - Peppermint candies, peppermint oil, and ginger can reduce nausea for some children able to use them.
  - Acupuncture, acupressure, and hypnosis may also work.
  - Based on oncology experience, 5-hydroxytryptamine antagonists (ondansetron and related drugs) have become very popular for treating nausea.
    - These drugs may be effective in combination with corticosteroids, which some use alone for nausea, particularly in patients with brain lesions.
    - For patients on drugs that may prolong the QT interval, 5-hydroxytryptamine antagonists may increase the arrhythmia risk.
    - In such instances, phenothiazines (e.g., perchlorperazine) and other antipsychotics (e.g., haloperidol) may be useful.
    - Metoclopramide, a dopamine receptor antagonist, can be useful, especially in patients with reduced GI motility.
    - Antipsychotics and metoclopramide may produce dystonic reactions.
    - Anticholinergic agents, particularly scopolamine patches, may benefit some patients, but may cause confusion or other unpleasant CNS symptoms, especially in children younger than 12 years.
    - Other useful medications include cannabinoids (dronabinol), octreotide, and BZDs, although the latter may work through sedation rather than a direct antiemetic effect.
    - The substance P antagonist aprepitant recently has come into use. It is only available in oral form.

Itching

Patients' underlying disorders as well as medications and other treatments may cause nausea, sometimes more disturbing to the child and family than pain.

- Many circumstances produce itching, including (among others)
  - Primary skin conditions
  - Medications
  - Liver and/or kidney failure
  - Paraneoplastic processes
- Severe skin involvement of graft-versus-host disease may produce especially difficult-to-control pruritis. Careful attention to skin care can make an enormous difference for patients *and* may engage family members meaningfully in applying moisturizing agents.
- Antihistamines have limited value, especially for itching from opioid administration.
  - Of the H1 antihistamines, dermatologists prefer hydroxyzine for its sedative effect.
  - Ondansetron at antiemetic doses may also work for opioid-induced itching.
- Patients with severe pruritis may require considerable sedation for control.

Constipation

Constipation is a frequent side effect of agents commonly used to manage pain.

- Constipation troubles many patients, especially older children and adolescents.
- Assume all patients receiving opioids for more than a few doses will develop constipation unless treated with a bowel regimen.
  - All patients on opioids should receive stool softeners (e.g., docusate), bowel stimulants (e.g., bisacodyl), and/or osmotic agents (e.g., lactulose, polyethylene glycol) to prevent or treat constipation.
  - Most palliative care practitioners recommend combining stimulants with stool softeners or osmotic agents.
    - Producing more liquid stool without propulsion predisposes to incontinence.
    - These agents treat constipation from most causes and usually render enemas and manual disimpaction unnecessary.
    - Bulking agents (fiber) have no role in palliative treatment of constipation.
    - More or less GI-specific mu-receptor opioid antagonists may prevent or treat opioid-induced bowel dysfunction, although few studies have addressed use in children. Methylnaltrexone is available for subcutaneous injection and typically works in minutes to hours. While naloxegol only comes in tablet form, the manufacturer has provided instructions for mixing with water for gastric tube administration. Details are available at http://www.azpicentral.com/movantik/movantik_med.pdf#page=1

Central Nervous System Disturbances

Primary disease processes, side effects of treatment, and emotional distress make central nervous system disturbances very common among patients in the PICU, perhaps especially those at the end of life.

- Agitation
  - There are multiple possible causes of agitation, sometimes in combination, including pain, sleep loss, encephalopathies (from infection, autoimmune phenomena, vascular lesions, graft-versus-host disease in stem cell transplant patients), anxiety/depression, and delirium
  - When known, treat underlying causes.
  - In general, normalize the environment by maintaining day/night distinctions, reducing noise, and maximizing touch from loved ones.
- Delirium (acute confusional state)
  - Delirium is characterized by fluctuations in severity, disturbances of consciousness, cognitive impairment, unwelcome sensations, and hallucinations. Hypoactive forms may be difficult to recognize
  - Patients with resolved delirium report the experience was very unpleasant and express considerable relief with resolution.
  - Delirium also has multiple causes, including dehydration, metabolic disturbances, constipation, hypoxia, fever, infection, nutritional deficiencies, medications or medication withdrawal, and paraneoplastic phenomena.
  - When known, treat the underlying cause. Rehydration alone is frequently sufficient.
  - Treatment
    - Normalize the environment and provide reassurance.
    - Rehydrate.
    - Medicate. Haloperidol is the drug of choice. Risperidone is a reasonable alternative, and other antipsychotics may work as well.
    - Avoid BZDs if possible (may exacerbate delirium).
- Dysautonomia after brain insult (paroxysmal sympathetic hyperactivity)
  - Most patients typically experience periods of increased heart rate, blood pressure, temperature, sweating, and pupillary dilation, but the reverse of these is possible as well.
  - Other features may include posturing, spasticity, teeth grinding, hiccups, tearing, sighing, and yawning.
  - Treatment is somewhat controversial.
    - All recommend a low-stimulation environment and treatment of triggers, such as infection and metabolic disturbances.
    - The medications recommended most include opioids and/or BZDs as well as α agonists (dexmedetomidine or clonidine)
    - Other experts recommend β blockade.
    - Gabapentin is being used increasingly for prophylaxis.
- Nonspecific irritability

- Nonspecific irritability is difficult to distinguish from the previously listed causes. If there is no cognitive impairment, then delirium is not present.
- Treatment starts with nonpharmacological measures, as mentioned earlier.
- Acute management, if needed, involves BZDs, barbiturates, and opioids.
- There is increasing evidence for a link to visceral hyperalgesia/neuropathic pain related to GI dysmotility and distention of bowel.
  - Responds quickly to gabapentin (within 24 hours in newborns), with the ability to reduce BZD and opioid use.
  - Dose requirements may be high (up to 70–75 mg/kg/d).
  - Need to taper gabapentin when discontinuing.

Withdrawing Life Support

If a family decides that withdrawal of life-sustaining treatments is an acceptable course of action, careful planning and preparation are essential to minimize patient discomfort, as well as family and staff distress. An explicit plan should include the following:

- Notification of social service, clergy, primary service clinicians, and the organ procurement organization, as appropriate
- Clear communication with the family about the steps to be taken and the child's likely response, including anticipated changes in the breathing pattern. Avoid estimates of the time the child will survive; such estimates are commonly inaccurate. It is essential that one assure family members the child will be kept as comfortable as possible.
- Provision of the quietest and most private space available
- Discontinuation of testing that has no role in comfort care (e.g., blood draws, X-rays). In some cases, monitoring may also be discontinued to remove other sources of discomfort; in others, its predictive value is important to family members.
- Assessment of the value of each intensive care unit therapy, including antibiotics, diuretics, renal replacement therapies, and vasoactive drugs, among others, including fluids and nutrition. In most instances, these treatments can be discontinued abruptly without patient discomfort.
- Discontinuation of ventilatory support. The optimal approach varies for individual patients. Children with severe neurological injury may not experience distress, but those with greater awareness may experience significant dyspnea. Recommendations regarding the value of first lowering the fraction of inspired oxygen or mechanical rate versus abrupt extubation vary. Regardless, the team should be prepared to provide anxiolytics and opioids to prevent and treat signs of respiratory distress. The use of neuromuscular blocking agents interferes with the assessment of patient comfort and is unacceptable (with the possible exception of times when a patient has been

receiving these agents in high doses for a prolonged period, and resolution of their effect is prolonged markedly, in which case higher doses of sedatives and opioids may be needed to ensure a patient does not experience dyspnea or other discomfort after extubation).

After a Patient Dies

After a child dies in the PICU, when emotion makes practical matters difficult to remember, there are numerous tasks that need to be completed to minimize later distress.

- Was the family present? Do any members need to be contacted?
- Has the organ procurement organization been notified of impending or actual death?
- Does the coroner/medical examiner need to be notified?
- Have clinicians discussed autopsy with the family, including the option of a limited postmortem examination? Does the family know that questions they may have later will have less chance of clear answers if no autopsy is conducted? If the family has agreed to autopsy, has the pathologist been made aware?
- Has the primary service or referring primary care provider been notified?
- Are there other doctors, staff to notify? Who else was deeply involved?
- Has a death note been written? Has a death discharge order been completed?
- Has a death certificate been completed?
- Has the family been made aware of bereavement services available to them?
- Has the family been offered an opportunity to meet in the future to discuss the results of the autopsy or ask questions about the child's course?

The death of a child is difficult not only for families, but also for clinicians from all of the healthcare professions. Providing those closely involved an immediate opportunity to gather their thoughts before moving on to the next patient is important. Debriefing meetings to discuss the care provided and caretakers' responses to a death are important for supporting and maintaining a compassionate staff.

Index

Date Due
